Taking the Clinical History

Eliciting Symptoms
Knowing the Patient
Ethical Foundations

William E. DeMyer

Professor Emeritus of Neurology (Child)
Indiana University School of Medicine

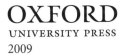
OXFORD
UNIVERSITY PRESS
2009

OXFORD

UNIVERSITY PRESS

Oxford University Press, Inc., publishes works that further
Oxford University's objective of excellence
in research, scholarship, and education.

Oxford   New York
Auckland   Cape Town   Dar es Salaam   Hong Kong   Karachi
Kuala Lumpur   Madrid   Melbourne   Mexico City   Nairobi
New Delhi   Shanghai   Taipei   Toronto

With offices in
Argentina   Austria   Brazil   Chile   Czech Republic   France   Greece
Guatemala   Hungary   Italy   Japan   Poland   Portugal   Singapore
South Korea   Switzerland   Thailand   Turkey   Ukraine   Vietnam

Copyright (c) 2009 by Oxford University Press, Inc.

Published by Oxford University Press, Inc.
198 Madison Avenue, New York, New York 10016

Oxford is a registered trademark of Oxford University Press

Library of Congress Cataloging-in-Publication Data

DeMyer, William, 1924-
Taking the clinical history : eliciting symptoms, knowing the patient, ethical foundations /
William E. DeMyer.
p. ; cm.
Includes bibliographical references.
ISBN 978-0-19-537377-6
1. Medical history taking. 2. Medical ethics. I. Title.
[DNLM: 1. Medical History Taking--methods. 2. Ethics, Medical. WB 290 D389t 2009]
RC65.D36 2009
616.07'51--dc22
2008035162

9 8 7 6 5 4 3 2 1

Printed in the United States of America
on acid-free paper

If you do not know what is wrong with a patient after you have taken a history, then take another history. If you still do not know, take a third history. If you do not know then, you probably never will.

Clifton K. Meador, M.D.

I do not ask what are your sins and transgressions or what is your value. I do not ask what is your religion or your politics. I ask only what is your suffering.

Paraphrased from
Louis Pasteur (1822–1895)

Contents

Foreword

After many years of planning and preparation, this book is the culmination of Professor William DeMyer's many contributions to his profession. In it, he has integrated the fundamentals and nuances of taking a medical history with the urgent goal, "to create ethical, compassionate physicians." He points out, "The physician can only know the patient as a person through the history. Above all, a masterful history leads to rapport, trust, and the selection of the best management by the patient." The reader is cautioned, "Be forewarned: My text presents some personal views." However, even if one has a different view, the careful consideration of Dr. DeMyer's reasoning will result in expansion of intellectual horizons and result in a greatly improved person and physician.

As the book was in its final stages of preparation, Dr. DeMyer became terminally ill. All therapy and his health progressively failed, but not his will to function and continue to contribute. In his 84th year, he continued to teach, see patients, and finish this text to the point of final editing. Days before his death, he asked me to do the final editing, check the references, and perform any minor rewriting for this book that might be required prior to publication. I was greatly honored and, of course, agreed. We would, 54 years after we published our first scientific work together, participate again in this, his final work.

It is unfortunate that this will be the last work of this remarkable man. His self-discipline was unbelievable. Even in play and in his personal life, he was focused and refused to settle for anything other than excellence. His accomplishments are varied and extensive.

Early in his career, Dr. DeMyer developed innovative techniques and stains as methods for identifying and counting nerve fibers. From this, he established the number and origin of axons and myelin sheaths in the rhesus monkey and human medullary pyramids. He was an international authority on median facial anomalies. With Dr. Alexander Ross, he conclusively established the side of symptoms related to the lesion in an isolated syndrome of the median longitudinal fasciculus in man. With his wife, Marian DeMyer, a distinguished child psychiatrist, he was among the first to define autism in children as an organic disease. These are just a few examples of his major original contributions to medical science.

In a department and school with many outstanding teachers, he was without doubt the premiere teacher of his time. Ten medical school classes voted him outstanding teacher in clinical sciences. He received the Golden Apple Award for best teacher in any area in the Indiana University Medical School for an unprecedented four classes. In 1981, he received the Frederick Bachman Lieber Me¬morial Award (All-Indiana University award for outstanding teaching). The class of 1972 established a special medical student scholarship in his name. For more than 50 years, neurology residents have considered his neuroanatomy course to be a highlight of their residency training.

His teaching contributions extend far beyond his direct contact with those trained at Indiana University. Through his publications, he taught and still teaches thousands whom he has never met. In addition to this, his final work, he has published four other single-author texts and more than 30 chapters in some of the most prestigious books in neurology. His *Technique of the Neurologic Examination* was the first programmed text written for neurology. It has been translated into a number of languages and has contributed to the education of countless physicians throughout the world. Currently in its fifth edition, it is the longest-running (41 years) neurology text by a single author. His other books concern neuroanatomy, self-assessment and review in psychiatry and neurology, and neurohistology for clinical medicine.

One would think with all these professional accomplishments that he would have had no time for any other activities. With amazing concentration and full utilization of every moment of his time, he was extremely, almost excessively, well-rounded. At the age of 27, he began playing tennis and rapidly became one of the top players in Indiana. At one time, he was nationally ranked as an amateur player. His trophy cabinet is overflowing with awards, plaques, and trophies. At the age of 50, he and Marian took up ballroom dancing and advanced to compete in amateur national championships.

Bill DeMyer was intellectually intact and effective to the very end. The text of this book is virtually unchanged in content from the final copy that he presented to me. However, at the end he was exhausted and physically unable to check with his usual meticulousness for detail. This was also confounded by his wide interest and citations from a variety of obscure sources and an inability to find the complete references for his many erudite quotes. Countless hours were spent searching and verifying. Critical to this were Dr. DeMyer's long time secretary, Teresa Wenzel, and our Medical History Librarian, Nancy Eckerman. Terry was able to trace many references to personal files at various locations. Nancy must be either a magician or a genius or both. She was able to trace original sources for brief excerpts from obscure longer quotations. Each spent many long hours searching for missing and incomplete references and confirmatory data. Largely due to them, we were able to find all the missing data with only a few minor exceptions. In these instances, we found alternates or were able to alter the text without changing Dr. DeMyer's intent. For me and for Dr. DeMyer, we thank them for their major contributions that make it possible for this book to be published without any major changes from the original intent.

On August 29, 2008, the last class in neuroanatomy ended. September 9, the final editing was decided. September 16, directions were sent to the publisher for final completion of the manuscript. September 19, the publisher confirmed the plans. On the morning of September 20, William Erl DeMyer exceptional teacher, distinguished scientist, outstanding clinician, superb athlete died.

—Mark L. Dyken, M.D.
Professor Emeritus of Neurology
Indiana University School of Medicine
November 2008

Preface

My text describes that indispensable process when a physician sits down privately with a patient to elicit a clinical history. The history offers no glamour, no oscilloscope flashes, no radiation counter clicks away. No MRI dinosaur swallows the patient, grunts and groans through its routine, and then disgorges the patient back into the world. Modern technology requires medical students to expend much time in learning how to operate and read the output from machines and computers, but these complex tests achieve full meaning *only* after integration with the patient's history. My text teaches how to elicit and read the output from the patient. The history provides the only way to diagnose the many disorders that produce symptoms but no signs. The physician can only know the patient as a person through the history. Above all, a masterful history leads to rapport, trust, and the selection of the best management by the patient.

Today, the most urgent goal of medical education is to create ethical, compassionate physicians. To that end, I integrate the technique of the history and ethics because I propose that the physician's ethics determine the form and content of the questions asked—and those not asked—thereby strongly directing the patient's choices. Thus, rather than postponing ethics to a course later in the curriculum, I propose that from the very first contact of the student with a patient, the student realizes that ethics, good or bad, will determine every technique and every action that we employ.

I start from a core ethic that should govern the entire practice of medicine: The physician must always act in the patient's best interest. Other medical ethics and the actions and techniques they mandate derive from this core ethic. Unless directed to the patient's best interest, the history can influence the patient to accept unneeded or unwise tests, operations, and management. To appreciate how ethics and goals slant a history, compare a clinical history to a police history, aimed at conviction, which employs lying, cajoling, bullying, and good-cop/bad-cop acting. Ideally, the clinical history uniquely brings one mind, the physician's—presumably free of ulterior or personal motives—into communion with the patient's, solely for the patient's benefit. In most other human interactions, both participants strive to promote a personal goal.

I include how to greet the patient, how to discover the patient's chief concern, how to elicit the symptoms and select the topics to explore—the word choice, phrasing, diction, and tone of voice—and how to recognize and manage the feelings generated as patient and physician interact. I review the actual questions for the physician to ask and the actual responses for the physician to make. I describe how to listen and discover the patient's real needs as a person, rather than as a repository of symptoms or a collection of organs. This text is neither a differential diagnosis text nor a series of algorithms, but I do include tables of some diseases to remind the student of the range of diagnostic vistas explored during the history.

Be forewarned: My text presents some personal views.

> Camerado, this is no book,
> Who touches this touches me.
>
> Walt Whitman (1819–1892)

Although I do write passionately about my profession and I do wander at times beyond the clinical history per se to show how commercialization and societal pressures distort the history, I have tried to avoid the arrogance of certainty. I realize that the young need to question the views and traditions of their predecessors. Assess my offerings, and then adopt those that will best serve your patients, the profession, and humanity at large—all of us.

A Brief Biography

When I read a text, I am curious about the author's background. My personal involvement in medicine extends over 60 years. It began in 1943, when, as a draftee at 18 years of age during World War II, I was trained as a venereal disease (VD) control aid in the U.S. Air Force. During my 3 years of military service, I assisted physicians in VD prevention programs, did laboratory tests to diagnose VD, and gave parenteral injections of arsenic and bismuth to treat syphilis. This experience provided career-long insights into public health problems. Postwar, in 1946, I entered premed and graduated from Indiana University School of Medicine in 1952. After internship at the University of Michigan, I completed a 3-year neurology residency at Indiana University and did a postgraduate year in a medical faculty training program at the University of Pennsylvania, under Dr. Julius Comroe.

Starting in 1957, I have spent my career on the faculty of the Indiana University School of Medicine, striving to learn how to practice clinical neurology, to teach neurology to students and residents, and to do research. I was board-certified in neurology in 1957, with subspecialty certification in child neurology in 1967. For 40 years, I served as the neurologic consultant to Larue Carter Memorial Hospital, a state mental hospital for adults and children. Since 1943, not a single day has passed that I have not studied, worked at, and puzzled over the practice of medicine.

I have been married to Marian DeMyer, M.D., for 55 years. A child psychiatrist, she has done notable research in autism while immensely contributing to my career. A daughter, Carolyn, is a teacher; one son, David, designs exercise equipment; our other son, Larry, is a musician. All of them—Marian, our children and grandchildren—and the thousands of medical students and patients I have seen have each in their own way filled my years with fascination and joy.

—William E. DeMyer, M.D.

Taking the Clinical History

Outline of the Clinical History

Definition and Scope of the Clinical History

The clinical history reviews the pertinent present and past information about the patient's health and the patient's health-related values and beliefs. The physician elicits the clinical history by orderly questions, addressed to the patient or to an informant, and from review of previous medical records. The physician phrases the inquiries in specific ways to elicit the characteristics, sequence, and severity of present or past symptoms. The history includes previous illnesses and treatments and all other health-related information, including the family history. For children, the physician questions the mother about the gestation, birth, developmental milestones, behavior, and school performance.

For an overview of the history, skim through Table 1–1 and leaf through the outline of the clinical history in the rest of the chapter. Then start to study the text with Chapter 2. Do not despair at the lengthy outline for the complete history. Chapter 7 discusses how to screen the categories efficiently.

Table 1–1. Brief Outline of the Clinical History

    I. Patient's name and identifying data (face sheet)
    II. Chief concern (also called the presenting concern or chief complaint)
    III. Present illness or current illness
    IV. Current medications and management
    V. Past clinical history: illnesses, injuries, hospitalizations, operations, and workups
    VI. Review of systems
    VII. Family history
    VIII. Psychosocial and mental status history
    IX. Pregnancy and developmental history (pediatric patients)
    X. Preventive history and wellness
    XI. Ethics, values, and spirituality history

Detailed Outline of the Clinical History

I. Identifying Data, the Face Sheet
  A. Page 1 of the medical record usually is the *face sheet* (see Table. 6–1). It lists personal data such as the patient's name, age, sex, occupation, address, referring source or doctor, next of kin, and insurance plan.

II. Chief Concern
  A. Reason for consulting the physician
  B. Record the source of information and reliability
    1. Patient
    2. Informant: parent, spouse, relative, or friend
    3. Medical records, radiographs, and laboratory reports

III. Present Illness
  A. Nature and location of discomfort
  B. Date of onset, frequency/duration
  C. Severity
  D. Triggering events, if any
  E. Alleviating events, if any
  F. Course of the present symptoms
    1. Temporal profile: acute/chronic, constant or intermittent
    2. Getting better, getting worse, or at a plateau

IV. Current Medications and Previous Management of the Present Illness
  A. Methods of self-therapy
  B. Physical therapy
  C. Prescription drugs
  D. Nonprescription drugs: analgesics, vitamins, laxatives, cold remedies, herbs, and street drugs
  E. Drug intolerances and allergies
  F. Previous medical evaluations and diagnostic studies

V. Past Clinical History
  A. Childhood and adult illnesses
  B. Injuries
  C. Hospitalizations
  D. Operations

VI. Review of Systems
  A. The head and nervous system
   1. Headache: standard types (see Table 6–9), including sinusitis, earache, toothache, and ocular pain (photophobia and glaucoma)
   2. Special senses: sight, hearing, equilibrium, smell, and taste
   3. Loss of consciousness, seizures, fainting
   4. General somatic sensation: pain, numbness, and tingling in face, hands, and feet
   5. Motor system
    a. Speaking or swallowing
    b. Breathing (see also under "Respiratory system")
    c. Gait: falls, imbalance, incoordination
    d. Fatigability, weakness, or paralysis
    e. Involuntary movements and tremors
    f. Cramps, stiffness, or exercise intolerance
  B. Skeletomuscular system
   1. Neck or back pain
   2. Joint pain, redness, and swelling
   3. Bone pain
   4. Trauma: fractures, sprains, and tears
  C. Hematopoietic system (spleen and bone marrow)
   1. Pallor, anemia
   2. Bruising or bleeding from the nose, gums, or rectum
   3. Unexplained fever and malaise
   4. Transfusions or receipt of other blood products such as platelets or gamma globulin
  D. Respiratory system
   1. Chest pain (see "Cardiovascular system")
   2. Shortness of breath
    a. Hyperventilation
    b. Exertional dyspnea
    c. Nocturnal dyspnea (orthopnea)
    d. Wheezing/asthma
    e. Snoring, sleep apnea
   3. Coughing, sputum production, hemoptysis
   4. Smoking
   5. Previous respiratory illness
   6. Exposures to people, birds, or other animals

E. Cardiovascular system
   1. Chest pain
   2. Blood pressure
   3. Palpitations, pulse irregularities
   4. Swelling of feet
   5. Varicosities
   6. Cyanosis, blanching,
   7. Intermittent claudication
F. Gastrointestinal system
   1. Appetite, diet, weight, and food intolerances
   2. Abdominal pain, food intolerance, heartburn, and abdominal discomfort related to meals
   3. Nausea and vomiting
   4. Belching, flatulence
   5. Previous liver disease, hepatitis, or jaundice
   6. Bowel habits
      a. Changes in habits, stool frequency, straining, constipation, diarrhea, or incontinence
      b. Character of bowel movements, volume, consistency, and color
      c. Rectal pain, bleeding, piles, or itching
      d. Enemas, laxatives, antacids
G. Renal system
   1. Flank pain, burning on urination, dysuria
   2. Episodes of cystitis or nephritis
   3. Continence, ability to start and stop the stream, dribbling, frequency and amount of urination, bed-wetting
   4. Ability to feel full bladder
   5. Urine color, clear or cloudy, pus or blood in urine
   6. Urinary odor
   7. Kidney failure and uremia
H. Reproductive system and sexuality
   1. Sexual performance (males and females)
      a. Sexual activity, satisfactions/dissatisfactions (self and partner)
      b. Interest, arousal, foreplay, orgasm
      c. Marital status, cohabitation, multiple partners
      d. Sexual orientation
      e. Masturbation
      f. Vaginal, oral, or anal sex

    g. Contraception

    h. Venereal disease

  2. Males

    a. Erectile insufficiency and premature ejaculation

    b. Penile discharge

    c. Fertility

    d. Testicular masses

  3. Females

    a. Breast pain, lumps, or nipple discharge

    b. Genital pain, itching, infections, dyspareunia

    c. Menstruation

      (1) Menarche

      (2) Frequency

      (3) Duration

      (4) Flow, interperiod bleeding, or spotting

      (5) Cycle-related changes in affect or behavior

      (6) Menopause

    d. Pregnancies (see also sections II and III of Chapter 10)

      (1) Fertility

      (2) Number of children

      (3) Nature of pregnancies, pregnancy illnesses, labor, and deliveries

      (4) Pregnancy loss, miscarriages, stillbirth, abortions

  4. Deviant sexuality (paraphilias, including child molestation as victim or pedophile)

  5. Rape

I. Endocrine system

  1. Habitus, stature: dwarfism/gigantism

  2. Puberty/menarche/menopause

  3. Hair texture, distribution, and beard

  4. Excessive thirst (*polydipsia*), food intake (*polyphagia*) or excessive urination (*polyuria*),

  5. Heat or cold intolerance

  6. Bronzing of skin and salt craving

J. Immune system/lymphatics

  1. Infections

    a. Frequency and type of infections

    b. Infectious disease exposures

    c. Unexplained fevers, chills, and night sweats

  2. Immunizations: record dates and agents protected against

  3. Allergies and sensitivities

      a. Sneezing, wheezing, hay fever, and asthma
      b. Hives
      c. Food intolerances
      d. Medication sensitivities
      e. Anaphylactic reactions
        (1) Bee stings
        (2) Snake venoms
        (3) Insect bites
    4. Lymphadenopathy
  K. Skin
    1. Eruptions, redness, rashes, itching, or wheals
    2. Infections: tinea, folliculitis, or acne
    3. Dryness
    4. Excessive sweating or loss of sweating (*hyperhidrosis* or *anhidrosis*)
    5. Ulcerations of skin or mucous membranes
    6. Changes in pigmentation: light spots (*vitiligo*) or brown spots (café au lait spots, moles, or freckles)
    7. Tumors: warts, growths, or cancer; sun exposure and tanning
    8. Nails: infections, brittleness
    9. Edema or puffiness of the skin, such as periorbital or of lips, arms, legs, or abdomen
  L. Environmental/toxic exposure history: review of exposure to toxic chemicals at home or in the workplace

VII. Family History
  A. Blood relatives with illness resembling the patient's
  B. Cancer, high blood pressure, stroke, heart disease, diabetes mellitus, asthma, arthritis, and mental illness or retardation
  C. Other familial diseases

VIII. Psychosocial History and Mental Status
  A. Psychosocial screening
    1. General mood and satisfactions/dissatisfactions
    2. Family relationships
    3. Peer relationships
    4. School or work performance/occupational history
    5. Play/hobbies/recreation
    6. Personal habits

      7. Sleep disorders (dyssomnias and parasomnias,
         see Table 9–6)
         a. Insomnia/quality of sleep
         b. Hypersomnia
         c. Sleep apnea
         d. Snoring
         e. Nightmares
         f. Night terrors
         g. Restless legs
         h. Cramps
         i. Bruxism
      8. Legal problems
   B. Mental status history/mental status examination
      1. General behavior and appearance
      2. Stream of talk
      3. Mood and affective responses
         a. Appropriate
         b. Depressed
         c. Euphoric
         d. Manic
         e. Labile
         f. Blunted
   C. Content of thought
      1. Reality perception
      2. Illusions
      3. Hallucinations
      4. Delusions
         a. Persecution
         b. Grandeur
         c. Bodily defects
      5. Phobias
      6. Obsessions and compulsions
   D. Intellectual capacity
      1. Normal range
      2. Superior
      3. Dull
      4. Retarded
      5. Demented
   E. Sensorium
      1. Consciousness
      2. Attention span

3. Orientation for time, place, and person
4. Memory: remote, recent
5. Fund of information
6. Insight, judgment, and planning
7. Calculation

IX. **Pregnancy and Developmental History (for Pediatric Patients)**
   A. Fertility history of mother
   B. Pregnancy history
      1. Prenatal care
      2. Bleeding
      3. Known illnesses
      4. Drug exposure: street drugs, alcohol, and prescription drugs
      5. Weight gain
      6. Quickening
   C. Perinatal events
      1. Duration of pregnancy
      2. Birth weight and head circumference
      3. Duration of labor
      4. Method of delivery
      5. Immediate postnatal events
         a. Spontaneous breathing, assisted ventilation, Apgar score
         b. Spontaneous feeding, sucking, and swallowing
      6. Mother's mental state and attitude toward the pregnancy
   D. Developmental milestones (ages birth to 2 years)
   E. Behavior (ages 2–5 years)
   F. School history (ages 5–18+ years)

X. **Preventive History and Wellness**
   A. Infant and child
      1. Immunizations
      2. Routine physical checkups, developmental screening, vision and hearing screening
      3. Accident prevention: guns, seat belts, and helmets
      4. Crib safety (sudden infant death syndrome [SIDS])
   B. Teen and adult
      1. Planning for routine physicals and laboratory tests
      2. Diet and physical fitness
      3. Occupational hazards
      4. Prevention of venereal disease and other infections

5. Accident prevention, including gun safety
6. Heredofamilial disease risk
7. Prevention of birth defects in offspring
8. Prevention of illness in international travel
9. Recognition of incipient mental illness
10. Wellness review

XI. Ethics, Values, and Spirituality History

Basic Definitions: Disease, Symptoms, Signs, Syndromes, and Diagnosis

2

I. What Is Disease?

A. Definition: *Disease* means any abnormality in a person that causes undue discomfort, deformity, dysfunction, or death (Humber and Almeder, 1997). Literally the term *disease* means a state of *dis-ease* (*dis* = negation or lack of, *ease* = ease— therefore a state of *lacking* ease or of *un*-ease). Many states of discomfort, such as grief, reactive depression, or anxiety, only qualify as a disease if they exceed normal limits.

B. The concept of "normality" and "abnormality": The concept of disease and its diagnosis rests on the assumption that human beings exist in definable states of health or disease, but health and disease exist in a continuum. No strict dichotomy separates them, particularly in regard to mental illness. Some unusual, often creative people, like the mathematician Paul Erdös (Hoffman, 1998), defy a simple normal/abnormal dichotomy. Nevertheless, we can assume that a standard healthy "normal" or "average" person exists, normal in mind and body, to the degree that we could enshrine the person in the Bureau of Standards in Washington, D.C., along with the standard meter bar and standard kilogram. By matching the findings in a given patient against normal persons of like age, race, sex, and culture, physicians recognize abnormal states of body and mind that constitute disease.

C. Characteristics that define a disease
   1. The disease affects some part of the body, the whole body, or the person's mind.
   2. The symptoms and signs and the natural history of the disease (its onset, course, and prognosis) are similar from patient to patient, but the disease, as a dynamic process, may change in intensity and manifestations from time to time.
   3. The disease has one proximate cause, although typically numerous contributory causes exist. The proximate cause may be one agent or a group of very closely related agents. For example, perhaps fifty rhinoviruses cause the disease that we call the "common cold" (coryza).

    4. Patients with the disease respond similarly to the same management or therapy.

D. Contributory and psychosocial determinants of disease

  1. A disease is embedded within a whole person. To understand the total impact of a disease or an illness, the physician has to understand the whole person who has the disease. To accomplish this, the physician has to view and define the disease within the context of the patient's family, culture, and environment.

  2. What we deem as a disease with a proximate cause represents only the last event in a long chain of interconnected or contributory events. To acknowledge the contributory events, George Engle (1980) spoke of disease as having a biopsychosocial context (Del Piccolo et al., 2004; White, 2005). For example, a specific bacterium causes tuberculosis, but overcrowding, poverty, malnutrition, and immunodeficiency contribute to its pathogenesis and prevalence. The prevalence of tuberculosis is greatly increased in Africa and India because of the large number of immunodeficient individuals with acquired immunodeficiency syndrome (AIDS). Dyslexia, a significant problem in literate culture, would not constitute a disease in a culture without a written language.

  3. When a new disease has a clear proximate cause, as in Lyme disease, legionnaires disease, and AIDS, we accept the disease as a biological entity. Without a clear proximate cause, a suspected new disorder may remain controversial, such as chronic fatigue syndrome (Abbey and Garfinkel, l991), fibromyalgia, posttraumatic stress disorder (Barglow et al., 2006), and sick building syndrome.

II. **Manifestations of Disease by Symptoms and Signs**

A. Definition of a symptom

  1. A *symptom* is any subjective manifestation of disease, that is, a change imposed on the patient's perceptions or mental state by a disease. Examples are pain, fatigability, and depression.

  2. Most patients recognize their symptoms and visit the physician because of them. Table 2–1 lists the commonest symptoms (apart from injuries) that cause patients to consult physicians.

Table 2–1. Commonest Symptoms (Apart from Injuries and Cuts) for Which Patients Consult Physicians

Adults
1. Headaches, including otitis and sinusitis
2. Backache
3. Pain in the abdomen, nausea, indigestion, diarrhea, or constipation
4. Pain in the chest, cough, or shortness of breath
5. Pain, numbness, or tingling in the extremities
6. Pain in the joints or cramps in the muscles
7. Fatigability, lack of energy, depression, or anxiety
8. Sleep disorders
9. Itching, skin rash, or skin infections
10. Dizziness (vertigo), lightheadedness, or unsteadiness in walking
11. Fever and malaise
12. Blurred vision
13. Weight gain or weight loss
14. Dysuria, incontinence, and enuresis
15. Episodic loss of consciousness
16. Cosmetic defects or appearance
17. Tremors and other involuntary movements
18. Reproductive organ concerns: pregnancy, childbirth, menstrual and sexual dysfunctions, and sexually transmitted diseases

Children (in addition to many of the above symptoms)
1. Developmental retardation—mental, motor, or both
2. Attention-deficit/hyperactivity disorder (ADHD)
3. Oppositional behavior, temper tantrums, and aggression
4. Learning disabilities
5. Seizures
6. Feeding disorders, aspiration
7. Hypotonia or spasticity

    3. Patients sometimes fail to recognize certain changes in their mental state as symptoms (e.g., paranoid delusions). Though unrecognized by the patient, the physician recognizes the symptom by taking the history.

  B. Definition of a sign

    1. A *sign* is any objective manifestation of disease, detected by physical examination or laboratory tests.

    2. A *physical sign* is any disease-induced abnormality in body structure or function directly detected at the bedside by one or more of the physician's senses (e.g., a lump, atrophy, unequal pupils, tremor, or unsteady gait). The methods involved in detecting physical signs consist of the following:

      a. Inspection (vision)

      b. Palpation (touch and proprioception)

   c. Auscultation (hearing, generally with the aid of a stethoscope)

   d. Olfaction (smelling)

   e. Percussion, with hand or reflex hammer

   f. Miscellaneous maneuvers, such as presentation of various stimuli, strength testing, and measurement of blood pressure

  3. A *laboratory sign* is any disease-induced abnormality detected by a test that requires special apparatus or chemicals. Laboratory procedures include the following:

   a. Chemical or immunologic tests; cultures; microscopic examination of fluid or solid tissue, such as sputum, blood, cerebrospinal fluid, and urine; or a biopsy

   b. Cytogenetic/DNA analysis

   c. Radiographic or sonographic imaging or Doppler flow studies

   d. Electrical recording of the activity of brain, heart, peripheral nerve, or skeletal muscles

C. Distinction between symptoms and signs

  1. Symptoms are the *subjective* manifestations of disease, the patient's personal experiences, as disclosed by the history.

  2. Signs are the *objective* manifestations of disease, disclosed by the physical examination and various laboratory tests.

  3. Physicians often use the term "symptom" to mean both signs and symptoms. However, by distinguishing the terms, we emphasize the important difference between the subjective and objective manifestations of disease.

  4. In addition to symptoms, the patient may, of course, perceive signs of disease, such as a lump, but the lump remains subjective or hearsay evidence (i.e., historical) unless currently perceptible to the physician. For example, the patient may report swelling of the abdomen, based on a feeling of fullness, even though no actual swelling ever occurred.

D. In summary, the physician recognizes disease

  1. By its symptoms, as discovered by taking the history

  2. By its physical signs, as discovered by doing a physical examination

  3. By its laboratory signs, as discovered by laboratory tests, including biopsy or ultimately autopsy

E. Diagnosis of the presence of a disease
1. If the history and physical examination do not disclose any evidence of disease, the physician may decide to forego laboratory tests or do only a few.
2. If the history and physical examination suggest disease, the physician proposes a single provisional or working diagnosis and lists differential or alternative diagnoses. The physician then outlines a management plan that includes any laboratory tests and consultations necessary to establish the correct diagnosis (see Fig. 4–1).
3. The final diagnosis depends on integrating the history, physical findings, and laboratory findings. Correct diagnosis is the key to optimal treatment.
F. Definition of a syndrome
1. A *syndrome* is a lawfully related set of signs and symptoms that in general result from more than one proximate cause. From the history and physical examination, augmented when necessary by laboratory procedures, the physician may recognize a specific disease state or only a syndrome (*syn* = with, *drome* = running—therefore, *running with*). In this sense a syndrome differs from a disease or disease entity, which by definition should have only one proximate cause or at most only a group of very closely related causes.
2. For example, a large number of viral and bacterial infections cause a syndrome of sore throat, fever, headache, anorexia, malaise, myalgia, nausea, and vomiting. From these symptoms and signs the physician recognizes a lawful reaction of the body to infection—hence, a syndrome. To diagnose the infection syndrome as a specific disease requires identifying the offending microorganism, for example, by doing a throat culture. If the throat culture discloses streptococci, the cause of the syndrome is a distinct disease, a "strep throat," or if the culture discloses a rhinovirus, the disease is a common cold (coryza).
G. Overlapping definitions of syndrome and disease
1. Teratogens, genetic defects, and prenatal infections can cause syndromes consisting of congenital malformations and functional defects. Many factors, genetic or teratogenic, can cause a syndrome of mental retardation, dysmorphic facies, and short stature. When the proximate cause is an excess of genetic material on the twenty-first chromosome,

the patient has Down syndrome. If alcohol has caused the disorder, the patient has fetal alcohol syndrome. Here, physicians interchange the terms "syndrome" and "disease." In the foregoing examples, Down syndrome and fetal alcohol syndrome might be called "diseases."

2. The proposal of some authors to call specific malformation syndromes "anomalads" or "sequences"—thus "Down anomalad"—rather than "syndromes" has not gained universal acceptance (Jones, 2006). The *Diagnostic and Statistical Manual of Mental Disorders* (DSM IV TR 2000) tiptoes around the issue of disease versus syndrome by using the term "disorder" (e.g., "passive–aggressive personality disorder"). Nevertheless, the distinction between a syndrome and a specific disease entity remains important, like the distinction between symptom and sign. A syndrome is generally not a final or specific diagnosis. The physician must complete further studies to diagnose the particular cause of the syndrome in the particular patient.

3. Although the overlapping use of "symptom"/"sign" and "syndrome"/"disease" may seem confusing, the context generally clarifies the intended meaning.

H. Overlapping manifestations of systemic and neurologic disease

1. The nervous system displays three types of functions: *mental, motor,* and *sensory.* Therefore, disease may express itself through mental, motor, or sensory dysfunction (Fig. 2–1).

2. Mental, motor, or sensory dysfunction may result either from primary disease of the nervous system or from the secondary effects of nonneurologic disease on the nervous system. For example, a nonneurologic disorder such as anemia can cause dizziness, as can a primary neurologic disorder such as a brain tumor.

3. Because the symptoms and signs of primary neurologic and nonneurologic disease overlap, primary neurologic disease enters the differential diagnosis of most of humankind's commonest symptoms, particularly headaches, backaches, other pains, blurred vision, dizziness, fatigability, and depression (Table 2–1). For example, pain in the left arm may arise from cardiac ischemia or from a herniated cervical disk, not disease within the arm itself. Fatigue felt over the whole body may arise from malabsorption of

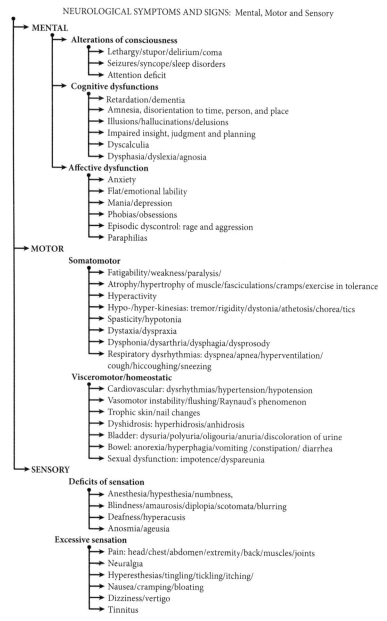

NEUROLOGICAL SYMPTOMS AND SIGNS: Mental, Motor and Sensory

MENTAL
- **Alterations of consciousness**
  - Lethargy/stupor/delirium/coma
  - Seizures/syncope/sleep disorders
  - Attention deficit
- **Cognitive dysfunctions**
  - Retardation/dementia
  - Amnesia, disorientation to time, person, and place
  - Illusions/hallucinations/delusions
  - Impaired insight, judgment and planning
  - Dyscalculia
  - Dysphasia/dyslexia/agnosia
- **Affective dysfunction**
  - Anxiety
  - Flat/emotional lability
  - Mania/depression
  - Phobias/obsessions
  - Episodic dyscontrol: rage and aggression
  - Paraphilias

MOTOR
- **Somatomotor**
  - Fatigability/weakness/paralysis/
  - Atrophy/hypertrophy of muscle/fasciculations/cramps/exercise in tolerance
  - Hyperactivity
  - Hypo-/hyper-kinesias: tremor/rigidity/dystonia/athetosis/chorea/tics
  - Spasticity/hypotonia
  - Dystaxia/dyspraxia
  - Dysphonia/dysarthria/dysphagia/dysprosody
  - Respiratory dysrhythmias: dyspnea/apnea/hyperventilation/ cough/hiccoughing/sneezing
- **Visceromotor/homeostatic**
  - Cardiovascular: dysrhythmias/hypertension/hypotension
  - Vasomotor instability/flushing/Raynaud's phenomenon
  - Trophic skin/nail changes
  - Dyshidrosis: hyperhidrosis/anhidrosis
  - Bladder: dysuria/polyuria/oligouria/anuria/discoloration of urine
  - Bowel: anorexia/hyperphagia/vomiting /constipation/ diarrhea
  - Sexual dysfunction: impotence/dyspareunia

SENSORY
- **Deficits of sensation**
  - Anesthesia/hypesthesia/numbness,
  - Blindness/amaurosis/diplopia/scotomata/blurring
  - Deafness/hyperacusis
  - Anosmia/ageusia
- **Excessive sensation**
  - Pain: head/chest/abdomen/extremity/back/muscles/joints
  - Neuralgia
  - Hyperesthesias/tingling/tickling/itching/
  - Nausea/cramping/bloating
  - Dizziness/vertigo
  - Tinnitus

Figure 2–1. Mental, motor, or sensory dysfunctions produced by primary neurologic disease or secondary to systemic disease. (Reproduced by permission from DeMyer W. Technique of the Neurologic Examination, 5th ed. New York: McGraw-Hill, 2004.)

vitamin B_{12} in the small bowel and the resultant anemia. These considerations lead to a profound general principle: *The symptoms and signs caused by a diseased organ may appear at a site distant from the organ and in a manner unrelated to the actual function of the diseased organ.*

III. **Diagnosis and Differential Diagnosis of Disease**

A. Definition of diagnosis: Literally translated, *diagnosis* means *through* (dia) and *knowing* (gnosis)—thus, to *know through* something, knowing through to the essence or cause.

B. Specificity of diagnosis: The specificity of diagnosis varies, depending on the information derived from the study of the patient and the current state of medical knowledge. A diagnosis may be descriptive, anatomic, pathologic, and etiologic.

1. *Descriptive diagnosis:* If the patient has some outstanding symptom such as a headache or a sign such as fever but no known cause, the physician can make only a descriptive diagnosis, such as headache of unknown origin or fever of unknown origin. When we do not know the cause of a disorder, we often precede the descriptive diagnosis by the term "essential" or "idiopathic" (*idio* = peculiar, related to itself, as in "idiosyncrasy"; and *path* = disease); thus, essential or idiopathic epilepsy means that the patient has epilepsy but without a known cause. Molecular biology has greatly reduced the number of idiopathic diseases. For example, an angiotensinogen gene on chromosome 1q42-43 may cause the disorder traditionally called "essential hypertension" (Caulfield et al., 1994).

2. *Anatomic diagnosis:* Sometimes the physician knows the site of the lesion but not the cause and can make a descriptive and an anatomic diagnosis.

   a. A patient may have paraplegia, a descriptive diagnosis meaning paralysis of the legs.

   b. The neurologic examination may localize the lesion to the tenth thoracic level of the spinal cord, thus giving an anatomic diagnosis of the site of the lesion.

3. *Pathologic diagnosis:* The lesion in the foregoing patient's spinal cord may be a neoplasm, infarct, inflammation, hematoma, or demyelination, among other possibilities. Such a list of diagnostic possibilities constitutes the *differential diagnosis.*

    4. *Etiologic diagnosis*

      a. Even when laboratory tests, such as radiographic imaging or biopsy demonstrate a lesion, the causal diagnosis may still be genetic, autoimmune, environmental, and so on. To establish a specific etiologic diagnosis may require a further step, such as a biopsy or identification of a virus in the spinal fluid by polymerase chain reaction.

      b. Ideally, the diagnosis is descriptive, anatomic, pathologic, and etiologic depending on the specific information provided by the history, physical examination, and laboratory tests, thus identifying the proximate cause.

C. Differential diagnosis

    1. Since more than one agent can cause most symptoms, signs, and syndromes, the physician constructs a list of differential diagnoses in every patient.

    2. The list of differential diagnoses may include a large number of possibilities—some common, others rare. A differential diagnostic dendrogram or algorithm illustrates how the diagnostic possibilities increase almost geometrically. Notice in going to the right in Figure 6–3 that the diagnosis gets more and more specific as the proximate causes under each large branch of the dendrogram are specified.

    3. When taking the history, the physician begins to review the different diagnostic possibilities and causes exemplified by dendrograms or algorithms and inserts questions to explore these possibilities. The diagnostic hypotheses not only direct the line of inquiry during the history but determine the focus of the subsequent physical examination.

IV. Summary

A. Physicians recognize disease by the deviation of the patient from physical and mental norms.

B. A disease has one proximate cause but often numerous contributory causes linked to the person's genetic background, environment, and culture.

C. Diseases manifest by subjective deviations called *symptoms* and objective deviations called *signs*. The clinical history discloses the symptoms, while the physical examination and laboratory tests disclose the signs. Symptoms and signs occur together in lawfully related patterns called *syndromes* or *diseases*.

D. Symptoms, signs, and syndromes can result from numerous causes. The physician tries to reach a single specific diagnosis that best explains the symptoms, signs, or syndrome. The clinical information may permit only a vague *descriptive* diagnosis such as recurrent abdominal pain of unknown origin, an *anatomic* diagnosis such as a mass in the left upper abdominal quadrant, or a pathologic diagnosis such as recurrent abdominal pain secondary to pancreatic carcinoma; and finally, if the cause of the carcinoma is known, a specific etiologic diagnosis can be achieved.

E. Confounding problems in diagnosis are as follows:

1. The symptoms and signs of disease may appear in a site distant from the site of the lesion or the diseased organ that causes them.

2. The manifestations of primary neurologic and nonneurologic disease overlap so much that the physician has to consider neurologic disease in the differential diagnosis of most symptoms, particularly the commonest symptoms of humankind, such as fatigability, dizziness, headache, backache, or pain in the extremities, chest, and abdomen. For example, headache may result from emotional stress, a primary intracranial lesion such as a brain tumor, or hypertension that arises outside of the nervous system.

References

Abbey SE, Garfinkel PE. Neurasthenia and chronic fatigue syndrome: the role of culture in the making of a diagnosis. Am J Psychiatry 1991; 148:1638–1646.

Barglow P, Bowman M, Friedlander J. Is post-traumatic stress disorder (PTSD) a valid psychiatric diagnosis? Sci Rev Alt Med 2006;10:36–44.

Caulfield M, Lavender P, Farrall M, et al. Linkage of the angiotensinogen gene to essential hypertension. N Engl J Med 1994;330:1629–1638.

Del Piccolo L, Putnam SM, Mazzi MA, et al. The biopsychosocial domains and the functions of the medical interview in primary care: construct validity of the Verona Medical Interview Classification System. Patient Educ Couns 2004;53:47–56.

DeMyer W. Technique of the Neurologic Examination. New York: McGraw-Hill, 2004.

Diagnostic and Statistical Manual of Mental Disorders, Text Revision, 4th ed. Washington DC: American Psychiatric Association, 2000.

Engle GL. The clinical application of the biopsychosocial model. Am J Psychiatry 1980;137:535–544.

Hoffman P. The Man Who Loved Only Numbers. The Story of Paul Erdös and the Search for Mathematical Truth. New York: Hyperion, 1998.

Humber JM, Almeder AF, eds. What Is Disease? Totowa, NJ: Humana Press, 1997.

Jones KL. Smith's Recognizable Patterns of Human Malformation. Philadelphia: Elsevier Saunders, 2006.

White P, ed. Biopsychosocial Medicine: An Integrated Approach to Understanding Illness. New York: Oxford University Press, 2005.

The Importance of the Clinical History

3

I. **Why the Clinical History Is the Most Important Event in the Practice of Medicine**
   A. The history discloses what the patient wants, needs, or expects.
   There are four questions which in some form or other every patient asks of the physician:
      1. What is the matter with me? This is diagnosis.
      2. Can you put me right? This is treatment and prognosis.
      3. How did I get it? This is causation.
      4. How can I avoid it in the future? This is prevention
   B. In response, the physician offers
      1. To diagnose and treat existent disease
      2. To prevent avoidable disease and death
      3. To promote a healthy life
      4. To always give comfort
      5. Compassion, humility, and grace in all acts (Schattner and Fletcher, 2004).
   C. The fundamental goals of the clinical history

II. **The Clinical History as a Mutual Process of Knowing Between the Physician and the Patient**
   A. The knowing process
      1. The knowing process and resultant trust is the pivotal and most important outcome of the clinical history. The clinical history enables the physician to know and empathize with the patient, but equally important is that the patient comes to know and decides whether or not to trust the physician (Inui, 2003). The result is a medical partnership of understanding, with as much unspoken as spoken between patient and physician (Frank, 2004). For the development of this trust, nothing can ever replace the history. *The quality of the history and physical examination determines the quality of the patient–physician relationship and the quality of the outcome for the patient.*

Table 3–1. Fundamental Goals and Importance of the Clinical History

1. The history discloses current symptoms and medically significant past events: previous illnesses, hospitalizations, operations, and injuries.
2. The history provides the basis for the appropriate diagnostic, therapeutic, and preventive management that match the patient's needs and values.
3. The history directs the physician to the essential steps of the physical examination and to the laboratory tests to order. The physical signs or laboratory results become meaningful only when integrated with the patient's history.
4. The history is the only way to diagnose the many diseases that cause only symptoms and no signs.
5. The history provides the only direct opportunity for the physician to learn about the hopes, needs, and beliefs of the patient as a whole person. It discloses how the patient feels about the illness and life itself. Neither technological wizardry nor checklists can ever substitute for the knowledge of the whole person provided by the history.
6. The most important outcome of the history, which nothing else can produce, is trust and understanding. From the quality of the history and the physical examination, the patient comes to trust or distrust the physician's ethics, competence, and offerings for management.
7. The questions asked by the physician in probing the patient's medical experiences, past and present, start the process of patient education as the patient comes to understand the purpose of the questions and the vistas they open.
8. The developmental history provides the basis for early recognition of mental, motor, and sensory dysfunctions and their remediation.
9. The family history is the basis for genomic medicine: recognition of familial diseases, assessment of the patient's risk of hereditary diseases, genetic testing, and genetic counseling. When eliciting the cause of death of family members, the physician gains insight into the patient's attitudes to end-of-life care.
10. The environmental history, along with the family history, discloses risk factors for the patient's health.
11. Because the history leads to the correct diagnosis of each individual, it also leads to accurate statistics of the type, frequency, and severity of disease in a population. Thus, it forms the basis for setting public-health priorities.

The same techniques for eliciting the history per se also serve to disclose whether the patient has the knowledge and mental status (sapience) to give rational, informed consent about management, particularly about terminal care (see Chapter 14).

2. Many factors impair trust in today's medical practice, particularly the restricted time allowed for taking the history (Anders, 1996; Horton, 2004).
3. Since disease may impair personality, mental competence, speech, movement, and employability, the physician must consider the patient's entire medical, social, and economic future in planning management. When unable to cure the patient, the physician must prepare to provide comfort and solace, the one eternal and universal goal of every patient–physician contact. To give such comfort and make such plans effectively requires a thorough, compassionate history

that discloses the patient's mental state, values, and life circumstances (Cassell, 1997).

> The competent physician, before he attempts to give medicine to his patients, makes himself acquainted not only with the disease which he wishes to cure, but also with the habits and constitution of the sick man.
>
> —Cicero (106–43 BCE), *De Oratore II*

4. Centuries later Hawthorne reaffirmed the principle.

> As not only the disease interested the physician, but he was strongly moved to look into the character and qualities of the patient. He deemed it essential, it would seem, to know the man, before attempting to do him good.
>
> —Nathanial Hawthorne (1804–1864), *The Scarlet Letter* (Hawthorne, p 124)

5. Some modernists assert that the principle of knowing the whole patient was just recently discovered (Odegaard, 1986). The foregoing quotations prove that the principle of knowing the patient extends far back into antiquity. The time-honored techniques for history taking enable the physician to achieve the kind of knowing that leads to the optimal management and the maximal benefit for the patient.

6. Optimal management goes far beyond just prescribing a pill. It requires the biopsychosocial approach (Engle, 1977; White, 2005). Consider Patient (Pt) 1, whom I saw in the Pediatric Neurology Clinic when she brought in two of her children because of failing in school. The children were neurologically normal. After checking school records and test results, I found that the children had normal intelligence but often were absent or distracted in class. The history clearly disclosed that the solution to the children's school problems required attention to the health of the mother and the family unit. Because my history disclosed significant health problems of the mother, I referred her to an internist who could pursue areas beyond my competence as a pediatric neurologist.

Please note: All 35 patients presented in this text are actual patients, except for the composite Pts 3 and 12.

B. *Pt 1* (abbreviated from the internist's report):
1. Identifying data: 30-year-old female, married, homemaker
2. Presenting concerns: several weeks of severe stomach pain after eating and extreme fatigability for several months
3. Review of systems: disabling daily headaches, persistent constipation, and *dyspareunia* (painful intercourse)
4. Family history: four children, two of whom are failing in school; husband and some of his family are alcoholic
5. Psychosocial history: dropped out of tenth grade because of pregnancy; overburdened with the four children and an abusive, alcoholic husband; never employed; hobby of flower gardening but no social activities
6. Mental status: no facial expression or animation, spirits low, unkempt appearance, recently began drinking daily and finally confided that she had thought about ending her life
7. Physical examination: appeared weary and considerably older than her stated age of 30 years but otherwise normal
8. Laboratory workup: routine blood chemistry, blood count, and urinalysis normal; stool negative for ova, parasites, and blood
9. Radiographic studies of her upper gastrointestinal tract and endoscopy disclosed a peptic ulcer and *Helicobacter pylori* infection
10. Clinical impressions
    a. Peptic ulcer
    b. Situational depression
    c. Incipient alcoholism
    d. Tension headaches
    e. Dyspareunia
    f. Constipation
11. Patient management based on knowing
    a. The internist could have considered the patient as a collection of symptoms and treated her headaches with acetaminophen (Tylenol), her belly pain and *H. pylori* infection with cimetidine and antibiotics, her depression with amitriptyline, K-Y jelly for dyspareunia, a stool softener for constipation, and disulfiram (Antabuse) for alcoholism. Such a parade of pills alone would not resolve basic problems and, if given simultaneously, could lead to adverse drug interactions.

b. The internist did start by treating her ulcer, since that was the quickest resolvable problem, but went beyond the symptoms to help the patient work out a long-term plan to reorganize her life. By taking a history as described in this text, the internist encouraged the patient to disclose the information about the husband's and her own alcoholism and her depression, information required for optimal management. Having also learned about her interest in flower gardening, he discussed whether she might want to take a course in flower arrangement and perhaps to get work in a florist shop or garden store as a means of developing satisfactions and self-sufficiency. The internist also asked the patient to bring in pictures of her flower garden. He referred her to Alcoholics Anonymous, and he made follow-up appointments to monitor whether she would respond or ultimately need referral for psychiatric treatment.

c. Several weeks later, when she returned to me for a follow-up visit regarding her children, her abdominal pain had stopped and she looked years younger. She had a part-time job in a flower shop, and the children's schoolwork had improved. She stated that she had returned to the internist because of his personal interest in her flower gardening and was impressed that he had actually asked to see pictures of her garden. Gardening was the one factor in her life that she could control and gain gratification from. The internist's personal attention to this topic, disclosed only by a careful history that inquired not only into her discontents but also into her hobbies and interests, fostered the successful therapeutic alliance—a marvelous example of the value of the physician's "personal touch" and interest in the whole person (Charon, 2004).

III. **The History Is the Only Way to Diagnose the Many Diseases that Produce Only Symptoms But No Signs**

A. Most diseases cause symptoms and many also cause corroborative signs. For the many diseases that cause only symptoms but no corroborative physical or laboratory signs, the diagnosis rests essentially on the history. Only an optimal history makes the diagnosis of these diseases possible.

However, laboratory tests may play an important role in excluding diseases on the differential diagnosis list. Examples of diseases diagnosable solely or mainly by symptoms include numerous mental disorders; most types of headaches, particularly migraine; some forms of syncope; nonepileptic seizures (*pseudoepileptic* seizures); breath-holding spells; irritable bowel syndrome with dyspepsia and other multiple discomforts in the chest and abdomen (Lynn and Friedman, 1993); and a large number of pain syndromes. Examples of the latter include trigeminal neuralgia, which causes excruciating jolts of pain in the face, and proctalgia fugax with knife-like rectal pains.

IV. The History Focuses the Physical Examination

A. You cannot and need not do every possible test on every patient. The history guides you to focus on the pertinent parts of the examination. Given a previously well-functioning 26-year-old patient with acute onset of pain radiating down a leg, the physician must test for a dermatomal type of sensory loss, but extensive tests for cerebral dysfunction are unnecessary. For an elderly patient suspected of dementia, sensory testing for dermatomal loss is useless, but you then must focus on tests for cerebral dysfunction. The primary role of the physical examination becomes the testing of hypotheses derived from the history.

V. Why No Physical or Laboratory Finding Has Meaning Until Integrated with the Patient's Full Clinical History

A. Consider *Pt 2:* A healthy, 21-year-old woman, pregnant for the first time, had a routine Venereal Disease Research Laboratory (VDRL) test for syphilis, which was positive. She and her husband, both of whom seemed honest, reliable, and duly concerned about the health of the fetus, denied any sexual contact with other partners. She had no stigmata of congenital syphilis, such as Hutchinson incisors, interstitial keratitis, saber shins, or neurosensory deafness. Review of old medical records disclosed that the patient and her mother had a negative VDRL test at the time of the patient's birth. These facts excluded congenital syphilis. The patient had spent her nineteenth year in the Peace Corps in Africa, where she had contracted malaria and had received treatment for it. She had no history or physical findings suggestive of any other diseases that cause false-positive serologic tests and no evidence of an immunoglobulin disorder.

I did a fluorescent treponemal antibody absorption (FTA-ABS) test, which was negative. Putting the information together, particularly the malaria exposure and the fact that sometimes pregnancy itself can cause a reactive VDRL, I concluded that the patient had a false-positive VDRL and required no further evaluation or treatment for syphilis. Thus, one positive laboratory sign does not make a diagnosis. That requires integrating the laboratory tests with the history and physical examination. For this reason, select-it-yourself tests offered now in walk-in clinics in shopping malls constitute poor medical practice. The "consumer" does not know the limits of accuracy of the test and the frequency of false-positive and false-negative results or their meaning. The result may mislead the patient into a false sense of security or into taking drastic, totally unwarranted actions, even to the degree of suicide. Self-referral for electron beam computed tomography is another case in point (Taylor and O'Malley, 1998). In fact, a careful history would safely obviate many routine laboratory tests, even for patients scheduled to undergo surgery (Roizen, 2000).

VI. **How the History Provides the Basis for Public Health Policy**
Because the history is indispensable for determining diagnosis and for disclosing the proximate and the contributory causes of disease, it also provides the basis for compiling accurate population statistics of disease type, prevalence, and cause. The statistics, compiled from accurate diagnosis of individual patients, then lead to rational priorities for public-health measures, particularly when epidemics threaten.

VII. **Summary**
   A. The history is the indispensable foundation for all diagnosis and for the mutual knowing of physician and patient.
   B. From knowing the patient as a whole person, the physician can formulate an optimal management matched to that patient.
   C. From an optimal, compassionate history the patient comes to trust the physician and to select the appropriate medical management.
   D. The history discloses what education the patient will need in order to follow the appropriate management.

E. The history provides the only means to diagnose the many diseases that cause only symptoms.

F. The family history and environmental history disclose risk factors for diseases that may afflict the patient.

G. The history enables the physician to focus on the pertinent aspects of the physical examination and to eliminate unnecessary steps.

H. No physical or laboratory sign achieves meaning until correlated with the patient's full clinical history. Only then can decisions be made about the meaning of positive or negative results.

I. Because the history is indispensable for diagnosis and estimation of the frequency of disease and the disability caused by it, it forms the basis to set priorities for public-health policy. All of the foregoing reasons, summarized in Table 3–1, make an optimal clinical history indispensable and irreplaceable in the practice of medicine.

References

Anders G. Health Against Wealth: HMOs and the Breakdown of Medical Trust. Boston: Houghton-Mifflin, 1996.

Cassell EJ. Doctoring: The Nature of Primary Care Medicine. New York: Oxford University Press, 1997.

Charon, R. Narrative and medicine. N Engl J Med 2004;350:862–864.

Engel G. The need for a new medical model. Science 1977;196:129–136.

Frank AW. The Renewal of Generosity: Illness Medicine, and How to Live. Chicago: Chicago University Press, 2004.

Hawthorne N. The Scarlet Letter. New York: Charles Scribner's Sons, 1919, p 124.

Horton R. The dawn of McScience. New York Review of Books 2004; 51(March 11):7–9.

Inui, T. A Flag in the Wind: Educating for Professionalism in Medicine. Washington DC: American Association of Medical Colleges, 2003.

Lynn RB, Friedman LS. Irritable bowel syndrome. N Engl J Med 1993;329: 1940–1945.

Odegaard CE. Dear Doctor. A Personal Letter to a Physician. Menlo Park, CA: Henry J. Kaiser Family Foundation, 1986.

Roizen MF. More preoperative assessment by physicians and less by laboratory tests. N Engl J Med 2000;342:204–205.

Schattner A, Fletcher RH. Pearls and pitfalls in patient care: need to revive traditional clinical values. Am J Med Sci 2004;327:79–85.

Taylor AJ, O'Malley PG. Self-referral of patients for electron-beam computed tomography to screen for coronary artery disease. N Engl J Med 1998;339:2018–2020.

White P, ed. Biopsychosocial Medicine: An Integrated Approach to Understanding Illness. New York: Oxford University Press, 2005.

How the Physician's Ethics and Goals Determine the Content and Techniques of the Clinical History

4

I. The Ethical and Operational Components of the Medical Model for the Patient–Physician Relationship
   A. The ethical component of the medical model
      1. The ethical code of the medical model (Table 4–1) requires the physician to act always for the patient's benefit (Wynia et al., 1999). This key ethic is the foundation for the entire the physician–patient relationship (Li, 1996). Most of the major medical organizations worldwide and most ethicists either explicitly accept this ethic and the derivative ethics listed in Table 4–1 or do not contradict them (Ahronheim et al., 2000; Beauchamp and Walters, 2003; Bernat, 2002; Hope, 2004; Weinberg, 2000).
      2. This chapter shows how applying the explicit ethics listed in Table 4–1 results in a history that best serves the patient. Educators today plead for incorporating ethics in the daily

Table 4–1. Traditional Ethical Guidelines for the Medical Model

1. *Primum non nocere:* first, do no harm.
2. Act only in the patient's interest and only for the patient's benefit. Do not profit from nor sell what you prescribe, nor select tests on the basis of profit.
3. Revere life, everyone's life (and perhaps all life).
4. Accept every patient nonjudgmentally, as equal to every other patient in deserving care.
5. Respond to every patient professionally, not emotionally. Do not exploit the patient to serve personal financial, emotional, or sexual needs.
6. Preserve the patient's privacy and maintain confidentiality.
7. Practice evidence-based medicine. Employ those procedures and treatments that have passed rigorous scientific tests for safety and efficacy.
8. Manage patients not by ordering them what to do but by explaining the medically acceptable options and their probable outcomes.
9. Insure informed consent for your management plan and procedures.
10. Attempt no more than your knowledge and manual skills justify.
11. Continuously study to improve your skills and competency.
12. Respect the views of colleagues and teachers.
13. Pass on medical knowledge and discoveries freely to students and other physicians.
14. Observe moderation in demeanor, dress, and fees.
15. Do not diagnose or treat yourself nor accept family members or close personal friends as patients.
16. Act always with courtesy, humility, grace, and consideration.

medical curriculum, to show how ethics affect all of the physician's attitudes and acts, especially the taking of the history (Inui, 2003; Tauber, 2006).

3. Physicians have recognized most of the ethics listed in Table 4–1 for centuries, even millennia (Bynum et al., 2006;Yarnofsky, 2004). Some of the historical precursors are found in the oath of Hippocrates (460–377 BCE) (Chadwick and Mann, 1950; Miles, 2004) and the Prayer of Maimonides [1135–1204 CE (Friedenwald, 1917, pp 260–261))].

The Oath of Hippocrates

I swear by Apollo Physician and Asclepius [Aseculapius] and Hygieia [Hygeia] and Panaceia [Panacea] [daughters of Aesculapius] and all the gods and goddesses, making them my witness, that I will fulfill according to my ability and judgment this oath and this covenant:

To hold him who has taught me this art as equal to my parents and to live my life in partnership with him, and if he is in need of money to give him a share of mine, and to regard his offspring as equal to my brothers in male lineage and to teach them this art—if they desire to learn it—without fee and covenant; to give a share of precepts and oral instruction and all the other learning to my sons and to the sons of him who has instructed me and to pupils who have signed the covenant and have taken an oath according to the medical law, but to no one else.

I will apply dietetic [therapeutic] measures for the benefit of the sick according to my ability and judgment; I will keep them from harm and injustice.

I will neither give a deadly drug to anybody if asked for it, nor will I make a suggestion to this effect. Similarly I will not give to a woman an abortive remedy. In purity and holiness I will guard my life and my art.

I will not use the knife, not even on sufferers from stone, but will withdraw in favor of such men as are engaged in this work.

Whatever houses I may visit, I will come for the benefit of the sick, remaining free of all intentional injustice, of all mischief and particularly of sexual relations with both female and male persons, be they free or slave.

What I may see or hear in the course of the treatment or even outside of the treatment in regard to the life of men, which on no account one must spread abroad, I will keep to myself holding such things shameful to be spoken about.

If I fulfill this oath and do not violate it, may it be granted to me to enjoy life and art, being honored with fame among all men for all time to come; if I transgress it and swear falsely, may the opposite of all this be my lot.

—Reproduced by permission from
Temkin O, Temkin CL, eds. Ancient Medicine:
Selected Papers of Ludwig Edelstein. Baltimore:
Johns Hopkins University Press, 1967, p 6.

The Prayer of Maimonides

May the love for my art actuate me at all times. May neither avarice, nor miserliness, nor the thirst for glory, nor for a great reputation engage my mind; for the enemies of truth and philanthropy could easily deceive me and make me forgetful of my lofty aim of doing good to thy children. May I never see in the patient anything but a fellow creature in pain. Grant me strength, time and opportunity always to correct what I have acquired, always to extend its domain: For knowledge is immense and the spirit of man can extend infinitely to enrich itself daily with new requirements. Today he can discover his errors of yesterday and tomorrow he may obtain a new light on what he thinks himself sure of today. O God, thou has appointed me to watch over the life and death of thy creatures. Here I am ready for my vocation.

4. The oath of Hippocrates remained unchanged over the centuries, until recently (Temkin and Temkin, 1967; Jouanna, 1999; Markel, 2004; Pruchnicki, 1997). Now, some versions omit the reference to pagan gods, the prohibition of euthanasia and abortion, and the advocacy of free education for medical students (Markel, 2004). In fact, Leake (1927, appendix II) quotes a version that substitutes Christian gods. The issue here is not tone of accepting pagan gods, abortion, euthanasia, and free education for medical students but one of historical honesty. Medical schools, whose students today graduate with debts of $100,000–$200,000, have long ignored the Hippocratic injunction to pass on medical knowledge without a fee.

5. The traditional ethics for everyday medical practice may not answer the challenges posed by research in functional brain imaging. Functional brain imaging seeks to discover the

neural circuitry underlying consciousness, "free" will, moral reasoning and conscience, the persistent vegetative state, "out-of-body" experiences (De Ridder et al., 2007), and the use of mind-enhancing drugs in normal as well as sick people. Neuroscientists now seek objective analysis of mental functions, based on how the brain actually works, rather than just invoking collections of rules and admonitions based on ancient manuscripts and legal precedents. For example, consider the immense potential for good or harm from manipulating and controlling the reward circuitry of the brain. A new branch of ethics, neuroethics, has arisen to oversee these new developments (Glannon, 2007; Illes, 2005; Neuroethics.org). In any event, neuroethics still has to start from the basic ethic: First of all, do no harm; medical actions should be for the benefit of the patient.

6. Above all, discussions of ethics should not degenerate into hurling simplistic slogans but should proceed with humility, grace, respect for varying viewpoints, and the necessity to face new challenges not covered by previous formulations (Steinbock, 2007).

B. The operational component of the medical model

1. The operational part of the medical model calls for objective, scientific validation of medical concepts and of the safety and efficacy of medical management—in a phrase, evidence-based medicine. No other method of evaluation—intuition, anecdotes, folklore, shamans—can even begin to match science to ascertain medical reality. The very questions asked in the history reflect scientific concepts of causality and scientific theories of disease pathogenesis. In relying on science I refer to true science, not science warped by commercial interests (Angell, 2004; Horton, 2004; Washburn, 2005).

II. Origin of the Ethical Code for the Practice of Medicine

A. Independence of the ethical code from parochial belief systems

1. The measure of a physician's ethics is whether they promote the patient's health, not whether they express a particular political, religious, or societal view. No Arc of the Covenant exists with medical commandments inscribed in stone. The ethical code in Table 4–1 represents the cumulative wisdom of the best physicians throughout the ages, derived

empirically from their day-to-day observations of what has worked best with patients. Rational persons, whether secular or devout, can agree with this code because it is empirically derived, independent of authoritarian dogmas (Bernat, 2002). Not only does the code transcend personal beliefs but it discourages debating these beliefs in the consulting chamber. In attending to the patient's needs, the physician encourages the patient to voice his or her concerns freely without fear of rebuff or argumentation. By adopting the particular attitudes, techniques, and analytic thought processes of the medical model, physicians and patients of diverse beliefs, whether secular or religious, can find a common ground to work together (Bernat, 2002).

> Simply telling patients about one's personal beliefs, let alone proselytizing, potentially influences the patient who has placed her trust in a physician and feels awkward (or ashamed) about taking a different position.
>
> —Aubrey Milunsky (1986, p 9)

2. Although not topics for debate in the consulting room, the physician needs to learn about and nonjudgmentally deal with the patient's personal beliefs (see Chapter 14).

III. How Each Ethic of the Medical Model Shapes the Clinical History

A. Note: The order of the ethics discussed matches that in Table 4–1.

1. *Primum non nocere* (first, do no harm): Whatever we do in the history, physical examination, and management should not cause harm. Avoiding harm in taking the history means discretion in the type, phrasing, and timing of inquiries and avoidance of sarcasm or ridicule. In some instances we do have to accept harm, when the benefits outweigh the harm, as in chemotherapy for cancer. The special application of this ethic to children is especially difficult (Burgio and Lantos, 1998). The history also aids in avoiding harm by disclosing hazards such as allergies to drugs or adverse reactions to previous tests or therapeutic efforts.

2. Act only in the patient's interest and only for the patient's benefit.

a. The physician cannot serve two masters. You cannot simultaneously serve the patient and act as an agent for outside interests, as a gatekeeper to contain costs or enhance profits, to recruit for a religion or cause, or to reflect the prejudices of the family or society at large (Burnum, 1984; Zuger, 2004). Serving these extraneous goals would drastically change the very technique of the history because physician and patient would become adversaries, jockeying for advantage, rather than collaborators. The participation of Nazi physicians in the killing of mentally ill or retarded persons exemplifies the ethical error of acting for governmental or societal goals rather than serving each patient's health needs. Paradoxically, in acting in the patient's best interest and no other, the physician also ultimately acts in the best interests of the family and of the society at large because it enables each person to function at his or her best.

b. Physicians should neither sell what they prescribe nor select tests on the basis of profit. Decisions that affect the physician's income will taint the objectivity of the management and slant the history to justify exploitation.

c. In serving only the patient's interest, the physician must not exploit the patient to achieve personal goals: financial gain, conversion to a creed, or sexual gratification. All ethical codes, from the oath of Hippocrates until today, forbid sex between physician and patient. The trust and emotional transference that the patient invests in the physician precludes informed consent (Johnson, 1993). The patient, vulnerable because of illness or self-disclosure, has surrendered power; and that lends itself too readily to exploitation by a self-serving physician.

May I never see in the patient anything but a fellow creature in pain.
—From the Prayer of Maimonides (1135–1204)
(Friedenwald, 1917, pp 260–261)

Never go to a doctor whose office plants have died.
—Erma Bombeck (1992, p 226)

... and respect for all that lives whether it goes in skin, scales, feathers, leaves, or fur.

—Harvey Stanbrough (Stanbrough, 2005, p 151)

a. The physician reveres, fosters, and furthers the life of every person, recognizing life's preciousness and fragility and the irreversibility of death. Life is the most basic of the rights, from which all other rights derive. If you, as a person, have no right to exist, other rights become totally meaningless. The physician's reverence for life derives from and extends the social agreement that permits our survival as a species. That agreement or contract states that I will recognize and insure your right to occupy space, to sustenance, and to life, liberty, and the pursuit of happiness if you recognize and insure my right. Repudiation of this social contract leads to indiscriminate killing of one individual by another; organized killings by gangs; pogroms of racial, religious, and cultural cleansing; and international war.

b. Reverence for the life of the patient requires that the physician try to discover ways to promote the best life, whatever the patient's current circumstances, not to find excuses to deny treatment or for the patient to die. Affirmation of each person's life has constituted a basic, traditional mind-set of physicians. Reverence for the value of each person profoundly affects the technique of the clinical history. Unless we retain a reverence for life, why worry about taking a history to obtain the patient's trust in order to maximize health? Why not pursue an ethical bias toward death that permits us to sift through the history to find justification for letting as many patients die as possible? If you have heard any of the chilling televised interviews of patients by Dr. Jack Kevorkian ("Dr. Death") as he searches to justify euthanasia and guides the questioning toward its acceptance, you will understand this point (presented on CBS's *60 Minutes*, November 22, 1998; Hewitt, 2008). His history failed to explore the positive aspects of the patient's life, the satisfactions and rewards that would encourage the patient to live in spite of a terminal illness. Kevorkian's history exemplifies how the ethical goal—in his case the attempt to justify euthanasia—influences the form and content of the history. By misusing the power of the techniques of the clinical history, some might see Kevorkian as one of the most prolific serial killers on record.

c. To obviate divisive debate in a history text on the ethic of reverence for life in regard to elective abortion, let us observe that thoughtful, decent, and considerate people disagree about it. Let us not reduce complex issues to sloganeering about the right of the zygote or conceptus to life versus the right of the woman to choose termination. Instead, let us seek incremental agreements. Almost everyone agrees that the basic problem is not abortion but to prevent unwanted pregnancy, by abstinence or contraception. The pivotal question after pregnancy occurs is "When does the conceptus achieve personhood?" Almost everyone agrees that at sometime between the fertilization of the ovum and the arrival of the baby in your hands at birth, we must grant the conceptus the rights of personhood and revere and protect its life. Each of us then has to decide at what stage of development—is it at conception or at 4, 8, l6, or 32 weeks or full term—the conceptus achieves the rights of personhood. When the conceptus achieves personhood, the social contract that enables us to survive as individuals and as a species goes into force and requires a reverence (or at least a tolerance) for its life. In any event I suggest approaching such issues with humility and grace: humility about the absolute correctness of your own beliefs, and the grace to examine differing viewpoints. Productive dialogue requires you to avoid the "arrogance of certainty," which insists that your belief can be the only correct one.

4. Accept every patient nonjudgmentally as equal to every other patient in deserving care.

a. When ill and in need, everyone should feel that the physician, if no other person on earth, will accept them graciously and respectfully as worthy of help and worthy of life. By avoiding depreciatory judgments that condemn patients for their transgressions, beliefs, and lifestyle, the physician can respond as helpfully as possible to each patient's health needs as these exist at the time of the engagement. patients of any persuasion—of any race, religion, sex, age, lifestyle, or ability to pay—must feel free to disclose their real needs and circumstances to their physician and to trust their physician to respond with the best management. How can you possibly accept a physician whose history will search for ways to declare you "ineligible" or unworthy and undeserving of care?

> I do not ask what are your sins or transgressions or what is your value. I do not ask what is your religion or your politics [or your insurance plan]. I ask only, "What is your suffering?"
>
> —Paraphrased from
> Louis Pasteur (1822–1895)

> Not until the sun rejects you do I reject you.
> —Walt Whitman (1819–1892) (1900, p 299)

b. To accept each patient nonjudgmentally, the physician relinquishes blaming illnesses such as obesity, drug addiction, or mental illness on lack of character, dissolute morals, or a weak will. Physicians do not search for excuses to blame or harangue patients. The patients already feel forlorn, disgusted with themselves, and ashamed. Instead, the history searches for causes and remedies. A pejorative physician entrenches the patient's feelings of unworthiness and destroys the possibility for a productive history and an effective therapeutic relationship.

c. To insure that you understand the principle of nonjudgmental acceptance of everyone, try to decide which of these two patients, patients 3 and 4, both of whom have lung cancer from heavy smoking, does or does not deserve full medical care. (Patient 3 is a composite of the several CEOs involved in a congressional hearing. All other patients cited are actual patients who I have personally attended.)

Pt 3: This hardworking, 50-year-old tobacco company president is urbane, college-educated with an IQ of l28, church-going, clean, and impeccably groomed. His salary and perks reward him with millions of dollars per year. He denies in sworn testimony to Congress and on live TV that tobacco is a health hazard and that nicotine is addictive. He aggressively and seductively advertises a product that each year kills hundreds of thousands of people and each year recruits tens of thousands of youngsters—your children and mine—into a lethal nicotine addiction. Because of the aggressive worldwide marketing of tobacco, his industry makes the United States the world's largest dealer in addictive drugs.

Pt 4: This 50-year-old chronic alcoholic street person is a semiliterate, garrulous man with an IQ of 80, profane, disheveled, and filthy. Unemployed, he lives off of garbage, petty theft, and panhandling. He refuses job training or any rehabilitative measures. He has tuberculosis. By refusing hospitalization or treatment, he infects other people.

Which of these two persons is more or less morally superior, and which one has more or less redeeming social value? Which one is more responsible for his actions? Which one does or does not deserve medical care?

Wise and thoughtful physicians empirically have realized that neither as individuals nor collectively as a profession have we the wisdom to judge patients as worthy or unworthy. We view our role as helpers, not judges. When either person, corporation president or derelict, enters the consulting room, the physician, knowing the fallibility of judgments about individual worth, accepts each patient with equal grace. The physician's ethic to act to benefit every patient preempts judgmental exclusion of anyone. The physician asks the patient neither "What are your sins and transgressions?" nor "What is your social value?" but only the poignant question posed by Louis Pasteur, "What is your suffering?" Although a nonsectarian medical ethic, many philosophies and religions also voice it.

For I was an hungered, and ye gave me meat: I was thirsty, and ye gave me drink: I was a stranger and ye took me in: Naked and ye clothed me: I was sick, and ye visited me: I was in prison, and ye came unto me.

—Matt. 25:35–36 (Bible)

5. Respond to every patient professionally, not emotionally.
  a. Whatever the patient's behavior, whether hostile or seductive, the physician should regard it as a purely clinical phenomenon, as the product of nerve impulses in neural circuits (DeMyer, 2004, 3–4). To reach rational clinical decisions, the physician relinquishes the freedom to love or hate or to become sexually entangled with the patient. The physician must especially forebear those patients whose disorder causes irrational, uncooperative, or oppositional behavior and outbursts of anger and aggression. The physician has to restrain emotionality for these reasons:
    (1) In order to make objective decisions that best serve the patient's interests
    (2) In order for the patient to trust that the physician will act rationally in formulating an appropriate plan of management
    (3) In order to have the mental and physical energy to survive the day. If you weep over this patient who has carcinoma, you won't have any tears left over for that patient, a child dying of leukemia. You will encounter the extremes of human experience: birth and death, profound illness and ultimate recovery, brilliant successes and abject failures. The practice of medicine involves the peaks and valleys of the human condition, but you cannot become a roller coaster, subject to recurrent heights and depths of human emotion, and still function.

One of the most difficult tasks put upon man is reflective commitment to another's problems while maintaining his own identity. The ways in which one person may react to another are infinite. A subtle and significant feature of a happy medical practice is to remain unencumbered by the patient's problems.

—Charles D. Aring, M.D. (1971, p 48)

b. Distinguishing empathy from sympathy

    (1) At issue is the difference between empathy and sympathy (Aring, 1971). The physician tries to experience empathy without the extremes of emotion demanded by sympathy.

    (2) *Empathy* means the ability to insert one's self into another's place to ascertain what the patient feels and what is required for a solution.

    (3) *Sympathy* means literally "feeling with," experiencing the feelings with or in the same way as the other person.

    (4) Empathy means understanding another person and then communicating back to the patient that you have achieved that understanding. Sympathy means sharing or personally experiencing the other person's feelings. The physician cannot survive constantly feeling each patient's pain and grief. Sympathy makes one the servant of the situation. Empathy enables one to understand and master it.

c. I can best sum up the reasons for emotional neutrality by stating that you can't reach rational clinical decisions while sobbing, nor can you get through the day that way. Nevertheless, at times you will and should shed tears (Crow, 2000), as when holding the hands of parents whose child has just died, and you will and should rejoice immensely when a patient passes a crisis and begins to recover.

6. Preserve the patient's privacy and maintain confidentiality.

a. The physician discloses nothing learned in the medical process to the family or the public at large, unless authorized by the patient (Angell, 1984). How can patients relate their histories freely if they fear that the physician will publicize the information or turn it against them? This contrasts sharply with the police procedure of warning an accused person that what they disclose will, indeed, be used against them. Each profession takes a history according to its own goals and ethical standards.

b. Rarely, the physician must bypass the confidentiality ethic upon learning something that poses a clear and present danger to others (Helminski, 1993; Zeman and Emanuel, 2000). For example, the law requires the reporting of certain contagious diseases, child abuse, or any patient disclosure of plans to murder someone.

c. Lax office procedures, keeping medical records electronically, and providing diagnoses on insurance forms vitiate the confidentiality ethic. Any hacker or clerk with access to a computer potentially may learn your diagnosis, that you have AIDS, syphilis, or a mental illness (Consumer Reports, 1994).

d. Violation of the patient's need for privacy and confidentiality can clearly damage the patient–physician relationship. Read how it distressed one patient:

> To the Editor, N Engl J Med: The professions make such a fuss about confidentiality that the naive layperson invariably believes that lawyers, doctors, and the members of the clergy would rather face any horror than breach the confidence of their clients. Theoretically, I do not doubt that this is often the case, but practically, medical confidence is not important. I sit in a shared waiting room and the booming, clear voice of the telephoning receptionist informs me that she requires some demographic and personal information of A; question after question is clearly presented. Next, I learn that B is pregnant and has a history of seizures; and C must visit the hospital for an electroencephalogram. The names of these patients roll mellifluously off the woman's tongue. This no sooner ends than here are the doctor and a patient discussing some ocular malady: Things will improve in two weeks, we are all informed. I am bristling, but the receptionist is beckoning me to the safety of the examination room. The door closes behind me and I am safe from all these confidences that do not concern me. But not for long, for echoing clearly through the wall are the doctor and a patient discussing some personal misery that I want desperately to ignore. Now the doctor is in the hallway, continuing to talk, and I could ignore his words only if I had come equipped with earplugs. Next, I am at the receptionist's counter discussing costs, payments, bills, and photocopying, nothing I want the large audience to overhear, so I stay on the official side of the counter and speak quietly. As I leave, they all stare at me as if they know every secret I have carefully protected. I am off to the pharmacy for some prescription drugs. The pharmacist stands behind a partition, far away, and asks me lots of questions. I must speak loudly so that he can hear name, address, date of birth and other demographic details. Next, he wonders whether I am allergic to anything.

I balk: "Not here in public," I angrily reply, while an audience thinks me mad. "I just need to know for my records," he clarifies helpfully. Does that warrant broadcasting my personal clinical history to the winds?

—Robert Hauptman, Ph.D.
(reproduced by permission,
N Engl J Med 1993;328:1128–1129)

e. Most physicians today believe in first giving full information to the patient about diagnosis and prognosis and then allowing the patient to decide about dissemination to others (Angell, 1984; Annas, 1994). The physician should discuss with the patient how much to tell the family about the patient's disorder, particularly if the physician needs to discuss the management with the spouse or other family members.

7. Practice evidence-based medicine. Employ those procedures and treatments that have passed rigorous scientific tests for safety and efficacy. The physician relies on the methods of science to make diagnoses and to select appropriate and effective diagnostic tests and therapy. Before acceptance, all claims for medical management must pass rigorous standards of proof (Angell, 2004; Horton, 2004). Chapter 15 discusses this issue in detail.

8. Manage patients not by ordering them what to do but by explaining the medically acceptable options and their probable outcomes.

a. Some students may suppose that physicians tell patients what to do. In fact, the physician should make recommendations but not demands, particularly not demands based on paternalism or a parochial sense of superior morality.

b. The physician outlines all of the acceptable medical options, and then physician and patient, in alliance, select the most appropriate management. Outright demands and threats don't help: "You better quit that drinking or it will kill you." The patient already knows that. The physician's attitude then adds another threat for the patient to face. In fact, a death wish may provide part of the motivation for drinking. The physician tries to discover, enlist, and strengthen patients' own resources for making decisions and for controlling their own lives.

Advice or demands, given at the expense of active, informed decisions by the patient, foster a helpless dependence on the physician, who "knows best." The cult members who tragically die at the instruction of charismatic leaders exemplify the danger of relying on others for life decisions.

> If I could lead you into paradise I would not do so, because if I could easily lead you in, someone else could just as easily lead you out.
>
> —Paraphrased from Eugene Debs
> (1855–1926) (Debs, p 265)

   c. The physician makes recommendations but generally avoids giving direct advice even when the patient actively asks for it. Chapter 13 describes how to respond when the patient asks directly for advice.

9. Insure informed consent for your management plan and procedures.

   a. The physician attempts to communicate to the patient the major risks and benefits of each option (Angell, 1984; Annas, 1994). When the risk/benefit ratio of one medically acceptable approach just about matches another, then patient preference settles the issue. When one alternative is clearly best, the physician tries to insure that the patient understands the expected difference in outcomes and opts for the superior management.

   b. Without valid information about the disease and its prognosis, the patient cannot make rational, informed decisions about therapy and the future. The physician conveys likely medical outcomes gently, compassionately, and in bearable steps, depending on the mental state of the patient (Angell, 1984; Annas, 1994), but with ultimate honesty. Most patients can face the realities of their illnesses if given honest information by a compassionate physician. Most patients already recognize whether they have a serious disease with a poor prognosis. For the physician to pretend otherwise demeans the patient's intelligence and destroys trust just when the patient most needs to trust the physician's honesty and integrity. In fact, we might argue that the more threatening the illness, the more important honesty and trust.

10. Attempt no more than your knowledge and manual skills justify. Only cut for the stone if you have the training to cut for the stone. Leave cardiac surgery to the cardiac surgeons. This rule applies also to the management of everyday disorders. If the history and examination disclose something out of your realm of competence, the medical model requires you to refer the patient. In doing medical research to discover new treatments, the physician does attempt more than current skills permit but only with the informed consent of the patient and within the framework of a scientific study that objectively judges outcome.

11. Continuously study to improve your skills and competency.

   a. The frontiers of medical knowledge advance each day. The physician must keep up or soon become obsolete.

   > Life is short and the art is long.
   > —Hippocrates (460–377, BCE) (1985, p 697)

   b. The physician must adopt the history to encompass each new advance in causality and each new disease. The continuing medical education programs of today address this need.

12. Respect the views of colleagues and teachers.

   a. Because the judgments of other physicians may differ from yours, ask the patient to summarize what the previous physician conveyed, but realize that the patient's memories and purposes may have distorted the message. Do not immediately assume that a disgruntled patient's narrative establishes the preceding physician as an incompetent fool. If you also fail to solve the patient's problem, you will in turn become the next incompetent fool when the patient visits yet another physician. Listen respectfully when another physician's viewpoint differs from yours and try to understand the origin of the disagreement, whether in the patient's interpretation or as an honest difference of opinion. Remember that humility and grace serve best in trying to resolve most disagreements. However, respect for colleagues, if misapplied, may cause physicians to fail to censure errant practitioners.

b. Respect for colleagues has included professional courtesy, such as the waiving of fees for treating another physician or physician's immediate family. This custom still more or less prevails (Levy et al., 1993), but insurance plans have altered it.

c. As a corollary of respect for colleagues, physicians have prohibited advertising that trumpets a physician or medical group as superior to another. In my own community of Indianapolis, several medical facilities advertise themselves as "the best." What does such blatant bragging do to the public perception of our integrity and honesty? Stripped of its niceties, advertising aims to propagandize, persuade, and indeed to deceive (Rogers, 1994). It is the antithesis of the patient-centered history based on trust because advertising fails to objectively present all of the options and presents only those offered by the advertiser (Brett, 1992). Also, advertising adds another layer of expense for medical care. Announcing the availability of one's services is one thing. Claiming to be the "best" is arrogant deceit.

13. Pass on medical knowledge and discoveries freely to students and other physicians.

a. In the past, academic physicians and scientists were expected to share their knowledge and discoveries freely for the benefit of all. Secret remedies and tests, exploited for private gain, were not the mission of science. Now, researchers even in academia are exhorted to produce patentable discoveries (Magnus et al., 2002; Stix, 2004; Washburn, 2005). The scramble for patents has led to bitter legal wrangling between institutions and individuals, for example, the wrangling between the U.S. Department of Health and Human Services and the Pasteur Institute of Paris over patenting a blood test for AIDS (Cohen, 1994); between postdoctoral fellows and their academic mentors (*Moore v. Regents of the University of California*, 1990); and between doctors and patients and the profession in efforts to patent cataract surgery and to patent and restrict the use of the human gene for breast cancer (Magnus et al., 2002; Washburn, 2005). The scramble to privatize does affect the clinical history by reducing the public's trust in the integrity and beneficence of the entire structure of medicine and science.

b. In contrast to the current commercialization of academic science, consider Edward Jenner, who discovered the vaccine against smallpox. He did not hustle out to found a new biotech company to demand a dollar for everyone vaccinated. Instead, he disclosed the details of his experiments, making the results freely available, with the following dedication:

> Thus far I have proceeded in an inquiry founded, as it must appear, on the basis of experiment; in which, however, conjecture has been occasionally admitted in order to present to persons well situated for such discussions objects for a more minute investigation. In the meantime I shall myself continue to prosecute this inquiry, encouraged by the hope of its becoming essentially beneficial to mankind.
>
> —Edward Jenner (1749–1823,
> (Jenner, 1798, p 83)

c. Just how "beneficial to mankind" was Jenner's discovery, so modestly announced and freely offered? Vaccination has saved far more lives than we have sacrificed in all of the wars in history. Instead of privatizing his work, he hoped that others "well situated" might improve upon it, which is precisely what has happened because now we have eliminated smallpox, the first such disease that humans have totally eliminated. Contrast Jenner's free dissemination of his discovery with the current rush to commercialize every discovery. Each "new" discovery is in fact built on and derives from the cumulative experience and contributions of countless colleagues and predecessors and is often financed by public money through governmental and philanthropic funding of research.

> If I have seen further than others, it is because I have stood upon the shoulders of giants.
>
> —Sir Isaac Newton (1642–1727)
> (Newton, 1959-1727, p 416)

Who owns the patent on this vaccine? Well, the people, I would say. There is no patent. Could you patent the sun?
—Jonas Salk, (Salk, 1955, April 12).
See It Now [Television broadcast].
New York: CBS-TV.

d. The contrary point of view holds that an innovator or discoverer has intellectual property rights that deserve compensation (McSherry, 2003; Nathan and Weatherall, 2002); in fact, Solomon (2006) offers an outright *apologia* for "commercial science." Some balance has to be reached between reward for individual creativity and social good.

14. Observe moderation in demeanor, dress, and fees. Obtrusive personality traits, bizarre dress, religious or political symbols, and exorbitant fees all impose barriers between patient and physician and impair the history, as discussed in Chapter 5.

15. Do not diagnose or treat yourself or accept family members or close personal friends as patients.

   a. You cannot be a competent physician to a close personal friend, a family member, or yourself. Strong emotional entanglements to a close friend, spouse, offspring, or relative will preclude a proper mental status history and physical examination. Are you going to do the vaginal and rectal examination on your mother or your sister? What if you are the cause of the family member's problem? Your role as a physician necessarily differs from that of your role as friend, spouse, or parent. Finally, never try to treat yourself. The age-old admonition "Physician heal thyself" becomes "Physician get to a healer."

   A physician who treats himself [or a family member or friend] has a fool for a patient and a bigger fool for a physician.
   —Clifton K. Meador (Meador, 1992, rule 291)

   b. This guideline also explains why laymen should not diagnose, do medical tests, or prescribe for themselves. No one can do a competent history or physical examination on himself or herself.

16. Act always with courtesy, humility, grace, and consideration.

B. An exercise in how negation of medical ethics would impair the clinical history and management. Consider the consequence for the history of negating each of the ethics enumerated in Table 4–1.

1. Ethic 1: Suppose our histories failed to explore the dangers of and contraindications to the medications and management offered.

2. Ethic 2: Suppose we slanted the history to promote our own beliefs and agendas.

3. Ethic 3: Suppose we revered death instead of life and promoted death for whomever we, the family, or the state deemed unworthy or undesirable, as in Nazi Germany.

4. Ethic 4: Suppose we rejected anyone whom we judged responsible for their own illness, such as the emphysemic smoker, the obese, or the addict.

5. Ethic 5: Suppose we reacted with overt anger, lust, or laughter or ridiculed our patients.

6. Ethic 6: Suppose we sold patients' histories to a tabloid—as has happened all too frequently with celebrities—or blackmailed our patients.

7. Ethic 7: Suppose we touted nostrums that had not passed scientific tests for safety and efficacy or prescribed treatments or management based on financial interest.

8. Ethic 8: Suppose we managed patients according to directives of a third-party payer or government or personal prejudices (Burnum, 1984).

9. Ethic 9: Suppose the history failed to disclose barriers to informed consent or a lack of a basis for it.

10. Ethic 10: Suppose we did surgical operations for which we were not trained?

11. Ethic 11: Suppose we failed to update our knowledge.

12. Ethic 12: Suppose we trumpeted ourselves, covertly or overtly demeaning other colleagues and other clinics?

13. Ethic 13: Suppose we maintained a medical monopoly by refusing to teach medical students or we patented and privatized all discoveries to maximize profit.

14. Ethic 14: Suppose we charged outrageous fees, dressed ostentatiously or slovenly, and acted rudely, without compassion and grace.

15. Ethic 15: Suppose we accepted family and close personal friends as patients. What happens to confidentiality and

objectivity? Who does the mental examination, sexual history, and the rectal and vaginal examination on your own child, sibling, or parent?

16. Ethic 16: Suppose we substituted arrogance and rudeness for humility and grace.

C. Ethics as the defining characteristic of physicians
If you understand how any of the foregoing violations would chill the history and the patient–physician relationship, you will understand, clearly and unequivocally, that these ethics define our profession and our behavior as members of it (Burnum, 1984; Tauber, 2005). Clearly, the technique of history taking and the ethics of the profession are indivisible. Nor can you choose a few of the ethics listed in Table 4–1 and dismiss the rest as inconvenient. They are an integrated, interlinked code of attitudes and actions.

IV. **Replacing Social Responses with Professional Responses**

A. Why does the burden of adjustment fall upon the physician?

1. Because of depletion of emotional resources and coping mechanisms, the sick patient should not have to worry about adjusting to the physician. The physician adjusts to the patient by replacing social responses with a whole new set of effective professional responses. By disciplining their own reactions, physicians provide the maximum freedom for patients to express themselves. Here are some overt examples of foregoing customary social responses.

   a. The physician who sees blood spurting from the mangled leg of an accident victim foregoes the freedom to vomit or faint.

   b. The surgeon who opens the patient's abdomen and finds metastatic carcinoma foregoes the freedom to break into tears of despair or pity.

   c. The physician who sees a gangrenous foot foregoes the freedom to cringe at the sight or stench of the rotting flesh.

2. Some less obvious but equally important freedoms the physician foregoes in order to act with maximum effectiveness include the following:

   a. The physician foregoes the freedom to ridicule, laugh at, or demean the patient's appearance, beliefs, or speech.

b. The physician foregoes the freedom to display hatred or love or even to intensely like or dislike the patient. Every patient should feel equally welcome and accepted. The physician does not say to an unkempt patient, covered with tattoos and scarred from drug injections, "God, I hate you damned filthy, drug addicts." Even though feeling that way in private, the physician, when in the consulting room, accepts all such phenomena nonjudgmentally as clinical phenomena and important clues to diagnosis. Any other attitude reduces the possibility of helping the patient.

c. The patient does not come to be praised as a saint or reviled as a sinner but for help. The physician recognizes the tattered clothes, tattoos, and scars as diagnostic signs of underlying feelings of despair, unacceptability, unworthiness, and self-destruction. If the patient felt acceptable, sufficient, and comfortable as a person, would he or she have defiled his or her skin, neglected personal hygiene, and surrendered himself or herself to drugs? Often, these signs reflect the patient's diseased state of mind as strongly as other signs reflect a diseased body.

d. As a physician, you forego the freedom to exploit the patient for personal ends, such as amusement or sexual titillation. You are not free, as at a cocktail party, to indulge in a social response, such as "You've got great legs!" In the consulting room, the perceptive patient reacts to such gratuitous compliments at best as patronizing or at worst as a forewarning of a seduction. Such remarks present you as vacuous or lecherous.

e. The physician foregoes the freedom to respond to hostility with hostility. In interpersonal relationships, the message sent will be the message returned. Regard the patient's hostility as a clinical phenomenon, indicative of a state of unease or disease, no more nor less than a cough, depression, a broken leg, or anxiety. The physician remains as ever operational, trying to discover causes rather than make judgments. What in the patient's background or current life circumstances, the organic state of the patient's brain, or your own demeanor has generated the anger? In other words, the issue is a question of differential diagnosis, hence a puzzle to solve, not a behavior to condemn.

f. The physician foregoes the freedom to consider the patient as interesting or uninteresting. No matter what symptom the patient presents, some physician, somewhere in the world, finds it fascinating and will have studied it extensively or even have devoted a lifetime to its analysis. If you, as a physician, lack interest, the problem lies with you, not the patient.

(1) You won't find yourself disinterested or bored if you retain the wonder of curiosity: What causes this symptom to appear in this patient at this time? What does it mean, or what is its mechanism? How can I analyze it and alleviate it? Your level of interest or disinterest will definitely affect the way you take the history.

(2) Often, the physician's disinterest arises from insecurity about how to question, diagnose, and treat patients with particular disorders, let us say headaches, backaches, or the passive–aggressive personality. You groan at the prospect of facing yet another patient who has such a disorder. To remedy disinterest in patients with particular disorders—for example, headaches—become a mini-expert. Get a current text or monograph on the subject and study it thoroughly for several weeks. As you begin to feel informed about the subject and competent to deal with it, you will find that it also has become interesting.

g. The physician foregoes the freedom to wear flashy diamond rings and alligator shoes or to wear beach clothes. Dress in unobtrusive clothing that the patient will neither particularly notice nor remember. When you go to Acapulco or step out onto the street, wear what you want. In the consulting room, match your attire to your role.

h. The physician foregoes the freedom to use the consulting room to espouse a partisan political, religious, moral, or economic agenda. The patient did not come to get your views on these subjects. Such intrusions polarize the patient–physician relationship, destroy the patient's trust, and make it impossible for the patient to relate any cares or concerns that may infringe on the physician's prejudices.

B. Appropriate professional responses required by the medical model

1. Do all of the prohibitions against the ordinary emotional and social responses listed above mean that during the history you sit there, sphinx-like, not feeling and not reacting? Initially, the answer is to some degree "Yes," until the history clarifies just what you should react to and how to react helpfully.

2. Suppose the patient states "I feel terrible, just terrible. I just can't go on with life." You should not break into a huge grin and say "Aw, don't feel that way. Everything will be all right tomorrow," offered with a hearty slap on the back. That is a social response, not a professional one. The disconsolate patient, having suffered an unrelenting sense of foreboding and doom for months, knows that everything will not be all right tomorrow. The glad-handing response, with its gratuitous, forced alacrity, patently offends the depressed patient.

3. Similarly, the physician avoids the opposite social response: "Oh that's terrible. That's awful!" The hypochondriacal patient reacts with a shudder and a chill, immediately assuming that the physician has confirmed his or her worst fears about a hopeless prognosis. Superficial amenities never substitute for correct, tempered professional concern.

4. Respond in such a way as to convey concern and interest and encourage the patient to continue: "I see. Tell me about this feeling that you can't go on with life," reflecting the patient's own words (Othmer and Othmer, 2002).

5. Ultimately, after having learned much more about the patient, you can introduce appropriate supportive remarks that reflect the requisite professionalism: "Now that I understand what you are going through, we'll work on some ways to help you feel better."

C. The history in patients involved in illegal activities: suspected rape, drug abuse, or suspected traumatic or sexual child abuse

1. Circumstances change when the history discloses illegal activities that force the physician to bypass the ethics of confidentiality and acting solely for the patient's benefit.

While the private interview still applies in principle, the necessity to notify law-enforcement agencies will affect the history—again illustrating that changing the goal of acting solely for the benefit of the patient changes the questions and content of the history. The age of the victim, whether a child or adult, also alters the standard approach. Most jurisdictions have multidisciplinary crisis teams involving physicians, nurses, social workers, psychologists, and law-enforcement officials to cope with the highly complex problems presented by victims of rape and child abuse (Hampton, 1995). However, the U.S. Supreme Court found that legal coercion to force pregnant cocaine users into treatment violated the woman's rights (Annas, 2001). When the history discloses illegal or questionable actions, the physician has to straddle a fine line between privacy and public interest.

2. For patients with legal entanglements, the physician must take and record the history very accurately and circumspectly. The defense lawyer for the perpetrator will exploit any vague points or possible discrepancies between the victim's report when highly agitated just after the acute attack and later testimony (Hampton, 1995).

V. **The Actual Operational Steps of the Medical Model for the Practice of Medicine**

A. Short summary of the operational steps of the medical model (Fig. 4–1)

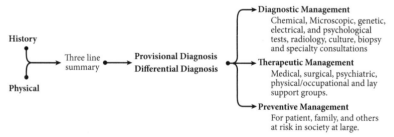

Figure 4–1. Short summary of the operational steps of the medical model. The history and physical findings lead to a provisional diagnosis and differential diagnoses that determine the management choices. (Reproduced by permission from DeMyer W. Technique of the Neurologic Examination, 5th ed. New York: McGraw-Hill, 2004.)

B. Expanded summary of the operational steps of the medical model
   1. Take a thorough clinical history
   2. Do a thorough physical examination
   3. Make a three-line summary of the clinical data that require an explanation
   4. Recite the analytic diagnostic catechism: It consists of *Is, Where, What,* and three *How Do I's* (Fig. 4–1)
      a. *Is* there a lesion or a disease? (Is the patient sick or well?)
      b. *Where* is the lesion? (Anatomic diagnosis)
      c. *What* is the lesion? (Etiologic diagnosis)
      d. *How* do I confirm or reject the presumptive diagnosis?
      e. *How* do I treat the patient?
      f. *How* do I prevent the disease in the patient or others at risk?
   5. Write down a provisional diagnosis or clinical impression and list the differential diagnoses
      a. Select the most likely diagnosis, the single one that best explains the clinical data
      b. Then devise a list of differential diagnoses
   6. Construct a problem list and propose solutions when desirable or appropriate, but do not allow it to obscure the basic disease that unites the symptoms and signs (Donnelly, 2005)
   7. Outline the diagnostic management
      a. Select the consultations and tests which best confirm or deny the provisional diagnosis
      b. Review and reduce the differential diagnosis list to reach a final diagnosis
   8. Outline the therapeutic management
      a. State the therapeutic goals or problems to be solved, including the prognosis or degree of disability, when pertinent
      b. Outline the therapy
         (1) Medical: drugs, diet, lifestyle changes
         (2) Surgical
         (3) Psychiatric: supportive office visits or referral to a specialist for long-term management
         (4) Physical, occupational, or speech therapy and vocational rehabilitation

    c. Refer the patient to any offices, organizations, or lay support groups that may improve the patient's therapeutic, social, or economic prospects

9. Outline the preventive management

    a. Plan how to prevent a recurrence of the disease in the patient or anyone else identified as at risk and how to prevent other diseases likely to afflict the patient

    b. Consider offering a wellness program (Chapter 11)

10. Plan a beneficence to end each visit

    After each contact with the physician, the patient should feel a sense of benefit and comfort. Comfort comes not from pity, false optimism, or condescending platitudes but from empathy, compassion, and competence. Each patient–physician contact remains incomplete, the ring remains open, and the physician remains but a technocrat until the patient feels this beneficence.

11. Make follow-up appointments. The follow-up visits serve to monitor the patient's progress, the success of the therapy, and the accuracy of the original diagnosis and to assure the patient of the physician's continuing interest.

VI. How the Medical Model Leads to the Maximum Benefit Permitted by the State of Medical Knowledge

Pt 5: This 36-year-old man reported persistent, almost daily, moderately severe, generalized headaches, beginning a year or so ago. The physical examination disclosed one sign, high blood pressure. The symptoms of headache and hypertension constitute a syndrome; that is, they may be causally related, not two separate findings, but they do not at this point constitute a specific disease.

    To discover the cause of the high blood pressure, the workup included chemical tests of the blood and urine and sonographic imaging of the abdomen. The chemical tests indicated impaired renal function, and sonography disclosed polycystic kidneys, which cause gradual kidney failure. The kidney disease caused the high blood pressure, which caused the headaches. Thus, the cause of the headaches was found in the kidney, not the head. The symptom of headache and the syndrome of headache and hypertension led to the discovery of a specific disease: polycystic kidneys.

Management of the kidney failure then involves dialysis or ultimately kidney transplantation. Since 10%–20% of patients with polycystic kidneys also have intracranial aneurysms that may rupture and cause severe disability or death, the patient's cerebral blood vessels were visualized by magnetic resonance imaging angiography. Angiography disclosed an aneurysm encroaching on the optic nerve. Visual field examination showed a corresponding defect that the patient had not noticed. Since the aneurysm was already symptomatic, a neurosurgeon then clipped it; but it might not have justified surgery otherwise (Suarez et al., 2006).

Polycystic kidney disease is the most common potentially fatal monogenic autosomal dominant disorder. Because of autosomal dominant transmission of polycystic kidney disease, other family members who desired it were given physical examinations, renal ultrasonography, and DNA analysis (Elias and Annas, 1994; Harris, 1994). Prophylactic treatment for the hypertension and proteinuria was instituted for the affected members (Taylor et al., 2005). Such comprehensive management shows how the correct diagnosis, which began in the consulting room with the individual patient's headache combined with the family history, led to benefit for the patient and preventive or palliative measures for the immediate population at risk, thus extending benefits to the family and to society at large (Johnson, 1993).

Consider the difference in outcome if the patient had made an autonomous self-diagnosis and simply bought over-the-counter analgesics; chose an acupuncturist, homeopath, or faith healer; or asked his pharmacist to recommend some pain pills—none of whom has the credentials to diagnose and deal with medical reality.

VII. Beyond the Consulting Room

You might wonder whether my focus on the individual doctor with the individual patient overlooks how external factors influence the flow of patients to physicians. Of course, physicians should lead in making medical care accessible to everyone (Farmer, 2003). Of course, physicians should not remain cloistered in their consulting rooms and treat the victims of addictive drugs, violence, pollution, infections, malnutrition, or war without asking "What public policies can prevent these scourges?" We can set rational priorities and policies for prevention only after the medical model has produced accurate diagnoses in individual patients.

VIII. Summary

A. The medical model consists of two integral and cohesive parts, the *ethical/attitudinal* part and the *operational/scientific* part. The techniques and format of the clinical history derive from and reflect the ethics of the full medical model.

B. The physician must act only in the patient's interest. To achieve this goal, the ethical code requires that the physician does no harm; acts in the patient's interest; reveres life; accepts every patient nonjudgmentally; preserves confidentiality; makes all medical decisions on the basis of patient need; employs scientifically proven methods; offers medically acceptable alternatives to the patient; obtains informed consent; attempts only what his or her skills permit; continuously studies; respects the views of colleagues; passes on medical knowledge freely; observes moderation in fees, dress, and demeanor; avoids diagnosing and treating self, family members, and close personal friends; and acts with humility and grace (Table 4–1).

C. These ethics and goals determine the technique of the history and the very questions asked or omitted. If our goals change to serve ends other than benefit for the patient, we have to redefine the role of the physician and recast the technique of the history. Two aphorisms perhaps best summarize the physician's approach to the history:

> I do not ask what are your sins and transgressions or what is your value. I do not ask what is your religion or your politics. I ask only, "What is your suffering?"
> —Paraphrased from Louis Pasteur (1822–1895)
> (Pasteur, 1968, p 979)

> May I never see in the patient anything but a fellow creature in pain.
> —From the Prayer of Maimonides
> (1135–1204)

D. The physician strives for *empathy*, which means ascertainment of the feelings the patient experiences, rather than *sympathy*, which means actually feeling what the patient feels. Sympathy emotionally drains the physician and impairs objective management decisions.

E. The physician replaces social responses with disciplined professional responses to patients. Professional responses encourage the patient to communicate significant health needs, whereas social responses serve an entirely different goal from patient benefit.

F. The medical model applies a series of formalized steps, almost a catechism, to analyze each patient (Fig. 4–1, see also section V, B). The steps begin with the history, physical examination, and laboratory tests. These measures lead to a "best fit" diagnosis that forms the basis for appropriate, scientifically validated treatment and to prevention.

G. Statistics that set priorities for public-health measures must rest on accurate diagnosis of the individual patient, a goal best achieved by the traditional medical model.

References

Ahronheim JC, Moreno JD, Zuckerman C. Ethics in Clinical Practice. Gaithersburg, MD: Aspen, 2000.

Angell, M. Respecting the autonomy of competent patients. N Engl J Med 1984;310:1115–1116.

Angell, M. The Truth About the Drug Companies. New York: Random House, 2004.

Annas GJ. Informed consent, cancer, and truth in prognosis. N Engl J Med 1994;330:223–225.

Annas GJ. Testing poor pregnant women for cocaine—physicians as police investigators. N Engl J Med 2001;344:1729–1732.

Aring CD. The Understanding Physician. Detroit,: Wayne State University Press, 1971, p 48.

Beauchamp TL, Walters L, eds. Contemporary Issues in Bioethics. Belmont, CA: Wadsworth-Thompson Learning, 2003.

Bernat JL. Ethical Issues in Neurology, 2nd ed. Boston: Butterworth-Heinemann, 2002.

Bible, King James Version, public domain. Matt. 25:35–36.

Brett AS. The case against advertising by health maintenance organizations. N Engl J Med 1992:326:1353–1357.

Brombeck E. In: Applewhite A, Evans T, Frothingham A. (eds), And I Quote: The Definitive Collection of Quotes, Sayings, and Jokes for the Contemporary Speechmaker. NewYork: Macmillan, 1992, p 226.

Burgio GR, Lantos JD, eds. Primum Non Nocere Today, 2nd ed. International Congress Series, vol 1171. Amsterdam: Excerpta Medica, 1998.

Burnum JF. The unfortunate case of Dr. Z: how to succeed in medical practice in l984. N Engl J Med 1984;310:729–730.

Bynum WF, Hardy A, Jacyna S, et al. The Western Medical Tradition: 1800–2000. New York: Cambridge University Press, 2006.

Chadwick J, Mann WN. The Medical Works of Hippocrates. Springfield, IL: Charles C. Thomas, 1950.

Cohen J. U.S.–French patent dispute heads for a showdown. Science 1994;265: 23–25.

Consumer Reports. Who's reading your medical records? 1994(October): 628–632.

Crow EW. Don't hold back tears. Pharos 2000(Spring);63:31.

Debs EV. Debs: His Life, Writings and Speeches. Girard Kansas: The Appeal to Reason, 1908, p 265.

DeMyer WE. Technique of the Neurologic Examination, 5th ed. New York: McGraw-Hill, 2004.

De Ridder D, Van Laere K, Dupont P, et al. Visualizing out-of-body experience in the brain. N Engl J Med 2007;357:1829–1833.

Donnelly WJ. Viewpoint: patient-centered medical care requires a patient-centered medical record. Acad Med 2005;80:33–38.

Elias S, Annas GJ. Generic consent for genetic screening. N Engl J Med 1994; 330:1611–1613.

Farmer P. Pathologies of Power: Health, Human Rights and the New War on the Poor. Berkeley: University of California Press, 2003.

Friedenwald H. The Physician's Oath and Prayer of Maimonides. Translated by Harry Friedenwald. Bulletin of the Johns Hopkins Hospital 1917:28: 260–261.

Glannon W. Bioethics and the Brain. New York: Oxford University Press, 2007.

Hampton HL. Care of the woman who has been raped. N Engl J Med 1995; 332:234–237 (see also D'Onofrio G, et al., Letter to the Editor, N Engl J Med 1995;332:1714–1715).

Harris P. The polycystic kidney disease 1 gene encodes a 14 kb transcript and lies within a duplicated region on chromosome 16. Cell 1994;77:881–894.

Hauptman R. Confidentiality. N Engl J Med 1993;328:1128–1129.

Helminski F. Near the conflagration. The duty to warn. Mayo Clin Proc 1993; 68:709–710.

Hewitt, D. (Executive Producer). (1998, November 22). *60 Minutes* [CBS News Transcript]. New York. Retrieved November 4, 2008 from http://web.lexis-nexis.com/universe.

Hippocrates. The Genuine Works of Hippocrates. Birmingham: Classics of Medicine Library, 1985, p 697.

Hope T. Medical Ethics: A Very Short Introduction. New York: Oxford University Press, 2004.

Horton R. The dawn of McScience. New York Review of Books 2004;51 (March 11):7–9.

Illes J. Neuroethics: Defining the Issues in Theory, Practice and Policy. New York: Oxford University Press, 2005.

Inui TS. A Flag in the Wind: Educating for Professionalism in Medicine. Washington DC: Association of American Medical Colleges, 2003.

Jenner E. An Inquiry into the Causes and Effects of the Variolae Vaccinae, a Disease Discovered in Some of the Western Counties of England, Particularly Gloucestershire, and Known by the Name Cow-Pox. London: Sampson Low, 1798, p 83.

Johnson SH. Judicial review of disciplinary action for sexual misconduct in the practice of medicine. JAMA 1993;270:1596–1600.

Jouanna J. Hippocrates, trans. J. Deveboise. Baltimore: Johns Hopkins Press, 1999.

Leake CD, ed. Percival's Medical Ethics. Baltimore: Williams and Wilkins, 1927.

Levy MA, Arnold RM, Fine MG, et al. Professional courtesy—current practices and attitudes. N Engl J Med 1993;329:1627–1631 (see also Letters to the Editor, N Engl J Med 1994;330:1085–1086).

Li JTC. The patient–physician relationship: covenant or contract? Mayo Clin Proc 1996;71:917–918.

Magnus D, Caplan A, McGee G, eds. Who Owns Life? Buffalo, NY: Prometheus Books, 2002.

Markel H. "I swear by Apollo" —on taking the Hippocratic oath. N Engl J Med 2004;350:2026–2029.

McSherry C. Who Owns Academic Work? Battling for Control of Intellectual Property. Cambridge, MA: Harvard University Press, 2003.

Meador C. A Little Book of Doctors' Rules. Philadelphia: Hanley and Belfus, 1992, rule 291.

Miles SH. The Hippocratic Oath and the Ethics of Medicine. Oxford: Oxford University Press, 2004.

Milunsky A. Genetic counseling: prelude to prenatal diagnosis. In: Milunsky A (ed), Genetic Disorders and the Fetus Diagnosis, Prevention and Treatment 2nd ed. New York: Plenum Press, 1986, p 9.

Moore v. Regents of the University of California, 51 Cal.3d 120, 271 Cal. Rptr. 146, 793P.2d 479 (1990).

Nathan DG, Weatherall DJ. Academic freedom in clinical research. N Engl J Med 2002;347:1368–1371.

Neuroethics.org, http://www.neuroethics.org

Newton I. Letter to Hooke, 5 Feb 1676. In: Turnbull HW (ed), Correspondence. Cambridge: Royal Society at the University Press, 1959–77, p 416

Othmer E, Othmer SC. The Clinical Interview Using DSM IV-TR. Washington DC: American Psychiatric Publishing, 2002.

Pasteur L. Speech at the opening of the Philanthroic Society' Refuge for Mothers, June 8, 1886. In: Strauss MB (ed), Familiar Medical Quotations, Boston: Little Brown, 1968, p 579.

Pruchnicki A. First do no harm (pending prior approval). N Engl J Med 1997;337:1627–1628.

Rogers DE. On trust: a basic building block for healing doctor/patient interactions. Pharos 1994(spring);57:2–6.

Salk J. CBS-TV interview, *See It Now* (1955, April 12). Quoted In:Gardner H, Csikszentmihalyi M, Damon W (eds). Good Work: When Excellence and Ethics Meet. New York: Basic Books, 2002, p 111.

Stanbrough H. Beyond the Masks. Albuquerque: Central Avenue Press, 2005, p 151.

Steinbock B. The Oxford Handbook of Bioethics. New York: Oxford University Press, 2007.

Solomon LD. The Quest for Human Longevity: Science, Business, and Public Policy. New Brunswick, NJ: Transaction, 2006.

Stix G. Working the system II. Corporate greed no longer remains the sole domain of the corporation. Sci Am 2004;290:41.

Suarez JI, Tarr RW, Selman WR. Aneurysmal subarachnoid hemorrhage. N Engl J Med 2006;354: 387-396.

Tauber AI. Patient Autonomy and the Ethics of Responsibility. Boston: MIT Press, 2006.

Taylor M, Johnson TM, Tison M, et al. Earlier diagnosis of autosomal dominant polycystic kidney disease: importance of family history and implications for cardiovascular and renal complications. Am J Kidney Dis 2005;45:415–423.

Temkin O, Temkin CL, eds. Ancient Medicine: Selected Papers of Ludwig Edelstein. Baltimore: Johns Hopkins University Press, 1967 p 6.

Washburn J. University Inc, the Corporate Corruption of Higher Education. New York: Basic Books, 2005.

Weinberg M, ed. Medical Ethics: Applying Theories and Principles to the Patient Encounter. Buffalo, NY: Prometheus Books, 2000.

Whitman W. Leaves of Grass. Philadelphia: David McKay, 1900, p 299.

Wynia MK, Latham SR, Kao AC, et al. Medical professionalism in society. N Engl J Med 1999;341:1612–1616.

Yarnofsky CS. A catalogue of physician's oaths, 2004, http://www.pneuro.com/publications/oaths.

Zeman A, Emanuel LL. Ethical dilemmas in neurology. In: Major Problems in Neurology, vol 36. Philadelphia: WB Saunders, 2000.

Zuger, A. Dissatisfaction with medical practice. N Engl J Med 2004;350:69–75.

Privacy, the Setting, and the Apparel for an Optimum Clinical History

5

I. Privacy and the Private Interview

> Whatsoever I shall see or hear concerning the life of men, in my attendance on the sick, or even apart there from, which ought not to be noised abroad, I will keep silence thereon . . .
> —Hippocrates (460–377 BCE)

A. The reasons for a private interview with the patient
   1. The circumstances for taking the history strongly affect the kind of information derived and the feeling tone produced. Without certain basic conditions, you lose any possibility of eliciting an optimal history. I advocate interviewing most adult patients in private. I start out by defending the necessity for privacy because many physicians ignore this rule. Although some patients do not require strict privacy, you do not know in advance when privacy may make a crucial difference (Petronio, 2002).
   2. First of all, the clinical history, by its very design, discloses the most personal and intimate details of the patient's life. Compile all of the medical questions that you would not want to answer with your spouse, parent, or child present: "Are you sexually active and have you ever had a venereal disease?" or "How much alcohol do you drink?" or "Do you use street drugs?" Suppose the husband did not father the child brought in by a couple for examination but does not know this fact. Then, a family history taken with both persons present will produce wrong genetic information. If the husband or live-in boyfriend is physically or sexually abusive, how can the woman tell the physician with the abuser present? Abusers want total domination and submission. With an abusive spouse present the abuser is continuing his total domination by inhibiting what the woman can say. Privacy allows patients to reveal their real concerns.
   3. Finally, the private interview allows patients to reveal thoughts that they cannot voice to anyone but a physician or

to discover feelings that they had never previously acknowledged (see Chapter 10, section I, D).

B. The legal necessity for privacy

The Health Insurance Portability and Accountability Act (HIPAA) passed by Congress in 1996 explicitly outlines privacy rules for keeping and disseminating medical records. Physicians are required to comply. Electronic storage and dissemination of patient data (Frasca, 1996) and DNA data (Welch, 2001) complicate the problem. For practical steps a patient may take to preserve privacy, see Consumer Reports (1999, p 7).

C. Dampening effect of a third party in the consulting room

1. The basic contract, explicit in the medical model, requires the physician to act in the patient's interest. Any fear that the physician may act in the interest of the spouse, family, or a third party or from some consideration other than solving the patient's health problem destroys the whole basis of the patient–physician relationship.

2. The presence of a third person requires the patient to consider the emotional needs of that person but at a time when illness may reduce her or his capacity to do so. Likewise, you have to shift your attention to consider the feelings of the third person and to censor the questions that should be asked. How can the physician function as the agent or confidant of the patient with someone else intruding?

3. A third party in the room must of necessity inhibit the range and nature of the questions the physician asks (Greene et al., 1994). The third party not only inhibits what the patient will reveal but reduces the ability of the patient to discuss freely any feelings and problems related to that person. Unless you do private interviews, you won't discover their importance because you won't get the kind of information a private interview provides or thanks from the patient for having respected the need for privacy.

4. Physicians who ignore private interviews argue that they can get a more accurate history with the companion, usually the spouse or parent, present because that person can amplify and confirm what the patient says (Lown, 1996). I say that this results in getting someone else's version of the history

rather than the patient's. Often, the companion and patient waste time haggling over irrelevancies:

> Patient: "It started on June second."
>
> Spouse: "No, don't you remember? It was June third when you were sitting on the porch."

5. Sometimes the companion simply takes over the interview and the patient feels excluded. If you need to verify or extend the patient's narrative, interview the third party *after* you interview the patient in private. After reassuring the patient that you will not divulge any sensitive information to the companion, ask for the patient's permission to question the companion. Then, interview the companion in private. That gives the companion a chance to describe freely the memory loss, personality change, temper outbursts, insomnia, or drinking problem that the patient may have concealed.

6. Another reason some physicians give for not conducting private interviews is that they learn how the patient and partner interact. I counter by saying that I learn as much by seeing how the patient and the partner accept the separation. Anyway, you can very quickly perceive how they interact by their voice tone and word choice. You can talk with both parties together later, after a private interview has disclosed the nature of the patient's problem and what subjects the physician should discuss or avoid.

7. After a private interview with a companion, you should usually describe to the patient what transpired. If the informant has irrational views or demands, you should generally inform the patient either directly or by having the informant voice these views later, with the patient present.

8. When the time comes to discuss the diagnosis and management, ask whether the patient prefers the presence of the companion.

D. Exceptions to the private interview rule

1. If the patient is retarded, is demented, or has unconscious spells and cannot describe what happens, always supplement the patient's narrative by interviewing an informant. Again, a private interview enables the informant to describe the patient's aberrancies, without embarrassment for the patient or informant.

2. Some circumstances forewarn you not to conduct a private interview, such as when a patient of the opposite sex is known to be psychopathic, litigious, overly seductive, or overtly mentally ill.

3. At least during the physical examination, the physician should arrange for an attendant (Gawande, 2005). Generally, the attendant should be a nurse or other professional, not a family member. Whether to require attendants for all physical examinations between adults of opposite sexes is debatable (Speelman et al., 1993). Female physicians receive sexual harassment frequently enough (Phillips and Schneider, 1993) that they may prefer an attendant present with most male patients. A male physician should have a female attendant when asking about sexual activities or molestation or doing a rectal or vaginal examination on girls or young teenaged females, or he should assign the examination to a female physician.

E. The private interview when the patient is a child accompanied by parents

1. When a man accompanies the mother and child, I may start the history with all present but at some point I may interview the mother alone. The mother usually knows much more about the pregnancy and course of the child than the man, whether father or companion. For many couples today, the man is a stepfather or simply live-in companion. In the man's presence, the mother may not want to answer questions relevant to the child's health, the paternity of the child, or her own health, sexual, or reproductive history.

2. Ages birth to three years: The physician may interview the parents with the infant present, but the mother will give a better history if relieved of the moment-to-moment demands of child care. A mother shifting a crying baby from arm to arm cannot closely attend to your questions. If possible, have someone take care of the infant outside of the consulting room. With young children you learn very quickly how the mother relates to the child when she undresses the child for the physical examination.

3. Ages three to 12 years:

   a. I often start with everyone present until I discover whether the concerns are behavioral or psychiatric.

To take a history of behavioral problems, I generally arrange for the child to stay in the waiting room with someone while I interview the mother. I cannot count how many mothers have said to me, after I have interviewed them privately, how relieved they felt after I had excused the child and how embarrassed they had been to try to describe the child's problems to other doctors with the child present. If you do private interviews, you will receive similar thanks from mothers. How can a mother feel free to describe a child's mental retardation and behavioral difficulties or the pregnancy and birth history with the child sitting there absorbing it all? Think of how an 8-year-old child feels listening as his or her mother, who is supposed to love and cherish him or her, describe his or her seizures—the jerking, slobbering, and incontinence—or clumsiness, learning disability, temper tantrums, oppositional attitude, or stealing and lying. Remember also that 4-year-olds get the gist of a conversation that reviews their deficits and problems.

b. Even if the father accompanies the mother, at some point I try to interview the mother alone and then mother and father together.

c. A child less than 6–7 years of age has difficulty relating a history. For patients more than 10 years of age, I may interview the mother alone first, excuse her, and then interview the child alone.

4. Ages 12–14 years and above:

a. For patients more than 12 years of age, I may start the history with the mother alone before interviewing the patient, but the patient may then view you as an agent of the parent rather than representing her or him. Adolescents and teenagers, particularly if troubled, always feel inhibited in the presence of the parents and embarrassed by the parents' words and actions. Think of how mortified you felt, as an adolescent, if someone discussed a simple pimple on your nose, much less complained about your behavior. I think you will understand immediately why at some point you should interview some adolescents and many older teenagers in private (Weisleder, 2004) in order to establish yourself in the mind of the patient as her or his advocate. To understand how patients feel about it, read Jessica Levin's letter:

> To the Editor, N Engl J Med: I am writing to express concern about what I understand to be a standard practice of physicians in dealing with minors. Before my operation, my anesthesiologist met with me (16 years old) and my parents to review the procedure. At that time, I was asked if I used recreational drugs, smoked, or drank alcohol. Fortunately, my answer put my parents and my doctor at ease.
>
> This apparent formality could prove to be very dangerous if an adolescent who takes drugs, drinks or smokes is unable to be frank with the doctor while the parents are listening. Kids have the same right of patient confidentiality as adults. I suggest that doctors review their practices so that minors can speak with them privately.
>
> —Jessica Levin (reproduced by permission, N Engl J Med 1990;323:1569)

b. So here a teenager pleads with the learned profession, reminding us of what we ought to know and practice. Most other teenagers feel the same way, and that feeling may interfere with their seeking medical care (Cheng et al., 1993). Again, we return to fundamental ethics: Arrange each interview to achieve maximal health benefit for the particular patient before you.

5. Sample statements to separate parents and children diplomatically for private interviews

   a. Say to a parent when behavioral issues arise concerning the child "Would you prefer we discuss this in private? We can ask Johnny to sit in the waiting room."

   b. Say to the child or teenager "Would you mind sitting in the waiting room while I talk with your mother? We'll call you back shortly." Sometimes standing up and gesturing toward the door helps.

F. How to arrange for a private interview diplomatically when an another adult accompanies an adult patient

   1. After greeting the patient, greet and shake hands with the companion. Say courteously, yet with a hint of authority and finality, "Make yourself comfortable here in the waiting room while I talk with Mr. [or Mrs.] Jones." Make a gesture with your arm toward a chair in the waiting room. Then

escort the patient into the consulting room. If the patient asks "Is it all right if my wife comes along?" respond with "Let me talk with you first, and I'll be glad to talk with both of you later." The patient may not really want the spouse along but may accede out of deference. If the patient flatly states "I would like her to be present," accept that and cordially invite the companion, "Yes, please come in." You can talk with the patient alone when you excuse the companion for the physical examination.

2. In summary, a private interview encourages freedom of expression, promotes disclosure, preserves confidentiality, and affirms the physician's role as the patient's advocate and agent.

3. Before leaving the topic of privacy, I urge you to skip forward and read the vignette for Patient 13 in Chapter 10, Section I, D.

G. Confidentiality and the family physician
Confidentiality problems may arise when one physician treats the whole family, as frequently happens in general practice. Note that half of all marriages end in divorce, and the family may consist of stepchildren and half-siblings of different ages and needs. The requirement for confidentiality may preclude one physician taking care of the current partners, the previous partners, and all of their dependents. In a bitter divorce or custody battle, each adult will try to manipulate the physician into taking his or her side. One blanket rule does not resolve this difficult issue, but the physician should remain alert to this problem.

II. The Room Design for the Medical Interview

A. How the design of hospitals and medical offices affects the history

1. I sometimes wonder whether architects have ever spent time in a hospital bed because they almost invariably make five mistakes. They always put bright lights in the ceiling, apparently not realizing that hospitalized patients, many of whom suffer from photophobia, recline on their backs most of the time, with the light directly in their eyes. They fail to appreciate that ordinary sounds disturb ill persons, day and night, and do not design adequate sound insulation (Grumet, 1993). They fail to design blinds that completely

darken a room for proper pupillary and funduscopic examinations and for the comfort of patients with photophobia, and they often fail to provide properly designed private rooms for medical interviews.

2. Unfortunately, in teaching hospitals, medical students become accustomed to trying to take a history while standing in the hall, while contending with visitors or relatives of the other three patients in a four-bed cubicle, or in a busy emergency room (Karro et al., 2005). A scoundrel, plotting to destroy any possibility to get an optimal history, would impose just such conditions.

3. The size, decor, and appointments of the waiting room and consulting room itself affect the outcome (Epstein, 1992; Shea, 1998). A tiny consulting room feels uncomfortably intimate, if not downright claustrophobic. A large room always seems formal, cold, and barren. The treatment room has dirty or blood-stained sheets. A large desk puts the physician too far away, a tiny one too close (Shea, 1998). Too much clutter on the desk suggests that you aren't well organized. Search out a place that offers at least a chance to elicit an optimal history.

B. Characteristics or feng shui of the consulting room
The consulting room should be moderate in size and decor, with a moderate-sized, uncluttered desk, some chairs, and little else. Adjust the lighting for comfort, not so bright as to suggest an inquisition or third degree nor so dim as to suggest a rite of mystery or séance. Avoid a bright light that shines directly from behind you into the patient's eyes. Eliminate distractions and intrusions: no telephone ringing, no beeper, and no overhead paging system blaring. Avoid grisly anatomical charts, skulls, or skeletons. Display no rare collector's items or fancy rugs that will intimidate some patients or impel others to make some comment to preen the physician's ego.

C. Privacy in the emergency room
Many emergency rooms today still have cubicles separated only by a flimsy wall or curtains, making privacy impossible. Often, physicians or other medical personnel, under the stress of the moment, discuss the patient loudly, for all to hear.

III. Personal Attributes of the Physician

A. The costume for the physician

> The dignity of a physician requires that he should look healthy, and as plump as nature intended him to be; then he must be clean in person, well dressed, and anointed with sweet-smelling unguents, that are not in any way suspicious.
>
> —Hippocrates (460–377 BCE)

> A leech [Yes, medical doctors were once called "leeches" because they applied them to patients to cure disease, in contrast to surgeons who cut to cure disease and were in fact barbers] ought also to have well cut clothes, dressing soberly, not like a clown or a poet. He ought too to have clean hands and well shaped nails which should not be black or filthy. He should behave himself courteously. He should hear many things but speak little; the wise man says "it is better to use the ears than the tongue."
>
> —Master John Arderne (1307–1380)

1. What to wear poses an eternal question, to go on your first date, to a dance, or just to school on a given day. What you select to wear, the garb of a clown or a poet, proclaims something that you consciously or unconsciously want known about yourself: you are cool or hep or in tune or a rebel. Why do police officers and soldiers wear a uniform, or why do priests wear robes? The costume gives a force and identity beyond nudity. It magnifies and projects the aura of the wearer. Dictators to a man—Stalin, Hitler, Mussolini, Saddam Hussein—try to magnify their tough-guy image by military costumes, often with a pistol displayed conspicuously, whereas elected leaders in the past invariably wore formal suits to match their fellow politicos and the businessmen who financed their campaigns. Now the candidates are likely to appear also in open collars and jeans, a costume designed to magnify their affinity with the people.

2. The physician should wear essentially neutral clothes or a white coat, the habiliment that signifies the profession (Stevenson, 1971). A dignified 83-year-old patient will visit the physician only after taking care to dress well. Albeit his best suit and tie or her dress are worn and frayed, the garments demonstrate the patient's respect for the occasion.

Having shown you this respect, the patient will feel very uncomfortable if you appear in a baseball cap, jeans, and open-toed sandals or, conversely, if you appear impeccably costumed in a sleek $1500 suit, with a silk handkerchief peeking out of the breast pocket, and large diamond cuff links sparkling at your wrists. At the end of the visit, the patient should hardly have noticed what the physician wore. Nothing worn—miniskirts, Bermuda shorts, or spectacular hairstyles—should intrude into the patient's consciousness.

Pt 6: In l993, while going to a neurology consultation at Carter Hospital (a psychiatric hospital for adults and children, then on the campus of the Indiana University School of Medicine), I happened to overhear a heated discussion between a resident physician and a 38-year-old paranoid female patient as they stood in the hall just outside of the nursing station. The resident physician was demanding that the woman take her medication. He hadn't shaved for a day or so. He wore a short-sleeved, flowered shirt with an open collar, blue jeans with red suspenders, and filthy sneakers. A missing button at the top of his fly revealed incomplete closure of his zipper. A bit of a potbelly protruded through the open notch caused by the missing button. His one concession to appropriate garb was the obligatory stethoscope, dangling around his neck. In the heat of the debate, the patient rather suddenly stopped, put her hands on her hips, screwed up her face, and shouted, "Why should I listen to you? How do I even know that you are a doctor?"

I thought, "Right on lady. I can't tell that this guy is a doctor either." But I said nothing. His costume, his confrontational attitude, and the public setting absolutely destroyed any chance of success. How much better if the resident, appropriately dressed and groomed, had sat down in a private room with the patient and calmly tried to discover why the patient resisted taking her medication.

3. Female physicians should insure that they dress modestly and avoid any hint of sexual invitation. Around 75% of female physicians get unwanted sexual advances from male patients (Phillips and Schneider, l993). Avoid low necklines, high skirt lines, excessive jewelry, excessive makeup, and pervasive perfumes. Remember Hippocrates' warning that

the unguents worn should not be "in any way suspicious." The message sent is the message returned. Men don't need much encouragement. The necessity to repel a sexual advance, whether made by patient or physician, disrupts the whole patient–physician relationship. Feminists may insist that they have the right to wear what they want and that men have to learn to behave. The "rights" doctrine applies to the social and political arena. In the consulting room, medical ethics become the highest authority. The physician has to act and dress as a physician, in ways that promote, not impair, the patient–physician relationship.

B. Avoid accoutrements that may polarize the patient

In suggesting that you wear unobtrusive clothes, I also advise against wearing adornments such as long chains, crosses or other religious symbols, political buttons, or even health advisories (e.g., "Stop Smoking"). Any such items will cause offense or downright distress for at least some patients. Think of a Palestinian waking up in an emergency room and looking up at a physician wearing a yarmulke or conversely an Israelite finding his physician kneeling to Mecca. In each instance the physician hopefully would treat the patient properly, but the encounter would start with polarized feelings. Eliminate from the consulting room and your costume political, religious, or social symbols and displays that may instantly polarize people. If you wish to promote a personal cause or recruit for your religion or political party, well and good, but do so outside of the consulting room, where it then becomes your right, not inside the consulting room, where it may interfere with your duties. Avoiding polarization becomes especially important today because the intermingling of diverse populations, cultures, and religions inevitably brings physicians and patients of diametric viewpoints into contact.

C. Other aspects of nonverbal communication

1. Many nonverbal behaviors communicate positive or negative impressions to the patient. Appropriate behavior mostly derives from common sense and simple good manners. Body posture and tensions, voice intonation, and facial expression all affect the outcome (Larsen and Smith, 1981). Drumming the fingers, fiddling with a pencil, sipping coffee, sighing, looking out the window, glancing at your

watch—all convey a disinterest that unctuous words cannot neutralize. After the initial handshake, the physician should generally avoid touching the patient during the history; but some exceptions will be appropriate, particularly for a grieving patient. Cleanliness, good grooming, and ordinary good manners go without saying. Don't pick your teeth or nose, chew gum, yawn, or scratch yourself. Don't eat or drink, and certainly don't smoke. I am embarrassed to have to review these elementary rules, but some students (and some graduate M.D.'s) need these gentle reminders.

2. As to posture, always sit down. Assume a position face-to-face, at eye level with the patient (Creagan, 1994). If you take the history standing up, it appears that you are in a hurry and about to scurry off or are imperiously towering over the patient. Sit upright, with your manubrium and chin up, a posture that conveys alertness and interest. Do not thrust the chest forward, military style; just lift the manubrium up. A slouched posture implies disinterest. Do not place an ankle on one knee with the other knee dangling out to the side. Such a casual posture looks as if you have settled in for a nap. Contrarily, if you sit with both feet planted firmly, you look as if you intend to jump up and sprint off. Cross your legs at the ankles or perhaps the knees, but keep your thighs together in any case. Please, no crotch displays by male or female physicians. All behavior has a meaning and serves a purpose. Insure that all of yours are gentle and promote the patient–physician relationship.

3. Of all factors, physicians tend to neglect voice tone and diction (Ambady et al., 2002). The medical school curriculum might well contain some formal training in speech production and diction, but your voice must sound natural, not manufactured.

4. You will best appreciate the role of nonverbal communication by awareness of its importance and by studying videotapes of your own interviews (Gallagher et al., 2005).

IV. **Use of the Telephone and Telemedicine**
Although the initial history is rarely taken by telephone, telephoning is particularly valuable in responding to emergency

calls and for following up an illness. Telephoning, particularly the use of cell phones, raises additional concerns about privacy, not the least of which is the actual identity of the person on the other end of the line. For the special problems in telephone communication with patients, see Katz (2001) and Reisman and Stevens (2001). So far, consultation by telemedicine with videoconferencing produces less satisfaction for the patient and more procedures (Chua et al., 2001) but may prove successful (Eikelboom et al., 2005; Norris, 2002). I doubt that taking the history by electronic media can ever produce the communion, empathy, and trust between patient and physician that can come from a face-to-face history (Onor and Misan, 2005).

Telemedicine, using the Internet and digitization, while fraught with the possibility of commercial exploitation (Stix, 2004), can result in great benefit. Teleradiology has already become commercialized and globalized (Wachter, 2006). Some forms of telemedicine have led to great benefits, such as the nonprofit Orbis International program (http://telemedicine. orbis.org). Sponsored by ophthalmologists, many of whom are retired, the program provides free consultation with colleagues in underserved countries to diagnose and treat eye disorders. This program, begun in Havana, Cuba, in 1999, is now worldwide. When pursued by physicians driven by the best ethics of the medical model, telemedicine could be a major advance in health care.

V. Summary
A. Conduct private interviews and eliminate the "third party" from the consulting room, whether the third party consists of another person or an economic, social, political, religious, or personal agenda.
B. The medical play has only two actors, the physician and the patient, and no audience. If the play is the thing, the stage is also part of it. Everything affects the success of the patient–physician interaction: room size, decor, lighting, posture, costume, voice production, and not least of all full attention to ordinary good manners, humility, and grace.
C. Insure privacy for most patients, including teenagers by diplomatically separating the patient from others who have come along.

References

Ambady N, Laplante D, Nguyen T, et al. Surgeons' tone of voice: a clue to malpractice history. Surgery 2002;132:5–9.

Cheng TL, Savageau JA, Sattler AL, et al. Confidentiality in health care. A survey of knowledge, perceptions, and attitudes among high school students. JAMA 1993;269:1404–1407.

Chua R, Craig J, Wootton R, et al. Randomized controlled trial of telemedicine for new neurological outpatient referrals. J Neurol Neurosurg Psychiatry 2001;71:63–66.

Consumer Reports. Rx for medical privacy. 1999 64:7(May).

Creagan ET. How to break bad news—and not devastate the patient. Mayo Clin Proc 1994;69:1015–1017.

Eikelboom RH, Mbao MN, Coates HL, et al. Validation of tele-otology to diagnose ear disease in children. Int J Pediatr Ophthalmol 2005; 69:739–744.

Epstein O. Clinical Examination. London: Gower, 1992.

Frasca TA. Issues of confidentiality in the information age. Pharos 1996 (winter);59:17–19.

Gallagher TJ, Hartung PJ, Gerzina H, et al. Further analysis of a doctor–patient nonverbal communication instrument. Patient Educ Couns 2005;57:262–271.

Gawande A. Naked. N Engl J Med 2005;353:645–648.

Greene MG, Majerovitz SD, Adelman RD, et al. The effects of the presence of a third person on the physician–older patient medical interview. J Am Geriatr Soc 1994;42:413–419.

Grumet GW. Pandemonium in the modern hospital. N Engl J Med 1993; 328:433–437.

Karro J, Dent AW, Farish S. Patient perceptions of privacy infringements in an emergency department. Emerg Med Australas 2005;17:117–123.

Katz HP. Telephone Medicine: Triage and Training for Primary Care, 2nd ed. Philadelphia: FA Davis, 2001.

Larsen KM, Smith CK. Assessment of nonverbal communication in the patient–physician interview. J Fam Pract 1981;12:481–488.

Levin J. Letter to the editor. When doctors question kids. N Engl J Med 1990;323:1569.

Lown B. The Lost Art of Healing. Boston: Houghton Mifflin, 1996.

Norris AC. Essentials of Telemedicine and Telecare. Chichester: John Wiley, 2002.

Onor ML, Misan S. The clinical interview and the doctor–patient relationship in telemedicine. Telemed J E Health 2005;11:102–105.

Petronio S. Boundaries of Privacy: Dialectics of Disclosure. Albany: State University of New York Press, 2002.

Phillips S, Schneider M. Sexual harassment of female doctors by patients. N Engl J Med 1993;329:1936–1939.

Reisman AB, Stevens DL, eds. Telephone Medicine. Philadelphia: American College of Physicians–American Society of Internal Medicine, 2001.

Shea SC. Psychiatric Interviewing: The Art of Understanding: A Practical Guide for Psychiatrists, Psychologists, Counselors, Social Workers, Nurses, and Other Mental Health Professionals, 2nd ed. Philadelphia: WB Saunders, 1998.

Speelman A, Savage J, Verburgh M. Use of attendants by general practitioners. BMJ 1993;307:986–987.

Stevenson I. The Diagnostic Interview, 2nd ed. New York: Harper and Row, 1971.

Stix G. Working the system II. Corporate greed no longer remains the sole domain of the corporation. Sci Am 2004;290:41.

Wachter RM. The "dis-location" of U.S. medicine—the implications of medical outsourcing. N Engl J Med 2006;354:661–665.

Weisleder P. The right of minors to confidentiality and informed consent. J Child Neurol 2004;19:145–148.

Welch CA. Sacred secrets—the privacy of medical records. N Engl J Med 2001;345:371–372.

The Patient's Chief Concern and Present Illness

6

I. The Initial Contact and the Face Sheet

A. The face sheet

1. Most physicians meet the patient after a receptionist has recorded personal and financial data on a "face sheet" (Table 6–1).

2. Perceptive analysis of face sheets raises many questions (Bluestone, 1996). The first contact with the physician's office should start the therapeutic process by making the patient feel welcome. Instead, the patient gets grilled by a disinterested receptionist who focuses on a computer screen, a process which annoys anyone, thus souring the very start of the visit. How much personal information should the patient have to disclose to a receptionist in a more or less public setting? To demand that sick persons fill out a form when they feel ill, may fear for their very life, and need to think about what they want to tell the physician seems thoughtless at best, if not heartless. Even if feeling well, many people resent disclosing personal information about their age, race, religion, employment, and marital status, particularly with other patients crowding the waiting room, eavesdropping.

3. Consider the difficulty for some patients in disclosing partner status if the receptionist asks "Married or single?" Should the cohabiting but unmarried partner be listed? How should the often married or the never married person, the separated and divorcing, or the same-sex couples respond (Makadon, 2006)? If the patient does not want the marital partner to know of the visit, should the patient withhold the home address and phone number? For some patients, questions about occupation provoke anxieties. How do you explain that you are unemployed? What if you are a prostitute, are a street person, or were recently released from prison? Asking a woman whether she works or has a job insults some, who may reply sarcastically, "No, I don't work. I'm a housewife." Even the patient's address and why

Table 6–1. A Commonly Used Type of Face Sheet for a Patient's Chart

OUTPATIENT FACE SHEET
NAME OF HOSPITAL, CLINIC, OR PHYSICIAN

PATIENT IDENTIFICATION DATA I PATIENT:	BIRTH NAME:
	I MRN:
REGISTRATION	I MAR STAT: SEX: ACCT TYPE:
LAST ACCT DATE	I BIRTH DATE: SUBTYPE:
ALTERED DATE	I ACCOUNT #:
ALTERED USER	I ATTENDING DOCTOR:

REASON FOR VISIT: REQUESTED BY:
DATE OF VISIT: SENT ON: AT:
————DOCTOR INFORMATION————————(PATIENT REGISTRATION)——————————
FAMILY/PRIMARY MD: PHONE:
ADDRESS:
REFERRING MD (1):   PHONE:
ADDRESS:
REFERRING MD (2)   PHONE:
ADDRESS:
——————————PATIENT INFORMATION——————————————————
SSN: RELIGION:
ADDRESS:
COUNTY: DAY/NIGHT PHONE:
OCCUPATION:
EMPLOYER: PHONE:
ADDRESS:
SPOUSE: WORK PHONE:
——————————NOTIFICATION INFORMATION——————————————
NEXT/KIN:
RELATION: DAY/NIGHT PHONE:
ADDRESS:
ALTERNATE CONTACT:
RELATION: DAY/NIGHT PHONE:
ADDRESS:
REGN COMMENT:
——————————GUARANTOR INFORMATION——————————————
NAME: SSN:
RELATION: PHONE:
ADDRESS:
OCCUPATION:
EMPLOYER: STATUS: PHONE:
ADDRESS:

Table 6–1. *(continued)*

─────ACCIDENT INFORMATION───────────────────────

CORONERS CASE: ACCIDENT LOCATION:
INJURY DATE/TIME   ACCIDENT TYPE:
ACCIDENT NATURE:

─────INSURANCE INFORMATION───────────────────────

PRI PLAN ID   PLAN NAME: POLICY NUM   GROUP NUM   EFF DT EXP DT   BC/BS PL CD

PRI/FC   INSURED NAME   INSURED ADDRESS (BILL TO)   VERIFICATION PHONE

he or she lives there may have medical significance. Living in a low-income neighborhood increases the risk of asthma in children several times over those living in affluent housing in the same city. Health risks are often embedded in particular environments.

4. Next comes the financial inquisition. It is particularly worrisome for a patient to have to divulge financial information before even seeing the physician and getting some idea of the financial burden the illness may impose. The physician's office or the hospital plots how to collect the bill before even attempting to help the patient. Does the financial information forewarn the physician, "Don't spend much effort on this one—she probably can't pay" or "This one has a lot of bucks—sock it to 'em, Doc." Even worse, a sign in the reception room may demand of the sufferer "Payment is expected at the time service is rendered." How can the patient come in with cash in hand without even knowing what the illness entails and what it may cost to investigate it? "Oh, this visit will cost me $500? Why sure, Doc, I always pack a spare $500 in my wallet." The patient may need to preserve the few dollars in pocket to feed the family during the illness. Now the patient not only has to face the illness and consequent loss of income and inability to support the family but doesn't know whether the physician will even accept him or her.

5. Then, the patient gets a record number, to keep jolly company with the social security number, the insurance policy number, the employer's number, sundry telephone numbers, the street number, and so on. The face sheet process has now dropped the patient into a statistical black hole, in the bowels of the computer, transformed from a named, real, suffering person into a string of digits, devoid of personality and dignity (Thomas, 1991).

6. The ultimate trial may come if the receptionist asks why the patient came in. Admitting to hemorrhoids is somewhat indelicate, but what if you fear gonorrhea or AIDS? Because of its sometimes sensitive nature, the receptionist should not ask anything more about the reason for the visit than what the patient offers.

7. In summary, the face sheet, with its worrying over personal data and billing, erects a barrier between patient and physician before they even meet. The process robs the patient of freedom of choice about personal disclosure and about the conditions of such disclosures. The process violates the whole basis of the medical relationship, which depends on trust and confidentiality between patient and physician. The face sheet custom shows what happens when the needs of the accounting system preempt the basic ethic of adapting all actions for the patient's comfort and benefit.

8. Other than the receptionist recording the patient's name, address, and phone number, I would suggest that the physician elicit most of the face sheet data because in the process the physician will learn much about the patient that is medically relevant but in the correct context of the patient-physician relationship (Bluestone, 1996). That custom would set the priorities straight: Consideration of the patient first, and all else second.

> In the bureaucracy of health care—whether in a private office, a clinic, or a hospital—individuals must conform to procedures of impersonal processing, modes of stylized identification, and rules of governance, often mysterious if not draconian. Persons become "clients" in this setting . . . losing their multidimensional identities as "persons."
> —Alfred I. Tauber (see Tauber, 2005, p 62)

B. Medical importance of ethnicity: nationality, geographic origin, religion, sex, and race

1. The patient's nationality and geographic origin may alert the physician to specific disease possibilities, such as parasitic infestations in immigrants or travelers from certain countries or the increased incidence of heredofamilial diseases in various inbred or ethnic groups (Shannon, 2001; see also www.omhrc.gov/, a site maintained by the U.S. Department of Health and Human Services, Office of Minority Health). Certain diseases and the necessary diagnostic workups do vary by age, race, and sex (Risch, 2006). For example sickle cell anemia would rank high in the differential diagnosis of an African American child with recurrent abdominal, pulmonary, or neurologic crises but very low for other children. Similarly, for some groups lactose intolerance (lactase deficiency) would be a much more likely cause of digestive and bowel symptoms than in other groups (Table 6–2).

2. Although a genomic basis for race is problematical (Hoover, 2007), ethnic stratification does show alarming discrepancies in health issues and health attitudes, for example, the appalling fact that the death rate for black

Table 6–2. Some Examples of Ethnic/Genetic Predilections for Disease

African American: sickle cell anemia and hypertension
Asian, African American, Hispanic: lactose intolerance
Finnish: infantile neuronal ceroid lipofuscinosis, myoclonic epilepsy
French Canadian: Morquio syndrome, agenesis of the corpus callosum, GM2 gangliosidosis
Native American: lactose intolerance, obesity, diabetes
Italian: thalassemia, cherry red spot (retinal degeneration) myoclonus syndrome
Japanese: galactosialidosis
Jewish:
    Ashkenazi: infantile Tay Sachs disease, recessive dystonia musculorum deformans, familial
        dysautonomia, abetalipoproteinemia, Niemann Pick disease, Gaucher disease
    Sephardic: cystinosis, ataxia telangiectasia
    Habbanite: metachromatic leukodystrophy
Pennsylvania Mennonites: maple syrup urine disease (frequency of 1 in 76 births but 1 in 220,000
    worldwide)
X linked diseases: hemophilia, Duchenne pseudohypertrophic muscular dystrophy,
    adrenoleukodystrophy, mucopolysaccharidosis II (Hunter syndrome), Pelizaeus Merzbacher
    disease, Albright pseudohypoparathyroidism, Lesch Nyhan hyperuricemia
    X linked dominant: Alport hereditary nephritis
Maternal transmission: mitochondrial myopathies and encephalopathies, Leber optic atrophy,
    Kearns-Sayre progressive ophthalmoplegia

infants is around 14/1000 compared to 6/1000 for white infants (Shannon, 2001).

3. Knowledge of the patient's culture (Lim, 2006) and religion alerts you to attitudes that may affect medical management apart from diagnosis per se (Pograis and Pellegrino, 2007). For example, Jehovah's Witnesses oppose blood transfusion, a Catholic woman may feel conflict over birth-control methods, and some patients who have depended on other beliefs may visit a physician only as a last resort (Simmons, 1991). For such patients or for atheists, agnostics, or deists, filling in the "Religion" blank on the face sheet may constitute a trial.

4. Although the differences cited are real, the physician should avoid stereotyping the patient on the basis of gender (Cooper et al., 2006; Hamberg et al., 2004), race (Garcia, 2004), religion, or culture (Juckett, 2005).

C. The medical importance of asking about occupation

1. If the patient states "I am a bus driver," the physician might respond with "How do you like the work?"—a response that a receptionist completing a form would not make. The answer gives insight as to the patient's overall adjustment to life and to its rewards or vexations. For a bus driver, a weak leg assumes an entirely different significance compared to an office worker.

2. If the patient's disorder impairs a major sensory avenue such as sight or the ability to move, as with severe back, hip, or knee pain, or the patient has fainting spells, again the knowledge of the occupation as a bus driver or machine operator might drastically alter decisions about management.

D. Source of referral

Learn whether the patient is self-referred or by whose recommendation and whether the patient expects you to have some special skills or abilities.

II. Format for the Clinical History

A. The order for the history

1. When dictating or writing down the history, adhere to the format in Table 1–1.

2. When taking the history, you more or less follow Table 1–1, but amend the order as needed. Continually refer back to Table 1–1 while studying the remainder of the text.

B. Sources of the history
The physician may derive historical information from the patient, relatives, acquaintances, and previous medical records. Write down the information source as follows: "The patient states ... ," or "The wife states ... ," or "Medical records from Dr._____ state...."

III. Technique for Meeting the Patient
A. Start each interview with a standard greeting.
1. Stand up to greet the patient. Ask for the patient's name and then introduce yours: "Hello. What is your name? I am Dr._____." Do not ask "How are you?"—an automatic, almost mindless social greeting. To answer that question may require the whole interview, and you aren't ready to address it yet. Make direct eye-to-eye contact. A smile usually helps, but do not come on like a toothpaste advertisement. A breezy greeting will alienate a grieving patient or one in pain.
2. The physician generally should shake hands with the patient.
3. Invite the patient to sit down. If the patient has acute pain, try to make her or him as comfortable as possible for the interview (Piasecki, 2003).
4. If your appointments are running behind, offer an explanation or apology and assure the patient that you have sufficient time for his or her examination.
B. What's in a name?
1. Address adult patients formally as Miss, Mrs., Ms., or Mr. A glance at the ring finger generally discloses marital status. Avoid addressing adult patients by their first name, certainly on the first visit. One patient felt compelled to compose this letter to her doctor.

> Dear Doctor: When I bring my gray hair, false teeth, sagging breasts, sick stomach, slipped disc, arthritic knees, varicose veins and fallen arches to your office, my self-esteem is so low I could trip on it. I would be a lot more comfortable if you called me by my married name.... When you call me "Dorcas" as I stand there in a cotton gown open at the back from neck to floor, I am a half-clad nobody, stripped of identity.... I have a

strong urge to greet you with "Hi Timmy" at next Thursday's appointment. D. H.

—From Ann Landers,
(*Indianapolis Star*,
April 4, 1979, by permission of
Esther P. Lederer Trust and
Creators Syndicate, Inc.)

2. Above all, never, never address elderly patients as "Pops," "Granny," or "Old-timer" or by their first name. Never, never address a woman as "Dearie," "Sweety," or "Honey."

3. Address and refer to children and babies by their given name. In January 1994, while outside a clinic desk in Riley Hospital, I saw a mother holding a baby whom she had brought for an appointment. An 11-year-old girl accompanied them. The receptionist had just said to the woman holding the baby, "Take it into the waiting room for now." The 11-year-old girl put her hands on her hips, tilted up her chin, and declared most indignantly, "How dare she call our baby an *it*." I can't think of a better way to emphasize the importance of addressing every patient correctly. The parents and the family regard the baby as a very real person. They have carefully and proudly selected a name. Don't refer to a baby as a neutral, nonentity like "it."

4. These introductory amenities constitute nothing mysterious or unique to medicine. They simply exhibit ordinary, basic good manners. Good manners are not a useless, archaic formality. By their very purpose, by their very design, good manners demonstrate your respect for the other person and convey your concern for that person's feelings and comfort.

5. In summary, a compounding of errors can start the medical interview off with tensions and frictions: The patient, feeling ill to start with, is irked, at least a little, by having to fill out a form that emphasizes personal details and financial information. Then, if the physician ignores the ordinary rules of dress, demeanor, and etiquette; fails to establish comforting physical contact by shaking hands; and fails to address the patient appropriately, the interview must start with a wary or resentful patient.

C. Introduce some chitchat.

1. After greeting and seating the patient, introduce some chitchat or small talk about the weather, the time of day,

or any neutral topic. If you happen to ask the patient, "Where are you from?" and the patient answers, "From the east side," you can respond, "Oh, did you grow up there?"—thus establishing a human bond. As chitchat for openers, do not offer compliments about the patient's appearance or clothing. That opener warns of the start of a seduction, not a medical interview.

2. Do not, in the vain hope of saving time, bypass the chitchat. In fact, regard the greeting and chitchat as commencing the diagnostic and therapeutic process. The chitchat will disclose much valuable information about the patient's attitudes and circumstances. The chitchat focuses on the patient as a person, not as a repository of disease. Most important of all, the chitchat eliminates any pressure on patients to reveal their most intimate concerns immediately to a stranger. These first moments of small talk that establish a human bond, a common touch, rank among the most valuable moments in the entire interview. First impressions are lasting impressions (Piasecki, 2003). Failure to insure this personal contact before launching into the history can result in outright disaster. See the case report by Brewster (1993), who was then a medical student.

3. Delay the start of the medical interview per se until the chitchat enables you both to begin to feel comfortable with each other. Your body language and the patient's body language signal this development—as both of you relax your shoulder girdles, unclasp your fingers, and settle back in your chairs.

D. Types of questions for the medical interview

1. The medical interview requires two types of questions, open and closed.

a. *Open* questions (e.g., "Tell me about your headaches") leave the patient complete freedom to answer with as little or as much information as he or she desires. Open questions increase the range and amount of information the patient produces (Takemura et al., 2005). Do not interrupt the patient until the flow of information from an open question stops.

b. *Closed*, or directive, questions restrict the patient to only one kind of answer: "When did the pain begin?" "How many brothers and sisters do you have?"

    c. Avoid asking leading questions that imply or force an answer or opinion: "You don't have headaches do you?"
2. Remain aware of the type of question asked. Particularly early in the interview avoid closed or leading questions.

IV. The Patient's Chief or Presenting Concern
  A. Why did the patient come?
1. Patients usually visit a physician because of some particular concern or worry that we label the "chief concern." You need to discover this chief concern in order to respond to it.
2. Most patients can express their concern directly: "I hurt my back the other day" or "I have a cough."
3. Other patients may feel too embarrassed to blurt out their concern: "I can't have bowel movements." Some patients may suffer vague fears or anxieties or unconscious motivations that they do not directly recognize and cannot recite outright. For these patients, the articulated chief concern (e.g., "I haven't been feeling well") serves only as the entree to the real concern (e.g., "I feel like killing myself"). Then only an artful interview will disclose the unvoiced, or "hidden," agenda. The quest for the patient's real chief concern requires the physician's skills and is the physician's responsibility (Baker et al., 2005; Sullivan and Wyatt, 2005). For this reason, the patient should not have to state it to a clerk or receptionist or by filling in a form.
4. Most textbooks label the patient's chief concern the "chief complaint." Over the years I and others (Benbassat and Baumal, 2004; Donnelly, 2005) have come to realize the pejorative implication of describing the patient's chief concern as a "complaint." One physician reacted this way:

> To the Editor: My chief complaint is with the "chief complaint," for, together with the process by which it is obtained, it is an organized put-down. Many things about it and the philosophy behind it are wrong. First of all, no one likes a complainer; therefore, to label every patient as having not only a complaint but a chief complaint is an unfortunate way to begin a visit. Secondly, from early in our medical education we are taught first to seek and then faithfully to record the chief complaint. This teaching has spread, so that now the clerk requests this information and places it within a box on the patient's record.

Thus, the search for the chief complaint has moved to the office desk, located near or within the waiting area, where the patient is asked to divulge (either publicly or over the telephone) this often sensitive and complicated information or to simplify falsely by answering "pain" or "rash" or "check-up" as the reason that he or she wants to see the doctor. Then, after being subtly identified as a complainer and forced into an evasion or a public revelation of fear, the patient is delivered—often humiliated, but always "one down"—into the presence of the physician. When it is discovered that the chief complaint is wrong, credibility and rapport crumble; patient and physician may even fall into an argument over whether the symptom or sign is present.

A patient needs an opportunity to "examine" the physician in order to decide whether he or she can express the true reason for coming to the doctor—the hidden agenda. ("Do I really want to spill my guts to this impatient, non-caring mechanic before me?") By a skillful and nonjudgmental interview, the physician must learn the patient's thoughts about the diagnosis as well as his or her expectations for investigation and management. Only then will the "chief complaint" be truly revealed and the expectations for diagnosis and treatment exposed so that they can be properly dealt with. Thus, if it is a chest x-ray film or a blood test that the patient seeks, how much better to know this, and to be able either to do it or to explain its need away, than to leave the patient with a nagging doubt about whether the doctor has even thought of performing the test, when the patient knows that that is how the cancer in little Johnny down the street was finally found.

My vote, therefore, is to banish the term "chief complaint" from our vocabulary, to recognize that it may be one of the last things to emerge in the course of the doctor–patient encounter, and to search for a comfortable way for the patient to see a doctor, a way that requires giving no particular reason in advance.

—Tom Frothingham, M.D. (reprinted by permission from N Engl J Med 1982;323;1569)

B. How to elicit the patient's chief concern
   1. What is an ideal question to start the medical interview?
     After the chitchat has allowed patient and physician to begin to feel comfortable with each other, the physician signals the time to get down to business by asking the most open question possible, "What did you come to see me about?"

or "What brings you to see me?" Notice that this question leaves the response entirely open. Perhaps the patient came in just to get a premarital blood test or a routine physical examination. Such a patient can answer directly, just as can a patient who has an overt symptom. If the patient cannot immediately blurt out the reason for coming, the wording of the question allows the patient an opportunity to temporize.

2. Incorrect or infelicitous opening questions:

   a. "What can I do to help you?" conveys condescension and implies that the patient knows what you can do.

   b. "What kind of trouble are you having?" conveys sinister implications (you are in trouble), when in fact the patient may merely want a routine checkup.

   c. "What's wrong with you?" has an accusatory tone and invites the patient to come forth with a conclusion, diagnosis, or speculation. The patient may reply to such a clumsy opening question by saying, "Doc, that's why I came, to find out what's wrong with me." By avoiding your question and calling you by the slightly derogatory term "Doc," the patient has subtly put you down a little and reminded you of a breach of technique.

   d. If the patient gives an evasive, uninformative, or sarcastic response, suspect that you have asked a gauche question or introduced it at an improper time. Then you have to waste time rescuing the interview. The patient expects you to proceed with professional aplomb. After a few errors in interview technique, the patient will lose faith in your professional competence.

C. Respond to the patient's voiced concern with an open invitation.

   1. If the patient voices a specific concern, make open, neutral responses that encourage the patient to elaborate on it: "Yes, go on" or "I see" or "Tell me about your headache" or whatever concern the patient has expressed.

   2. Before introducing closed questions that require specific answers, the physician uses several standard techniques to extend the patient's spontaneous narrative.

      a. Direct invitation: "Describe the dizziness to me."

      b. Repetition: You may quizzically repeat the patient's last words, "You feel very dizzy?"

    c. Facilitation or encouragement by voice and body language: You may lean back and relax slightly and say "mmm . . . yes go on" or "Tell me about that." Or you may choose to lean forward slightly, to signal interest.

    d. Remaining silent: Sometimes silence, perhaps with a nod of the head to indicate "Yes, go on," facilitates a response from the patient.

    e. Touching: Occasionally, a touch encourages a depressed or grieving patient to go on, but the patient must not perceive it as condescending or overly familiar. Touching may become appropriate later in the interview if the patient becomes upset.

D. Reflecting the patients vocabulary

    1. The foregoing open invitations by the physician leave the length and type of response to the patient's discretion, allowing free expression of their concerns, at their own pace and in their own words. In framing these responses, the physician uses, indeed parrots, insofar as seems appropriate, the patient's own vocabulary. Try to elicit the patient's spontaneous responses and concerns, free from any programming, prejudices, or medical jargon that you might inadvertently impose. Do not editorialize, moralize, or sympathize. Intrusion of your own personality, even overly solicitous receptivity, programs the patient to attend to you: "Look at me, patient, see what a wonderful, kindly physician I am." The physician has attempted to sell an image, rather than attending to the patient's needs.

    2. In reflecting the patient's own words, avoid the pitfall of premature conclusions or accepting the patient's diagnosis. The patient may complain of fainting spells, but whether they are faints (syncope), *fits* (seizures), *feigns* (either malingering or nonepileptic seizures), or *fugues* remains at this point unknown (see section VII, B of this chapter). The neophyte physician may respond with "When did your fainting spells begin?" While that reflects the patients own words, it implies acceptance of the patient's diagnosis. In such instances, you should use neutral phrasing: "Tell me more about these episodes." "Episodes" a neutral term, replaces "fainting," which implies a mechanism or, in a sense, a diagnosis that may be erroneous.

3. The patient who reports "sinus headaches" may or may not have sinus disease. You would reflect "headache" but not the diagnosis "sinus headache" in your response: "Describe these headaches." Ultimately, you should ask why the patient thinks sinus disease has caused them.

4. Because of differing lexicons, always clarify each patient's definition (Barr, 1971). "My nerves are bad" can mean almost anything. "I'm losing my nature" generally means a loss of sexual interest. "I'm having sick spells" may mean anything from vertigo or nausea to hallucinations of visitations by spirits or demonic forces.

E. Physician miscues that squelch the patient's responses

1. Avoid using the word "little." Avoid saying "Tell me a *little* more about that." "Tell me more about that" is perfect, but inserting "little" drastically alters the connotation. It implies, "OK, I've got to listen to this stuff but keep it brief. I'm far too busy to listen to a lot, so just tell me a little."

2. Avoid superficial condolences. If the patient states "I don't think my husband loves me," a perfect squelch would be "Well, we all need to be loved more." That response conveys disinterest rather than inviting the patient to talk about the problem. An appropriate reply would be "Tell me what's making you feel that way."

3. Avoid responses that accuse. Avoid questions such as "Why in the world did you do that?" or "Why did you let it go so long?" Such implications of wrongdoing or censure will make the patient defensive or angry. Instead, your responses should encourage introspection that will disclose the reasons for the patient's delays and will lead to therapeutic abreaction and patient education.

4. Avoid impatient body language. Do not fiddle with a pencil, glance at your watch, yawn, scratch yourself, sigh, or look bored. Nothing you say will counteract those messages. We return again to the issue of simple good manners.

F. Responding to unusual presenting concerns
Over the years, each physician will accumulate a number of unusual presenting concerns that seem bizarre or medically impossible or inexplicable (Carson et al., 2000). Don't dismiss a symptom simply because it seems bizarre. Here are some from patients of mine.

1. *Pt 7:* "I hear a swishing sound in my head," stated a 26-year-old man. If the patient complains of a swishing sound in the head, apply a stethoscope to the calvaria; and as in this patient, the physician will hear the swishing sound also. In this patient the sound, a so-called bruit, arose from the blood flowing through an intracranial arteriovenous malformation, as proven by angiography.

2. *Pt 8:* "After I have a bowel movement, I just don't feel satisfied." When I was a senior medical student, that statement emerged as a "hidden agenda," after I had struggled for an hour and a half to extract a history from a corpulent, middle-aged, overly talkative woman in whom every inquiry elicited endless vague symptoms. She was just the type of patient (fat, female, and fiftyish) whom young physicians tend to dismiss as just another complainer who would be well if she would just lose some of that blubber. After an hour and a half into the interview, I finally got the answer about unsatisfying bowel movements by bluntly asking, "Can you tell me any one thing that has caused you to come in today?" When I relayed the chief concern of dissatisfaction with bowel movements to the attending physician in the clinic, I thought he might just smirk a little, dismiss it, and go on to the next patient. But he knew better. He requestioned the patient and found out in 2 minutes that indeed she had experienced a change in her bowel habits and was having more and more difficulty and producing less and less stool. By listening to the patient and believing her story, he elicited the details that I had missed. Subsequent examination disclosed an annular carcinoma of the rectum. That patient left me with an indelible, career-long lesson.

3. *Pt 9:* "The top of my head feels too hot." That was the voiced concern of a 58-year-old woman. At first, I didn't know whether to take her seriously; but this time, as an intern, a year wiser than as a senior student, I believed the patient's history. Skull radiographs showed Paget disease of bone (osteitis deformans). The active metabolism of the bone greatly increases blood flow, accounting for the feeling of warmth.

4. *Pt 10:* "My face is getting ugly." In addition, this 38-year-old woman reported that she had to get bigger

shoes and bigger gloves. She had acromegaly from a pituitary adenoma. That disorder causes a gradual coarsening of the facial features and enlargement of the hands and feet. Coarsening of the features may also occur in hypothyroidism and leprosy.

5. *Pt 11:* "I have a snake in my bowels," stated this 23-year-old man, brought in by his mother. I had asked him whether he had any medical problems. Numerous other bizarre delusions and misperceptions quickly established a diagnosis of schizophrenia.

V. **Listening: The Essential Technique of the Clinical History**
   A. Nathanial Hawthorne offered the best description of the technique of listening that I can find:

> So [Dr.] Roger Chillingworth—the man of skill, the kind and friendly physician—strove to go deep into his patient's bosom, delving among his principles, prying into his recollections, and probing everything with a cautious touch, like a treasure-seeker in a dark cavern. Few secrets can escape an investigator, who has opportunity and license to undertake such a quest, and skill to follow it up. A man burdened with a secret should especially avoid the intimacy of his physician. If the latter possess native sagacity, and a nameless something more, let us call it intuition; if he show no intrusive egotism, nor disagreeably prominent characteristics of his own; if he have the power, which must be born with him, to bring his mind into such affinity with his patient's that this last shall unawares have spoken what he imagines himself only to have thought; if such revelations be received without tumult, and acknowledged not so often by an uttered sympathy as by silence, an inarticulate breath, and here or there a word, to indicate that all is understood; if to these qualifications of a confidant be joined the advantages afforded by his recognized character as a physician—then, at some inevitable moment will the soul of the sufferer be dissolved, and flow forth in a dark, but transparent stream, bringing all its mysteries into the daylight.
>
> —Nathanial Hawthorne (1804–1864)
> (Hawthorne, p 126), *The Scarlet Letter*

   B. Especially note the two most powerful lines that describe the physician's technique, "if he show no intrusive egotism of his own" and "if such revelations be received without tumult, and acknowledged not so often by an uttered sympathy as by silence, an inarticulate breath, and here and there a word, to indicate that all is understood." The more that patients talk and reveal their concerns and problems and the less the physician talks, the better the interview.

C. Out of sight, out of mind

Psychoanalysts recognize the same principles because to avoid "intrusive egotism," to avoid contaminating the patient's stream of consciousness, they may choose to sit behind their patients, completely out of sight. And finally note that, as documented by Hawthorne, the principles of nonjudgmental acceptance and neutrality of response in the medical interview have remained the same over the centuries.

D. The uniqueness of the interview process for the patient

> Hannah More wondered why people should be so fond of the company of their physician till she recollected that he was the only person with whom one dared to talk continually of one's self, without interruption, contradiction or censure.
>
> —(Roberts, 1841, p 317)

1. Few people have had the unique experience of sitting down with someone who focuses entirely on their concerns and needs and accepts them nonjudgmentally, as they are.

2. Working through the clinical history with a skilled physician amounts to an exercise in self-discovery for the patient and a tutorial in health education. As the physician builds the inventory of health-related information, the patient gains insight into the diverse factors that affect health and into the information that the physician needs. Ultimately, any unvoiced agenda that the patient cannot initially articulate will emerge, discovered by both the patient and the physician: too much stress in life, bereavement, social isolation, or simply a need to establish a nurturing and caring relationship with another human being (Barsky, 1981). If the latter is the patient's true agenda, how could he or she have articulated it as the "chief concern" or "chief complaint" in filling out a form or telling it to the receptionist?

VI. **Technique for Analyzing the Presenting Concern and Current Illness**

A. Try to learn when and how the illness started

After the flow of spontaneous information about the chief concern stops, elicit the chronological sequence of the illness. I often find it useful to ask, "When did you last consider yourself well? Let's start there." Or, as a means of focusing on the first events of the illness, "What was the first change you noticed about yourself?" Most patients recognize immediately that you want to review the time course of the illness; however, the patient may be able to neither supply an exact date of onset nor recognize which life events stem from the illness. In any event, try to learn whether the patient has a recent more or less continuous illness, a chronic illness, or an illness that comes in attacks interspersed with asymptomatic intervals.

B. Analyze the more or less recent or continuous symptoms by means of a symptom catechism.

1. After the patient's responses to open questions about the chief concern run down and you know what the symptom is, explore it and each additional symptom with closed, adverbial questions of *what, when, where, how* long, and *how* severe, according to Table 6–3.

2. To complete the catechism, ask about factors, circumstances, or actions that make the symptom better or worse. Ask whether any daily events such as meals, going to sleep or awakening from it, exercise or other daily activities, or social or emotional circumstances trigger the symptom.

3. Ask whether any particular symptom or attack restricts daily activities. If the patient reports a very severe symptom but it does not affect activity, such as going to school or to work, that throws some doubt on its severity. Contrarily, the symptom may serve as an excuse not to go to school or to work.

Table 6–3. A Catechism for Analyzing Each Symptom or Symptom Complex

1. What is the symptom under analysis?
2. When did the symptom start?
3. Where is it experienced in the body (locally or whole body)?
4. How long does it last? Is it intermittent or constant?
5. How severe is it? Ask the patient to grade it with a number. Does it make the patient go to bed? Does it interrupt play, school, work, or other activities?
6. What events or circumstances make it appear and disappear or get better or worse?
7. What is its overall course? Is it getting better or worse, or is it at a plateau?

4. Some authors question such catechisms as forcing the patient's history into a preconceived mold, but that objection confuses cause and effect. Physicians developed the catechism for the clinical history empirically, out of necessity because of the consistencies in one patient's history and another's. Current nosology, while continually evolving, fairly well reflects the reality of disease or the "natural order," not simply cultural bias. Although no pathognomonic signs or laboratory tests verify migraine, physicians did not invent it. Migraine has a remarkably consistent symptom pattern, even beginning in children 4–5 years old. This pattern consists of aura; throbbing, excruciating, often unilateral pain; visual changes; nausea and vomiting; extreme irritability; the necessity to retire to a quiet, dark room (photophobia and phonophobia); and alleviation of the pain by sleep. Although it merges with other types of headaches, it appears to exist as a way station or nodal point on a continuum of headache patterns. Physicians require a nosology that separates a malformation from an infection, a neoplasm, etc. because in the real world it makes a great difference for management, prognosis, and survival. These categories cannot be dismissed as arbitrary cultural biases.

5. The *Diagnostic and Statistical Manual of Mental Disorders* (DSM-IV) is most vulnerable to the accusation of cultural bias because of the difficulty in separating some mental illnesses from others and from normal limits. Nevertheless, for example, schizophrenia is not a conversion disorder. Successful treatment for the two differs drastically. In this sense, the classification of mental illness into separate categories receives empirical justification.

C. Analyzing a history of pain

1. Always start the analysis of any symptom with an open remark.

    a. Whatever the pain, an excellent opening remark is "Tell me about the pain" or "Describe the pain to me."

    b. After the patient's spontaneous response to the open invitation stops, systematically ask about the pain's *location, quality, quantity,* and *triggering* or *alleviating factors* (Table 6–3) (Weiner, l993).

2. Localizing the pain
   a. "Describe where you feel the pain. If possible use a hand or finger to show me where it is." Do not press the patient to localize the pain any more than corresponds to what the patient actually feels. An observant patient may localize some pain, particularly radicular or peripheral nerve pain, more accurately by describing it than you can disclose it by formal sensory testing during the neurologic examination.
   b. The location of the pain may or may not correspond to the diseased organ, nerve root, or nerve. Visceral pain in particular may be referred to a site distant from its origin. Classical examples include pain in the left arm arising from the heart and pain in the shoulder or neck region arising from irritation of the diaphragm.
   c. Abdominal pain
   (1) Pain arising in the abdominal viscera may feel sharp but often has a dull, intermittent, crampy character, relatively poorly localized. The pain from acute peritoneal inflammation tends to localize and to be sharper. The pain from an inflamed appendix localizes to the right lower quadrant, and its exacerbation by "rebound," so-called rebound tenderness, exemplifies this type of pain. When inflammation causes pain, the patient usually has a fever and an elevated white blood cell count with a shift to the left. Chronic right lower abdominal pain may also reflect Crohn disease, which involves the ileum and right colon (Rudolph, 2003).
   (2) Pain from upper gastrointestinal tract disorders such as esophagitis and peptic ulcers tends to localize in the upper part of the abdomen and to have a typical burning or gnawing character. Ingestion of food usually relieves such pain, whereas ingestion of food tends to trigger biliary or pancreatic pain. Pain in the left upper quadrant, particularly when exercising after meals, reflects contraction of the splenic capsule to increase the volume of circulating blood to fuel both the digestive tract and the muscles. After splenic rupture, the patient experiences some generalized

abdominal pain that tends to localize to the left upper quadrant.

(3) Patients with functional or psychogenic abdominal pain tend to describe it as being around the umbilicus. That corresponds to the "mental image" one has of one's abdomen and follows the rule that patients describe functional or nonorganic pain according to the mental image of the body part, not the wiring diagram of the nervous system (DeMyer, 2004). However, bowel obstruction also may cause periumbilical pain. Abdominal pain or headache that awakens the patient at night suggests, but does not assure, a definable organic cause.

(4) Explore any complaint of abdominal pain by asking specifically about fever, nausea, vomiting, hematemesis, melena, diarrhea, and constipation. Review any symptoms that could implicate the urinary and reproductive systems as the source of pain (see Chapter 7).

d. Nerve compression pain

Pain in the extremities from nerve root compression or other compression neuropathies tends to radiate distally, in the neuroanatomical distribution of the root or nerve (DeMyer, 2004; Wiener, 1993). The patient may also experience tingling, pins and needles, and numbness, which generally do not accompany pain referred from the viscera. Also an action, such as changing position or coughing, tends to trigger the pain of a compressive radiculopathy or neuropathy.

3. Characterizing the quality of the pain

a. "Describe how the pain feels." If this open question results in a vague response, you can then give the patient alternatives to select from, such as "constant," "localized," "radiating," "pounding," "throbbing," "dull," "sharp," "boring," "burning," "excruciating," or "cramping."

b. However, you should avoid programming the patient to give a more precise description than the sensation experienced warrants. Do not get impatient if the patient, even though intelligent and articulate, cannot describe pain very precisely.

4. Characterizing the quantity of the pain
   a. "How bad is the pain?" Many syndromes or diseases typically produce unbearable pain. Moderate or tolerable pain virtually excludes vascular headaches, such as from subarachnoid hemorrhage, migraine, cluster headaches, and temporal arteritis. Tolerable pain also virtually excludes many neuropathies, such as trigeminal neuralgia, postherpetic pain, causalgia (complex regional pain syndrome), and some visceral pain such as from gall bladder disease, renal colic, and gout (podagra).
   b. "Does the pain restrict your daily activity?" Pain of great severity will affect the patient's mobility and activity.
   c. Severe pain requires the patient to splint the affected part of the body. Pleuritic pain sharply arrests breathing movements. The patient cannot take a deep breath. The pain of backaches causes splinting of the back due to paravertebral muscle spasm. Patients with acutely herniated intervertebral disks try to avoid movement or jarring. To the contrary, some types of pain cause the patient to pace the floor, as with renal colic or with carpal tunnel syndrome in which severe nocturnal wrist pain awakens the patient, who then gets up and paces the floor. By carefully assessing the quantity, quality, and location of the pain; the exacerbating factors; and the effect of the pain on activity as well as the effect of activity on the pain, you can often infer the organ affected and the lesion.
   d. True migraineurs must, of necessity, go to bed in a quiet, dark room when they have an attack. That is one universal, inevitable feature of classical migraine attacks. If a patient with headaches does not have, of necessity, to retire to a quiet, dark room during the attacks, the patient probably does not have migraine; but exceptions occur.
   e. With other severe, ongoing symptoms, such as acute, true vertigo, the patient must, of necessity, remain in one position. The patient does not even want to turn over in bed because movement intensifies the vertigo or triggers a new attack. The fact that the illness demands immobilization or interferes with daily activities is a diagnostic feature of these illnesses.
5. Scaling the severity of pain and other symptoms

   a. Even the articulate, observant patient may fail to express the severity of pain very well. You may then suggest some descriptors:
      (1) Mild
      (2) Moderate
      (3) Bearable
      (4) Unbearable
   b. When reciting descriptors, you must avoid influencing the patient's judgment or forcing the patient into a pseudoaccurate or pseudospecific response.
   c. The physician can also ask the patient to grade the pain on a scale of 1–10, with 10 being the worst (unbearable) pain. Use numerical scales cautiously because the inquiry can degenerate into a game of picking out the number rather than focusing on the events that need attention. Some patients will pick 10 in an effort to impress the physician. Nevertheless, Beecher (1959) and many others have shown the value of scaling subjective responses.
   d. As another measure of severity, ask how much time the symptom has caused the patient to miss from work or school or how often the symptom has caused the patient to suspend activity to go to bed. Grading the severity of the symptom plus assessing the functional disability offers a better measure of the impact of headaches or pain in general (Jacobsen et al., 1994; Von Korff et al., 1994).
   e. Wherever appropriate, ask the patient to express the history in numbers: "How fast or slow was your pulse?" "When you felt hot, did you actually measure your temperature with a thermometer?" "How many times a day do you have to urinate?" "How often do you have headaches?" If necessary, ask the patient to keep an actual diary and record the numbers.
6. Triggering/alleviating factors for pain
   Of prime importance is to ask about specific events that may trigger the pain—movement, sneezing or coughing, eating, defecating, exercising, etc.—and any postures or actions that relieve it.
7. Relation of severity of pain to prognosis
   The degree of pain does not necessarily reflect the threat or prognosis of the underlying disease. Some intensely painful

syndromes, such as proctalgia fugax, which causes severe, knife-like or cramping pain in the rectum, pose no threat at all to the patient's overall health. Myocardial infarction may cause unbearable, vice-like pain but sometimes remains silent or asymptomatic.

D. Some characteristic temporal profiles of chronic diseases

    1. Gradual retrogression, a steadily declining course

        a. Various chronic diseases show similar temporal profiles of gradual onset and steady worsening. Malignant neoplasms usually cause a steady decline in health, consisting of weight loss, malaise, pain, and anorexia. Specific symptoms depend on the organ or organs affected. The patient gradually worsens over weeks, months, or years (Fig. 6–1A).

        b. So-called degenerative neurologic diseases, such as Alzheimer dementia, usually start insidiously with minor changes in mentation and cause a gradual, relatively smooth decline, extending over many years.

        c. Even diseases that usually worsen gradually may in some patients cause precipitous changes. For example, the onset of seizures in dementia or the sudden hemorrhage into a brain tumor or gastrointestinal hemorrhage from esophageal varices or peptic ulcer may cause a sharp change in the patient even though the disease per se has not suddenly worsened.

    2. Intermittent exacerbating-remitting but nonretrogressive course

        a. Some diseases such as migraine headaches, contact dermatitis, breath-holding spells, or mild asthma cause only intermittent symptoms or signs. The patient returns to normal or near normal between attacks and overall does not decline (Fig. 6–1B).

        b. Allergies tend to show seasonal exacerbations, depending on the allergens in the air at various times of the year.

    3. Intermittent exacerbating-remitting diseases with an overall retrogressive course

        a. Some diseases, such as multiple sclerosis or rheumatoid arthritis, cause intermittent attacks, with exacerbations and remissions; but the patient may not return completely to normal in between attacks. The overall course shows a stepwise, cumulative decline, in contrast

A

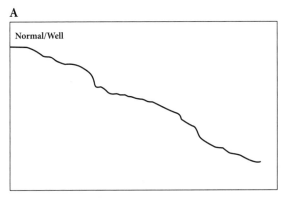

Time: days, months or years.

B

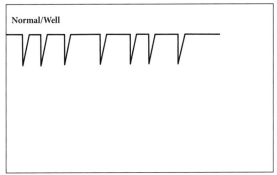

Time: days, months or years.

C

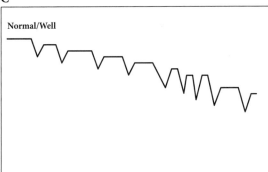

Time: days, months or years.

Figure 6–1. Time course of various diseases (temporal profiles). *A* Gradual retrogression, as in neoplasms, dementia, or any disease that worsens with time. *B* Intermittent attacks with complete return to normal during the symptom free intervals, as in migraine or epilepsy. *C* Stepwise retrogression, as in diseases with exacerbations and remissions, but incomplete recovery between attacks, as in multiple sclerosis or rheumatoid arthritis.

to the rather smooth curve of the decline in neoplastic and degenerative diseases (compare Fig. 6–1B and C).

   b. Exacerbating and remitting diseases sometimes reach a plateau, with little change for years, and then flare up again.

4. Typical temporal profiles in chronic developmental disorders of children

   a. Figure 6–2A shows the curve of normal development for numerous anatomic parameters, such as height, weight, and occipitofrontal circumference or the acquisition of skills.

   b. The history and physical examination will disclose whether a child's developmental progress matches or departs significantly from the normal curve or normal timetable.

   c. Figure 6–2B shows how an infant with a static brain lesion, destined to be retarded, may appear normal at birth but then lag more and more behind normal, ultimately paralleling the normal curve but never catching up. The ultimate peak plateau falls at a significantly lower level than the peak plateau for the normal child.

   d. Figure 6–2C shows how the infant or child with a degenerative disease or brain tumor may show a completely normal early period of development and then drop off of the curve. Again, the history establishes this characteristic declining course: "Tell me what the child could once do that he cannot do now?" or "What abilities has the child lost?"

E. Changes in preexisting symptoms or baselines

Always explore worsening of old symptoms or symptoms of new onset, such as changes in headaches, mild mental aberrations, changes in sleep patterns, or changes in bowel and bladder habits. A new disease may have started or an old disease may have flared up. Any change in customary life patterns, such as the onset of constipation or weight loss in a previous healthy person, requires investigation.

F. Differences between psychogenic and organic disease profiles

1. The symptoms of organic diseases tend to change with time and with triggering or alleviating circumstances (i.e., they get better or worse). Absolutely constant headache or

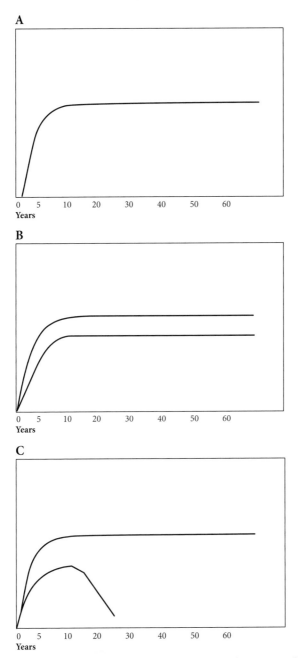

Figure 6–2. Time course of developmental disorders. *A* Normal curve of development for many physical measurements, such as head size, height, and weight. *B* With a static brain lesion, the gap between normal development and mental retardation increases initially, then parallels the normal curve but does not close. *C* With a progressive degenerative disease, the patient may develop normally initially but then fall further and further below the normal curve.

backache, present every day for weeks or months with no mitigation or change and no triggering or alleviating maneuvers, usually signifies nonorganic disease or a nonorganic, functional overlay.

2. Functional symptoms do not reflect the anatomic arrangement and physiologic functions of the body. Rather, they imitate the patient's mental image of how a part functions (DeMyer, 2004).

3. No corroborative physical and laboratory signs appear that should accompany the symptom.

4. Functional illnesses result in primary and secondary gains. The primary gain is relief from anxiety. The secondary gain consists of manipulative control over the emotions, attention, and actions of other persons and relief from responsibilities. The patient, who may have both organic and psychiatric disease, makes the rounds of physician after physician, responds little if at all to therapy, and generally ends up in a chronic pain clinic.

VII. **Historical Analysis of Recurrent Attacks That Are Similar**

A. Determining the pattern of recurrent attacks

1. Many disorders such as headaches and renal stones cause recurrent, intermittent attacks. Each disorder presents attacks with their own characteristics but that more or less follow the same pattern, with symptom-free intervals (Table 6–4).

2. To learn whether the attacks do indeed have a similar pattern of onset and evolution, ask the patient to describe in detail the first attack and the last attack. Usually, the patient remembers the last attack vividly. Also ask for descriptions of the worst attacks and of a typical attack. Comparison of the first, last, worst, and typical attacks will show whether the attacks more or less match, thus suggesting one disorder. However some disorders, such as porphyria, multiple sclerosis, and collagen diseases, cause intermittent attacks that may differ in expression.

3. After the patient finishes the spontaneous description of the attacks, the physician systematically analyzes the attacks by more or less following Table 6–5. Any sudden attack, especially an epileptic attack, is called an *ictus*.

Table 6–4. Some Common Disorders Characterized by Intermittent Attacks and Symptom-Free Intervals

Headaches	Dizziness
Backaches	Insomnia
Chest or abdominal pain: spontaneous, anginal, or pre or postprandial	Panic/anxiety attacks
Numbness, tingling or pain in the extremities	Earaches and sore throats
Loss of consciousness	Fever and malaise
Fainting (syncope)	Nausea, vomiting
Epilepsy	Diarrhea or constipation
Nonepileptic seizures	Asthma and hay fever
Breath-holding spells	Skin rashes/wheals/itching
Hyperventilation attacks	Exercise intolerance: cramps or claudication
Blurred vision or double vision	Transient ischemic attacks

Analyze these attacks in three phases: the pre-ictal, ictal, and post-ictal phases (Table 6–5).

4. By following the outline in Table 6–5, you will discover the physical activity and the social circumstances of the patient at the onset, the first symptoms of the attack, and the time of day. The details of the beginning of the attack or of the activity preceding the attack provide the most useful information for the diagnosis of intermittent disorders because they may disclose the triggering factor or suggest the organ involved and type of lesion. For example:

   a. In some children, fever triggers seizures or anger triggers breath-holding spells (DeMyer, 2005); or in adults, hunger, alcohol, certain foods, or withdrawal of caffeine may precipitate headaches or abdominal discomfort or diarrhea. Elimination of the triggering factor then provides the best treatment.

   b. A fainting spell that occurs when the patient arises suggests orthostatic hypotension (Low et al., 1995; Streeten, 1995), while one that occurs after hyperventilation suggests hyperventilation syncope and one that occurs after urinating suggests micturition syncope. Fainting after emotional turmoil suggests psychogenic syncope (Fig. 6–3).

   c. Retrosternal discomfort after meals and pain in the left arm after exercising suggest coronary artery disease.

Table 6–5. A Catechism for Analysis of Recurrent Attacks that Have a Similar Pattern (Although Specifically for Attacks that Impair Consciousness, the Principles Apply to All Recurrent Attacks)

I. First and last attacks and typical attacks: Ask the patient to describe the first or last attacks because these are likely to be remembered best, particularly the last. Ask whether all attacks are similar.

II. The pre-ictal stage. Ask about:
   A. Triggering factors: any relation to time of day, meals, sleep–wake cycle, physical activity, posture, or social circumstances?
   B. Physiological changes: pulse, respiration, pallor or cyanosis, sweating, hyperventilation, or breath-holding?
   C. Changes in mental state: immediate premonitory symptoms or aura. Ask about:
      1. The first change that heralds an ictus
      2. Any change in affect, mood, or thought processes
      3. Any changes in vision, hearing, smell, or taste
      4. Any nausea, vomiting, or other thoracoabdominal sensation
      5. Any numbness, tingling, or pain

III. The ictal stage
   A. If the attack does not involve loss of consciousness, get a full beginning to end description of what the patient experiences during the attack.
   B. If the patient loses consciousness, ask "What is the last thing you remember before the attack?" and "What is the first thing you become aware of when recovering from an attack?" Ask someone who has witnessed an attack for the following details:
      1. Facial appearance, skin color, eye movements, pupillary size, facial twitching, lip smacking, and vocalizations
      2. Response to voice or other stimuli during the attack
      3. Falls or retains posture
      4. Becomes stiff or limp
      5. Twitches or jerks: Are the jerks focal, lateralized, or generalized?
      6. Alterations in breathing
      7. Incontinence of urine or stool
      8. Injury
      9. Tongue biting

IV. The post-ictal stage. Ask about:
   A. Rapidity of recovery
   B. Stage of confusion, lethargy, or sleep
   C. Awareness of having had the attack
   D. Stiffness or soreness in the muscles and joints

V. Ask about the duration of each stage.

    5. Ask selected patients to keep a diary that documents the timing, preceding events, frequency, and characteristics of their attacks. The concatenation of events may disclose specific trigger factors or explain the nature and cause of the attacks.

  B. The history in epilepsy and syncope: How to get an accurate description of recurrent attacks that alter consciousness

    1. Three common intermittent disorders—seizures, syncope, and headaches—provide models for investigating recurrent

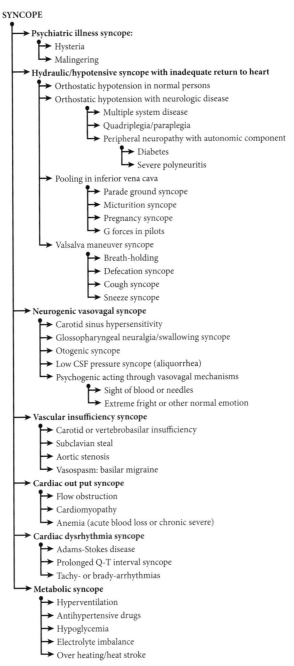

SYNCOPE
- **Psychiatric illness syncope:**
  - Hysteria
  - Malingering
- **Hydraulic/hypotensive syncope with inadequate return to heart**
  - Orthostatic hypotension in normal persons
  - Orthostatic hypotension with neurologic disease
    - Multiple system disease
    - Quadriplegia/paraplegia
    - Peripheral neuropathy with autonomic component
      - Diabetes
      - Severe polyneuritis
  - Pooling in inferior vena cava
    - Parade ground syncope
    - Micturition syncope
    - Pregnancy syncope
    - G forces in pilots
  - Valsalva maneuver syncope
    - Breath-holding
    - Defecation syncope
    - Cough syncope
    - Sneeze syncope
- **Neurogenic vasovagal syncope**
  - Carotid sinus hypersensitivity
  - Glossopharyngeal neuralgia/swallowing syncope
  - Otogenic syncope
  - Low CSF pressure syncope (aliquorrhea)
  - Psychogenic acting through vasovagal mechanisms
    - Sight of blood or needles
    - Extreme fright or other normal emotion
- **Vascular insufficiency syncope**
  - Carotid or vertebrobasilar insufficiency
  - Subclavian steal
  - Aortic stenosis
  - Vasospasm: basilar migraine
- **Cardiac out put syncope**
  - Flow obstruction
  - Cardiomyopathy
  - Anemia (acute blood loss or chronic severe)
- **Cardiac dysrhythmia syncope**
  - Adams-Stokes disease
  - Prolonged Q-T interval syncope
  - Tachy- or brady-arrhythmias
- **Metabolic syncope**
  - Hyperventilation
  - Antihypertensive drugs
  - Hypoglycemia
  - Electrolyte imbalance
  - Over heating/heat stroke

Figure 6–3. Dendrogram of causes for syncope. (Reproduced by permission from DeMyer WE. Technique of the Neurologic Examination. New York: McGraw-Hill, 2004.)

attacks affecting any part of the body. Attacks that alter consciousness (blackout spells) may consist of *faints* (syncope), *fits* (seizures), *feigns* (malingering or nonepileptic seizures; Patel et al., 2007), or *fugues* (a temporary altered mental state of walking around but with no memory of the event). About 5% of the population will have one or more seizures, and a larger percent will have fainted at sometime in their lives.

2. Definitions of seizures and epilepsy:

> And who are you who draws his veil across the stars?
> —Langston Hughes (1902–1967)
> (Hughes, 1994, p189)

a. By definition, an *epileptic seizure* is any change in motor, mental, or sensory function caused by an excessive or hypersynchronous discharge of central nervous system neurons. An electroencephalogram (EEG), by recording the electrical activity of the brain, confirms the abnormal, hypersynchronous discharge of neurons.

b. Mention any—yes, *any*—motor act, mental experience, or sensory complaint and in some patients it will have occurred as a manifestation of a seizure. The various expressions of seizures continue to astonish even the most seasoned clinician (Tables 6–6 and 6–7).

c. *Epilepsy* is recurrent seizures. The interval between the seizures may vary from seconds to years. Most seizures stop after seconds to minutes, but in status epilepticus or partial continual epilepsy, seizures may continue without interruption for hours, days, or years.

d. To accurately describe and classify the type of seizure, see Tables 6–5 to 6–8. Such classifications, whether of epilepsy, syncope (Fig. 6–3), headache (Table 6–9), or sleep disorders (Table 9–6), remind the physician what to ask about during the history. Systematic questioning not only provides the necessary diagnostic information for the physician but also teaches the patient and family how to observe the attacks more accurately. Because the physician usually does not directly see a seizure, an accurate history that allows classification of the seizure type is essential (Tables 6–7 and 6–8). causes, medication

Table 6–6. Mental, Motor, and Sensory Manifestations of Seizures: To Characterize the Seizure, Ask the Patient About the Items Listed

I. Mental manifestations of seizures
   A. Loss of consciousness, with amnesia for the ictus
   B. Changes of mood: anxiety, fear, elation
   C. Forced thinking, déjà vu or deja pensé, etc.
   D. Transient disorientation
II. Sensory manifestations of seizures
   A. Numbness or tingling in the face, tongue, or extremities
   B. Formed or nonformed visual hallucinations, changes in the size of objects seen (macropsia or micropsia) or of loudness of sounds
   C. Formed auditory hallucinations
   D. Visceral sensations of water or wind moving in chest or abdomen, vague feeling of something rising in the body
III. Motor manifestations of seizures
   A. Somatomotor
      1. Single focal jerk of a part of the body (myoclonic jerk) or the whole body (salaam seizure)
      2. Clonic jerks (series of myoclonic jerks), focal or general
      3. Tonic contractions
      4. Akinetic or inhibitory seizures (drop attacks)
      5. Automatisms: chewing, walking, running (cursive epilepsy), laughing (gelastic epilepsy), complex acts, such as picking at clothes, singing, or even driving a car
   B. Visceromotor and autonomic
      1. Changes in blood pressure, respiration, and pulse rate, including cardiac arrhythmias
      2. Sweating, skin pallor, or flushing
      3. Pupiloconstriction or dilation
      4. Changes in gastrointestinal or genitourinary motility: incontinence
      5. Piloerection

required, and prognosis differ drastically for the various types of seizures.

  e. In taking the history of recurrent attacks of any type, always ask, "Can you describe the first change you notice when an attack comes on?" (see Table 6–5). A seizure initiated focally by tingling in a thumb suggests a focal lesion of the contralateral sensory cortex. A seizure starting with a sensation of smell or taste suggests a focal lesion in the uncus of the temporal lobe. The very first manifestation localizes the lesion or gives insight into the mechanism of the event, whereas the generalized jerking and loss of consciousness that may ensue do not localize the origin of the seizure. The generalized seizure reflects a gross disturbance of cerebral function that can be the end result of a variety of preceding types of seizures.

Table 6–7. Comprehensive International Classification of Epileptic Seizures

I. **Partial (focal) seizures**
   A. Simple partial seizures
      1. With motor signs
      2. With sensory hallucinations, somatosensory or special sensory
      3. Mental (psychic) changes
      4. Autonomic signs
   B. Complex partial seizures (psychomotor)
      1. Simple partial onset followed by impaired consciousness
      2. With impaired consciousness at onset
   C. Partial (focal) seizures evolving secondarily to generalized motor seizures (GMS)
      1. Simple partial seizures evolving to GMS
      2. Complex partial seizures evolving to GMS
      3. Simple partial seizures evolving to complex partial seizures evolving to GMS
II. **Generalized seizures (convulsive and nonconvulsive)**
   A. Absence seizures
      1. Typical absence seizures = petit mal seizures
      2. Atypical absence seizures = atypical petit mal seizures
   B. Myoclonic seizures
   C. Clonic seizures
   D. Tonic seizures
   E. Tonic-clonic seizures = GMS
   F. Atonic seizures (akinetic seizures or drop attacks)
   G. Unclassifiable seizures

Based on Epilepsia 1981;22:489–501.

Table 6–8. Clinical Features of the Commoner Epileptic Seizures as Derived from the History

1. Generalized motor seizures (grand mal): typically consist of an aura, loss of consciousness, cry, fall, tonic contractions followed by clonic contractions of the trunk and all four extremities, and often incontinence. The ictus lasts several minutes, followed by post ictal stupor.
2. Focal motor seizures: typically start in one part of the body such as the face, hand, or foot. The movements may spread ipsilaterally and then bilaterally and may end as a generalized motor seizure with loss of consciousness. Often, the patient has transient post ictal hemiparesis (Todd paralysis) after a unilateral seizure.
3. Focal sensory seizures: may manifest as somatic, visceral, visual, auditory, olfactory, or gustatory symptoms; may or may not proceed to a motor seizure and loss of consciousness.
4. Myoclonic seizures: manifest as sudden, single, shock like jerks of parts of muscles or muscle groups, affecting the neck, trunk, or extremities; may occur alone or with other seizures, particularly in infantile spasms, consisting of myoclonic jerks, staring spells, drop attacks, and salaam movements.
5. Absence seizures (petit mal): no aura but an abrupt arrest of activity with loss of consciousness, staring, and sometimes facial movements, without convulsive movements elsewhere, fall, or incontinence. The ictus lasts less than 30 seconds, followed by abrupt, complete recovery and abrupt resumption of preseizure activity.
6. Akinetic seizures (drop attacks): typically no aura, but an abrupt loss of consciousness and muscle tone cause the patient to plummet to the floor. The ictus may last seconds to minutes, followed often by post ictal confusion.
7. Psychomotor seizures (temporal lobe or complex partial seizures): typically consist of an aura, loss of consciousness, often with aversive head and eye turning, vacant facial appearance, performance of automatic acts such as walking or chewing; may end with a generalized motor seizure and sometimes incontinence. The ictus lasts minutes, followed by confusion and gradual resumption of consciousness.

Table 6–9. Classification of Headaches

Primary headaches
    Migraine
    Migraine without aura
    Migraine with aura
    Migraine with focal neurologic signs
    Hemiplegic, ophthalmoplegic, hemiparesthetic, hemianopic, or aphasic migraine
    Childhood precursors of migraine
    Cyclic vomiting
    Abdominal migraine
    Benign paroxysmal vertigo
    Chronic migraine, merges with chronic daily headache and chronic tension-type headache
        (Silberstein et al., 1996)
    Tension-type headache
    Infrequent or frequent episodic headache
    Chronic (daily) tension-type headache
        Associated or not associated with pericranial tenderness
    Cluster headache and other trigeminal autonomic cephalalgias
    Cluster headache
    Paroxysmal hemicrania
        With conjunctival injection and tearing, other autonomic signs
    Other primary headaches
        Stabbing headache (ice-pick headache)
        Cough headache
        Postexertional headache
        Coital/orgasmic headache
        Hypnic headache
        Primary thunderclap headache
        Hemicrania continua
        New daily persistent headache
Secondary headaches
    Headache attributed to head and/or neck trauma
    Acute or chronic posttraumatic headache
    Acute or chronic headache attributed to whiplash injury
    Traumatic intracranial hematoma, epidural or subdural
    Postcraniotomy headache
    Headache attributed to cranial or cervical vascular disorder
    Ischemic stroke
    Subarachnoid or intracerebral hemorrhage
    Unruptured vascular malformation, aneurysm, malformation, or fistula
    Carotid or vertebral artery pain from dissection
    Giant cell arteritis/angiitis
    Cerebral venous thrombosis
    Headache attributed to other vascular disorders, hereditary or mitochondrial
    Headache attributed to nonvascular intracranial disorder
    High cerebrospinal fluid pressure
    Idiopathic intracranial hypertension
    Metabolic, toxic, or hormonal causes
    Intracranial hypertension secondary to hydrocephalus
    Low cerebrospinal fluid pressure
    Postdural puncture headache/post–lumbar puncture headache

(continued)

Table 6–9. *(continued)*

Secondary headaches *(continued)*
    Idiopathic
    Noninfectious inflammatory disease
    Neurosarcoidosis
    Aseptic meningitis
    Other noninfectious inflammatory diseases
    Intracranial neoplasm
    Postseizure headache (specify seizure type)
    Headache attributed to a substance or its withdrawal
    Headache induced by acute exposure
    Nitric oxide
    Carbon monoxide
    Alcohol
    Food components and additives
    Street drugs
    Prescription medications
    Organic solvents
    Medication overuse headache
        Ergotamine
        Triptan
        Over-the-counter analgesics
        Opioids
        Exogenous hormones/contraceptive hormones
    Medication withdrawal headache
        Caffeine
        Opioids
        Estrogen
    Headache attributed to infection
        Meningitis
        Encephalitis
        Brain abscess or empyema
        Systemic infection
        HIV/AIDS
    Chronic postinfection headache
    Headache attributed to disorder of homeostasis
    Hypoxia or hypercapnia
    Arterial hypertension
    Fasting
    Headache or facial pain attributed to disorder of cranium, neck, eyes, ears, nose, sinuses,
        teeth, mouth, or other facial or cranial structures
        Disorders of cranial bone
        Cervicogenic headache
        Ocular disorders
        Glaucoma
        Refractive errors
        Ocular misalignments (heterophoria/heterotropia)
        Inflammations
        Iritis
        Conjunctivitis
        Ear infections/otitis media/mastoiditis
        Sinusitis
        Dental pain, caries or abscess
        Temporomandibular joint

Table 6–9. *(continued)*

Secondary headaches *(continued)*
 Headache attributed to psychiatric disorder
  Somatization disorder
  Psychotic disorder
 Cranial neuralgias and central causes of facial pain
  Trigeminal/glossopharyngeal/occipital neuralgia
  Cold stimulus headache
  Optic neuritis
  Herpes zoster
  Poststroke pain
  Burning mouth pain
 Other headache, cranial neuralgia, central or primary facial pain
 Headache not otherwise classified
 Headache unspecified

Headache Classification Subcommittee, 2004 (reproduced by permission from Cephalalgia 2004; 24(Suppl 1):16–22).

  f. Ask what the patient remembers about the attacks. Generalized motor seizures commonly cause falls and injuries, tongue biting, incontinence of urine or feces, post-ictal soreness of the muscles, and lethargy or sleep. Patients with nonepileptic (pseudoepileptic) seizures do not usually show any of these features (Bowman, 2000; Patel et al., 2007).

  g. Nonepileptic (pseudoepileptic) seizures imitate epilepsy. They commonly occur in patients during life stresses in which the episodes provide a strong secondary gain. A key point in the history is that the attacks usually appear in the presence of an emotionally significant person or to avoid some responsibility. Apart from this "social trigger," the attacks may imitate true epilepsy so closely that even experienced clinicians cannot differentiate them by means of the history or even by directly viewing the attacks. One important distinction is that patients with nonepileptic seizures almost always close their eyes, whereas the eyes remain open in true seizures, although the eyeballs may deviate. Differentiation of epileptic and nonepileptic seizures may require prolonged ambulatory monitoring or combined EEG and video monitoring in a laboratory. If the patient has an episode, as documented by the video camera, but the EEG does not record a hypersynchronous neuronal discharge, the episode is generally not a true seizure. In fact, epileptic and nonepileptic seizures may coexist, which confounds the history and the management.

h. Especially for attacks that alter consciousness, ask about changes in breathing, pupillary size, eye position, pulse, sweating, and skin color, either pallor or cyanosis. Patients with organic causes for lapses of consciousness commonly show one or more of these objective changes.

3. The diagnosis of syncope

Syncope, or fainting, has psychogenic and organic causes. The history generally differentiates the two by disclosing that psychogenic fainting corresponds to psychogenic stress, whereas most organic types of fainting have other trigger factors (Grubb, 2005; Miller and Kruse, 2005). The physician must separate neurogenic from cardiogenic syncope (DeMyer, 2004). Cardiogenic syncope may cause sudden death, particularly in the prolonged QT interval syndrome (Moss, 2003; Roden, 2008). The differential diagnosis of syncopal attacks may require combined video–EEG–electrocardiographic–respiratory (polygraphic) monitoring.

4. Corroborative history of recurrent attacks that cause loss of consciousness

When recurrent attacks cause loss of consciousness, always question a witness who can describe details not known to the patient. Lay observers can describe episodes of unconsciousness accurately if the physician asks the applicable questions from Table 6–5 or uses a more formal structured interview (Ottoman et al., 1993). In absence (petit mal) seizures and some psychomotor (complex partial) seizures, the patient may fail to realize that an attack has occurred and cannot give an accurate account of the frequency or of the features of the attack.

C. Why the headache history is the most difficult of all histories

1. Nowhere in medicine is the history more crucial or more difficult than in the differential diagnosis of headaches, the commonest affliction of humankind. The correct diagnosis of headache is often more difficult to secure than most diagnoses. You always have to worry about missing a serious

underlying organic disease or whether the headache reflects a serious psychiatric disorder, such as depression. A trap always awaits the unwary: yes, the patient may have tension headaches; yes, that diagnosis may be correct, but that does not exclude a brain tumor. In fact, brain tumor headaches cause no pathognomonic features. They may resemble tension headaches, but the patient tends to have nausea and vomiting and often some neurologic sign that would not appear in routine tension headaches (Forsyth and Posner, 1993). Because many headaches are the apotheosis of a biopsychosocial disorder, with cultural, psychological, and physical contributions, a brief, designated "headache" history is insufficient. Because headaches require the most perceptive and thorough history, reserve an hour for the history for each new headache patient. You have to take a lifestyle history. Then, you have to expect to requestion the patient and extend the history on subsequent visits.

> One should be able to recognize those who have headaches from gymnastic exercises, or running, or walking, or hunting or any other unreasonable labor, or from immoderate venery.
> —Hippocrates (460–377 BCE)
> (Kelly, 2006, p 94)

2. The details from the history, elicited by following the catechisms of Tables 6–3 and 6–5, enable the physician to classify the type and probable cause of the headache (Table 6–9).
3. Always ask about the circumstances that precede each headache. Hippocrates forewarned that various factors trigger headaches, including exercise and overheating and, yes, venery—headaches triggered by orgasm (Silbert et al., 1991). The plea "Not tonight dear, I have a headache" becomes "Not tonight dear, it will give me a headache." Trigger factors vary from hormones to rebound from analgesics to stress from a visit by an unwanted relative. Table 6–10 lists factors that may trigger migraine.
4. Distinguishing primary from secondary headaches, as listed in Table 6–10, is important because primary headaches are essentially idiopathic, while a definable lesion or disease underlies the secondary. The lesion then may threaten life, such as with a subarachnoid hemorrhage (Brazis et al.,

Table 6–10. Factors that may Trigger Migraine Headaches in Some Patients

Beverages
  Alcohol
  Caffeine, excess or withdrawal
Foods
  Chocolate
  Dairy products
  Citrus fruits
  Onions
  Beans
  Nuts
  Fatty foods
Chemical agents/food additives
  Monosodium glutamate (taste enhancer added to many canned soups and processed foods
      such as Chinese, frozen dinners, sauces, and salad dressings)
  Artificial sweeteners (Nutrasweet, Equal)
  Sodium nitrite (preservative in hot dogs and lunch meats)
  Tyramine (found in cheeses, dried fish, wine, fatty food, yogurt, and yeasts)
Hormonal (hormonal changes may have variable effects)
  Related to the menstrual cycle, pregnancy, or menopause
  Oral contraceptives
  Drugs/toxins
  Many prescription medications
  Overuse of analgesic medication
  Nitroglycerine
  Histamine
Environmental/sensory stimuli
  Bright or flickering lights
  Eye strain
  Loud noises
  Strong odors
  Changes in altitude, humidity, air quality, and weather
Lifestyle/stresses
  Sleep cycle changes: too much or too little sleep
  Stress: anger, frustration, chronic worries, deadlines, and tests
  Letdown periods after exertion or effort
  Overexertion/overheating or excessive fatigue
  Smoking
  Irregular eating, missing meals
  Family strife

2007). In contrast to primary headaches, which occur over years or decades, many secondary headaches occur only once or only during an active illness, such as meningitis.

5. A particularly ominous secondary headache, the "thunderclap" headache, comes on abruptly. The patient usually describes it as "the most severe pain I have ever felt." This headache suggests subarachnoid hemorrhage and prompts questioning for risk factors, such as hypertension

or cocaine use, and neuroradiologic imaging to document intracranial bleeding. About 80% of the time angiography discloses a ruptured intracranial aneurysm (Dodick, 2002;), but the history alone cannot distinguish between bleeding and so-called benign thunderclap headache (Linn et al., 1998). Neuroradiologic imaging is required.

6. For chronic or recurrent headaches, the diagnosis depends on whether the patient's history corresponds to one of the well-categorized, common types of headaches, such as migraine, tension-type, or cluster (Table 6–11), or matches one of the rarer types (Diamond, 1990; Dodick, 2006; Olesen et al., 2006; Silberstein et al., 2001).

7. *Migraine* is an episodic, usually familial, disorder characterized by headaches as well as gastrointestinal, mental, and neurologic dysfunctions. The diagnosis depends entirely on the history. The symptoms follow a pattern of pre-ictal, ictal, and post-ictal stages (Table 6–5). Some patients have definable triggers (Table 6–10). Many patients can predict a migraine attack by a prodromal change in mood or affect. Prophylactic medication for the attack is most effective if taken early, during the aura, before the pain has reached a maximum. Migraine occurs without aura (common migraine) or with aura (classical migraine). The aura may last up to an hour or more and consist of personality changes, particularly irritability, focal neurologic signs, or visual disturbances. During an attack, focal signs may include transient hemiplegia, ophthalmoplegia, hemiparesthesia, hemianopsia, or aphasia and often have a traveling or crawling evolution. Nausea and vomiting are common. Visual changes include photophobia, flashing lights, and various scotomas that may have a fortification (zigzag pattern) or horseshoe shape. After asking an open question—"Do you have any changes in your vision with the headaches?"—you may need to ask about the specific visual changes just listed, being careful not to suggest that the patient must have any of them. Because of photophobia, phonophobia, and incapacitating pain, the patient must retire to a quiet, dark room. Sleep usually ameliorates the symptoms, but the patient feels "drained out" during the post-ictal phase. The pain, frequently throbbing, often causes the patient to cry, particularly children. Most

Table 6–11. Historical Features for the Differential Diagnosis of Some Common Primary Headaches

	Migraine	Tension-Type Headache	Cluster Headache	Chronic Daily Headache
Age at onset	2–30 years	Teens and adults	20–40 years	3rd–4th decades
Pain character	Incapacitating, pulsating, unilateral or bilateral	Moderate, aching, tight, band-like	Severe, boring	Variable, often severe
Pain location	Uni- or bilateral; may shift, tends to be frontal	Front, front-to-back, or generalized	Unilateral, periorbital; frontotemporal	Generalized
Pain frequency	Variable: daily/weekly/monthly intervals; may be related to menstrual periods	Rare to daily	Clusters for days to months, then periodic remissions	Nearly constant, daily
Pain duration	Usually 3–24 hours; peaks in minutes to hours	Hours to days	Rapid onset, lasts 30–90 minutes	Constant
Time of onset	Anytime, usually daytime	Builds during day	Onset at same time of day or night, awakens	Usually present on awakening
Nighttime onset	Sometimes	Rare	Very frequent	
Sex	F>M	F>M	M>F	F>M
Family Hx	Common	Common	Rare	Variable
Associated findings	An aura, focal neurologic signs, nausea, vomiting, photo- and phonophobia; must retire; exercise worsens pain	No aura; no systemic symptoms, neurologic signs, or dysautonomia; nausea infrequent	Dysautonomia: ipsilateral tearing, rhinorrhea, sweating, miosis, ptosis, conjunctival injection; paces floor	Often evolves from migraine or other periodic tension-type headache; no aura

migraineurs have one or more close relatives with migraine. The pedigree usually suggests an autosomal dominant pattern (see the analyses of headache patients in Chapter 13, section V, C).

8. Chronic daily headaches may represent transformed migraine (Silberstein et al., 1996, 2001), drug rebound (Dodick, 2006; Moore and Shevell, 2004), or tension-type headaches or may not clearly have a definable precursor.

9. Sinus headache may occur for days at a time, but the patient generally may have little or mild headache upon awakening. The headache tends to be localized to the affected frontal or maxillary sinus. The headache builds from a dull ache to a peak of pounding pain as the morning advances and recedes again by evening. Exercise or straining, as in the Valsalva maneuver, increases headaches due to sinusitis or other intracranial infections. The sinusitis patient frequently has a yellow nasal discharge, has fever, and feels systemically ill. Sinus infections are most common in the patient who suffers from nasal allergies, often seasonal, that result in swelling of the nasal mucosa and block sinus drainage.

10. The physician has to be patient in eliciting the headache history from children because they usually do not articulate or describe the pain readily (Abu-Arafeh, 2002; Guidetti et al., 2002; Winner and Rothner, 2001). Headaches, presumptively migraine, may start as early as the first year of life (Barlow, 1994) and not uncommonly by the age of 5 years.

D. Separation of psychogenic (functional) pain from organic headaches

1. No absolute rule separates putatively psychogenic headaches from organic headaches. However, most organic headaches or organic pain syndromes show some rhyme and reason, with discernible patterns of evolution, varying intensity in relation to time of day and activities, and varying frequency.

2. Some psychogenic headaches follow one of two extremes, constant or completely *random*.

   a. At one extreme is absolutely constant pain, day after day, week after week, and month after month, with little or no variation or relation to daily contingencies, particularly if the patient describes the pain in hyperbole or, conversely, with a soft voice and wan, automatic smile.

Unfortunately, intermittent, seemingly organic headaches may evolve into chronic daily headaches (Dodick, 2006, Moore and Shevell, 2004; Silberstein, et al., 1996).

b. At the other extreme are recurrent daily headaches that come on randomly and immediately reach an excruciating, incapacitating peak, with little or no evolution or relation to circumstances.

c. Known organic diseases or organic causes of headache or any pain uncommonly produce the foregoing two patterns.

VIII. **Current Medications and Previous Management**

A. Complete the history of the present illness by reviewing how the patient tries to obtain relief.

1. Ask an open question, "What have you done to get relief?"

2. Then ask specifically about:

a. Maneuvers or actions such as lying down, using cold compresses, and relaxation techniques

b. Nonprescription drugs (over-the-counter and home remedies): analgesics, vitamins, cold remedies, and herbs. At this point, you may choose to ask about psychoactive drugs–alcohol, tobacco, cocaine, heroin, and stimulants (caffeine and amphetamines)—or you may defer these questions until the psychosocial history (see Chapter 9).

B. Ask about treatments by other physicians.

1. Record prescription drugs from other physicians. Ask the patient to sign a release of information form to obtain any previous diagnostic studies and workups.

2. Ask about visits to alternative practitioners. patients may not volunteer this information spontaneously, but about a third do make such visits. patients most likely to do so usually have chronic pain (backache, headache, or arthritis), often mixed with depression, anxiety, and insomnia, and often express dissatisfaction with previous physicians. Some alternative medications have significant adverse effects and pharmacologic interactions with prescription drugs (see Dr. Stephen Barrett's website, http://www.quackwatch.com).

3. End this part of the history by asking the patient to review which medications or treatments seemed to work best and which failed or had adverse effects.

IX. Closing the Present Illness History in Preparation for the Past Clinical History

A. Summarize the chief concern and present illness.
To close the first part of the history and to insure accuracy, summarize the chief concern and present illness: "Alright, let's review what we've been over. You have had bad headaches almost daily for the last three weeks. You feel the pain over the front of your head, particularly when bending over or straightening up. . . ." Continue or correct the narrative as the patient indicates.

B. Indicate the transition to the past history (see Chapter 7).

X. Summary

A. The therapeutic process should begin the moment the patient contacts the physician's office. Set up all office procedures to make the patient feel welcome and to insure confidentiality. Throughout the contact, the physician and office staff should follow the ordinary rules of good manners and etiquette because, by design, these practices communicate respect and concern for the other person's comfort.

B. After greeting and seating the patient and addressing the patient properly by name, the physician indulges in some chitchat about neutral topics to create a break-in period for the patient and the physician to get comfortable with each other. Then, the physician elicits the reason for the visit by asking a neutral, open question: "What did you come to see me about?" Most patients can articulate a clear reason or "chief concern" for coming. Other patients have an unvoiced or unrecognized agenda that they conceal because of timidity or embarrassment or that they fail to recognize themselves. Sometimes disclosure of the real reason for coming requires a prolonged history. For these reasons, the patient should not have to state to anyone but the physician the chief concern or reason for coming.

C. The physician starts to analyze each symptom or concern by asking open questions. Open questions give the patient freedom to answer as little or as much as she or he can at that moment. Open questions encourage patients to describe their symptoms in their own words, free from any programming, preconceptions, or prejudices imposed by the physician. The physician listens without interruption or redirection.

D. After the patient's response to the open question stops, the physician asks a series of *what, when, where, how much,* and *how long* questions to fully characterize each symptom of the present illness (Table 6–3). When appropriate, the physician uses the patient's vocabulary and descriptions in talking about symptoms and asking questions about them.

E. Above all the physician reacts nonjudgmentally and professionally to the patient's revelations. The physician receives all disclosures "without tumult," criticism, or condemnation.

F. The physician elicits the temporal profile of the illness, whether acute, chronic, exacerbating and remitting, or recurrent attacks with symptom-free intervals. In analyzing recurrent attacks, the physician follows a catechism that seeks to disclose any triggering or alleviating factors, the sequence or evolution of symptoms, and the recovery phase from the attacks (Tables 6–5 and 6–7). Tables subdividing common disorders such as headache, epilepsy, and syncope aid the physician in remembering the range of manifestations and the kinds of questions to ask (Tables 6–6 to 6–11).

G. The physician asks about past efforts to treat or diagnose the present illness to find out what has worked and what has failed.

H. The physician closes the history of the present illness by summarizing it for the patient to check its accuracy.

I. Some eternal truths or cosmic laws emerge about the clinical history:

1. Believe the patient's history, unless clear evidence contradicts it.

2. The history often screams out the diagnosis, if the physician simply listens to the symptoms and remains curious as to their meaning and possible explanations, rather than dismissing, ridiculing, or denying them (Carson et al., 2000).

3. The more the patients talks and the less the physician talks, the better the history.

References

Abu-Arafeh I, ed. Childhood Headache. London: MacKeith Press, 2002.

Baker LH, O'Connell D, Platt FW. "What else?" Setting the agenda for the clinical interview. Ann Intern Med 2005;143:766–770.

Barlow CF. Migraine in the infant and toddler. J Child Neurol 1994;9: 92–94.

Barr R. Folk nosology: when textbook medicine isn't good enough. Hosp Phys 1971;6:28–55.

Barsky AJ. Hidden reasons some patients visit doctors. Ann Intern Med 1981;94(part I):492–498.

Beecher HK. The Measurement of Subjective Responses: Quantitative Effects of Drugs. New York: Oxford University Press, 1959.

Benbassat J, Baumal R. What is empathy and how can it be promoted during clinical clerkships? Acad Med 2004;79:832–839.

Bluestone NR. Identifying data. Pharos 1996(winter);59:20–23.

Bowman ES. The differential diagnosis of epilepsy, pseudoseizures, dissociative identity disorder and dissociative identity disorder unspecified. Bull Menninger Clin 2000;64:164–180.

Brazis PW, Masdeau JC, Biller J. Localization in Clinical Neurology, 5th ed. Philadelphia: Lippincott Williams & Wilkins, 2007.

Brewster A. A student's view of a medical teaching exercise. N Engl J Med 1993;329:1971–1972.

Carson AJ, Ringbauer B, Stone J, et al. Do medically unexplained symptoms matter? A prospective cohort study of 300 new referrals to a neurology outpatient clinic. J Neurol Neurosurg Psychiatry 2000;68:207–210.

Commission on Classification and Terminology of the International League Against Epilepsy. Proposal for revised clinical and electroencephalographic classification of epileptic seizures. Epilepsia 1981:4(4): 489–501.

Cooper LA, Beach MC, Johnson RL, Inui TS. Delving below the surface. Understanding how race and ethnicity influence relationships in health care. J Gen Intern Med 2006;21(Suppl 1):S21–S27.

DeMyer WE. Technique of the Neurologic Examination, 5th ed. New York: McGraw-Hill, 2004.

DeMyer WE. Breath-holding spells. In: Maria BL (ed), Current Management in Child Neurology. Hamilton: BC Decker, 2005, pp 353-355.

Diamond S, ed. Migraine Headache: Prevention and Management, 3rd ed. New York: Marcel Dekker, 1990.

Dodick D. Thunderclap headache. J Neurol Neurosurg Psychiatry 2002;72: 6–11.

Dodick DW. Chronic daily headache. N Engl J Med 2006;354:158–165.

Donnelly WJ. View point: patient-centered medical care requires a patient-centered medical record. Acad Med 2005;80:33–38.

Forsyth PA, Posner JB. Headaches in patients with brain tumors. Neurology 1993;43:1678–1682.

Frothingham TW. The chief complaint. N Engl J Med 1982;307:194.

Garcia RS. The misuse of race in medical diagnosis. Pediatrics 2004;113: 1394–1395.

Grubb BP. Neurocardiogenic syncope. N Engl J Med 2005;352:1004–1010.

Guidetti V, Russell G, Sillänpää M, et al. Headache and Migraine in Childhood and Adolescence. London: Martin Dunitz, 2002.

Hamberg K, Risberg G, Johansen EE. Male and female physicians show different patterns of gender bias: a paper-case study of irritable bowel syndrome. Scand J Public Health 2004;32:144–152.

Hawthorne N. The Scarlet Letter. New York: C. Scribner's sons, 1919, p 126.

Headache Classification Subcommittee. The international classification of headache disorders, 2nd edition. [Guideline] Cephalalgia. 2004: 24 (Suppl 1):16–22.

Hoover EL. There is no scientific rationale for race-based research. J Natl Med Assoc 2007;99:690–692.

Hughes, Langston. Let America be America Again in The Collected Poems of Langston Hughes, edited by Rampersad A, Roessel D. New York: Knopf: Distributed by Random House, 1994, p 189.

Jacobsen GP, Ramadan MN, Aggarwal SK, et al. The Henry Ford Hospital headache disability inventory (HDI). Neurology 1994;44:837–842.

Juckett G. Cross cultural medicine. Am Fam Phys 2005;72:2267–2274.

Landers A. Indianapolis Star, April 4, 1979 (with permission of Esther P. Lederer Trust and Creators Syndicate, Inc.).

Kelly, EC. The Genuine Works of Hippocrates. Translated by Francis Adams. Whitefish, MT: Kessinger Publishing, 2006, p 94.

Lim RF. Clinical Manuel of Cultural Psychiatry. Washington DC: American Psychiatric Publishing, 2006.

Linn FHH, Rinkel GJE, Algra A, et al. Headache characteristics in sub-arachnoid hemorrhage and benign thunderclap headache. J Neurol Neurosurg Psychiatry 1998;65:791–793.

Low PA, Opfer-Gehrking TL, McPhee BR, et al. Prospective evaluation of clinical characteristics of orthostatic hypotension. Mayo Clin Proc 1995;70:617–622.

Makadon HJ. Improving health care for the lesbian and gay communities. N Engl J Med 2006;354:895–897.

Miller TH, Kruse JE. Evaluation of syncope. Am Fam Phys 2005;72: 1492–1500.

Moore AJ, Shevell M. Chronic daily headaches in pediatric neurology practice. J Child Neurol 2004;19:925–929.

Moss AJ. Long QT syndrome. JAMA 2003;289:2041–2044.

Olesen J, Goadsby PJ, Ramadan N, et al. The Headaches, 3rd ed. Baltimore: Lippincott Williams and Wilkins, 2006.

Ottoman R, Lee JH, Hauser WA, et al. Reliability of seizure classification using a semistructured interview. Neurology 1993;43:2526–2530.

Patel H, Scott E, Dunn D, Garg B. Nonepileptic seizures in children. Epilepsia 2007;48:2086–2092.

Piasecki M. Clinical Communication Handbook. Malden, MA: Blackwell, 2003.

Pograis L Jr, Pellegrino ED. African American Bioethics: Culture, Race and Poverty. Washington DC: Georgetown University Press, 2007.

Risch N. Dissecting racial and ethnic differences. N Engl J Med 2006;354: 408–411.

Roden DM. Long-QT interval syndrome. N Engl J Med 2008;358: 169–176.

Rudolph CD. Gastroenterology and nutrition. In: Rudolph CD, Rudolph AM (eds), Rudolph's Pediatrics, 21st ed. New York: McGraw-Hill, 2003, pp 1305–1468.

Roberts, W. Memoirs of the Life and Correspondence of Mrs Hannah More. New York: Harper & Brothers, 1841, p 317.

Shannon JB, ed. Ethnic Diseases Sourcebook. Detroit: Omnigraphics, 2001.

Silberstein SD, Lipton RB, Sliwinski M. Classification of daily and near-daily headaches: field trial of revised IHS criteria. Neurology 1996;47: 871–875.

Silberstein SD, Lipton RB, Dalessio DJ. Wolff's Headache and Other Head Pain. New York: Oxford University Press, 2001.

Silbert PL, Edis RH, Stewart-Wynne EG, et al. Benign sexual headache and exertional headache: interrelationship and long term prognosis. J Neurol Neurosurg Psychiatry 1991;54:417–421.

Simmons T. The Unseen Shore. Boston: Beacon Press, 1991.

Streeten DH. Variations in the clinical manifestations of orthostatic hypotension. Mayo Clin Proc 1995;70:713–714.

Sullivan F, Wyatt JC. Why is this patient here today? BMJ 2005;331: 678–680.

Takemura Y, Sakurai Y, Yokoya S, et al. Open-ended questions: are they really beneficial for gathering medical information from patients? Tohoku J Exp Med 2005;206:151–154.

Tauber AI. Patient Autonomy and the Ethics of Responsibility. Cambridge, MA: MIT Press, 2005, p 62.

Thomas L. House calls. In: Reynolds R, Stone J (eds), On Doctoring: Stories, Poems, Essays. New York: Simon & Schuster, 1991, pp 203–214.

Von Korff M, Stewart WF, Lipton RB. Assessing headache severity: new directions. Neurology 1994;44(Suppl 4):S40–S46.

Wiener SL. Differential Diagnosis of Acute Pain. New York: McGraw-Hill, 1993.

Winner P, Rothner AD. Headache in Children and Adolescents. Hamilton: BC Decker, 2001.

The Past Clinical History and the Review of Systems

7

I. **Eliciting the Past Clinical History**

A. Definition: The *past clinical history* includes illnesses, injuries, hospitalizations, workups, and treatments prior to the onset of the present illness.

B. The open, transitional question
Upon completing the history of the present illness and summarizing it, the physician signals the switch to the past clinical history by an open question: "I understand about your health at present. Let's see about your health in the past. Have you had any serious illnesses or hospitalizations?"

C. The closed questions: After the response to the open question ends, ask specifically about the following:

1. Usual and unusual childhood illnesses

2. Previous adult illnesses

3. Hospitalizations or operations. Arrange to get the results of previous medical workups, examinations, and laboratory tests.

4. Serious accidents or injuries

5. Any intolerances, allergies, or adverse reactions to past medications

6. Foreign travel and military service. Foreign travel raises a different spectrum of diseases, particularly parasitic diseases.

7. Occupational and environmental history. The workplace and environment may expose the patient to a large number of toxins and physical hazards (Newman, 1995). Some diseases may have a long latency between exposure and clinical expression. Especially consider an occupational or environmental disease if the patient's clinical condition does not fit a conventional diagnosis.

D. Pregnancy and developmental history
While unnecessary for most adults, a detailed pregnancy and developmental history is crucial for the diagnosis and management of infants and children (see Chapter 10).

II. The Review of Systems (ROS)

A. Definition: The *ROS* consists of a series of questions designed to disclose any additional symptoms referable to specific organ systems but not reviewed in the chief concern, present illness, and past clinical history.

B. The transition statement to the ROS
Signify the transition to the ROS by stating "I am going to ask you a series of questions about your health." For the rare reluctant patient who seems hesitant or worried about further questions, state that you routinely ask every patient these questions. The systems for review are as follows:

1. Nervous system
2. Musculoskeletal system
3. Hematopoietic system
4. Respiratory system
5. Cardiovascular system
6. Gastrointestinal system
7. Genitourinary system
8. Endocrine system
9. Immune and lymphatic system
10. Skin

C. As a mnemonic, mentally dissect out the patient's organ systems and body parts and proceed through them in rostrocaudal order

1. Without an orderly approach you will inevitably omit some important questions. One fail-proof approach is to mentally dissect out each organ system, visualize its anatomic parts and their functions in rostrocaudal order, and ask the questions that each part evokes (Fig. 7–1). Note: For the ROS in this text, I state only the open question for the organ system or part of the body. I then list the technical terms for the specific dysfunctions that you should ask about. Even though I use technical terms in the text for clarity and precision of communication, always substitute vernacular terms when questioning the patient. Do not ask "Do you have dysuria?" but "Do you have trouble emptying your bladder?"

2. In reviewing systems, you generally should ask about dysfunctions rather than using an "organ recital" approach. Ask "How is your appetite and digestion?" not "How is

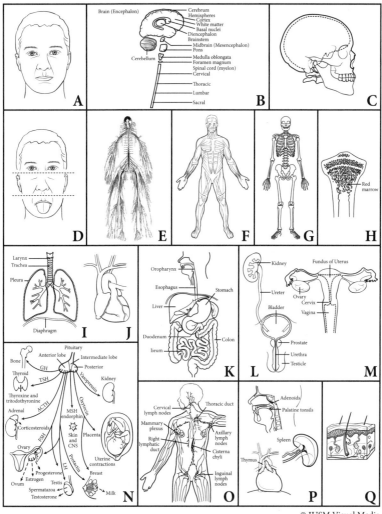

© IUSM Visual Media

Figure 7–1. Montage summarizing the rostrocaudal mental anatomic dissection method for remembering how to do the review of systems (ROS). *A* Commence the ROS by visualizing the head and ask about headaches. *B* Visualization of the components of the central nervous system. *C* Visualization of the skull cavities that can be infected and act as the source of headache and head pain, as seen in a lateral radiograph of the skull. *D* Visualization of the organs of special sense: eyes, ears, nose, and mouth. *E* Visualization of the peripheral nervous system, as dissected free from the body. (Reproduced courtesy of Dr. P. Amenta, Hahnemann University School of Medicine, Philadelphia, Pennsylvania.) *F* Visualization of the muscular system. *G* Visualization of the skeletal system. *H* Visualization of the hematopoietic system, the bone marrow and spleen. *I* Visualization of the respiratory system. *J* Visualization of the cardiovascular system. *K* Visualization of the gastrointestinal system. *L* Visualization of the renal and male genitourinary system. *M* Visualization of the female genitourinary system. *N* Visualization of the endocrine system. *O* Visualization of the lymphatic system. *P* Visualization of the remaining lymphatic and hematopoietic systems. *Q* Visualization of the skin.

your stomach?" or "Do you have any problems with bowel movements?" not "How is your colon working?"

3. In analyzing symptoms that arise from visceral disease, recall the most likely causes: inflammation, obstruction, perforation, bleeding, infarction, and neoplasm.

D. Start each part of the ROS with an open question.

1. Depending on the patient's state of health, intelligence, and medical knowledge, a single open question about each function or organ may suffice. For example, "Do you have any problems with your vision?" Depending on the patient's responses and the diseases suspected, you then introduce explicit questions, as detailed in section III.

2. To best analyze each positive response or symptom, use the symptom catechisms and techniques already described in Chapter 6.

III. The Head and the Nervous System

A. Preliminary observations on the neurologic and mental status during the history and the ROS

1. Certain observations, made almost automatically about the patient's nervous system and mental status during the regular history and ROS, save the experienced physician much time. For this reason, I often defer formal questioning about the mental status until the end of the ROS or even after the neurologic examination. From this information, you can best decide whether detailed questioning about the mental status is needed. Chapter 9 reviews the questions for the mental status history and how to weave them into the regular history and ROS.

2. In the first place, you will have learned about the patient's spontaneous behavior at a time the patient does not realize that observations are being made. The spontaneous behavior of the patient may differ from that seen during the formal examination.

3. Inspect the patient's face for dysmorphic features, emotional expression, and asymmetry of facial movements.

4. Inspect the patient's eyes for drooping of the eyelids, ocular misalignment, and the range of ocular movements.

5. Appraise how the patient swallows, breathes, sits, stands, and walks and look for tremors or other involuntary movements.

6. Appraise speech articulation, prosody, and word selection.

7. If the patient has no neurologic symptoms and thinks, talks, sits, stands, walks, sees, hears, and feels normally—that is, has no symptoms or signs of mental, motor, or sensory dysfunction—then in all probability, the patient does not have significant neurologic disease. A brief screening neurologic exam will suffice (DeMyer, 2004). If the history has disclosed mental, motor, or sensory dysfunction, this preliminary neurologic information will help to determine what to emphasize on the neurologic examination and how extensive it should be. The better the history and ROS, the shorter and more productive the physical examination.

B. First, visualize the patient's head and ask about sensory symptoms, starting with headaches (Fig. 7–1A).

1. To review the nervous system, recall its three functions—mental, motor, and sensory (see Fig. 2–1)—and start with the head and its sensory dysfunctions.

2. Open question: "Do you have headaches?" If the patient answers "Yes," analyze the pain as described in Chapter 6.

3. If the history suggests secondary headaches, start at the surface of the head and think through the anatomic sites where lesions may cause headaches: the scalp, skull, eyes, ears, meninges, and the brain and its ventricles and blood vessels (Fig. 7–1B, C).

   a. Scalp: temporal arteritis and various types of noninflammatory vascular headaches.

   b. Skull:

   (1) Bone tumors, primary or metastatic

   (2) Visualize the skull cavities—the frontal, maxillary, ethmoid and sphenoid sinuses and mastoids—and ask about pain in these regions (Fig. 7–1C).

   (3) Ask about skull fractures and previous head injuries.

   (4) Pain in the teeth and gums

   (5) Temporomandibular joint pain (pain when chewing)

   c. Meninges: subdural and epidural hematomas and meningitis

   d. Brain: encephalitis, vasculitis, intra- and extra-axial tumors, idiopathic intracranial hypertension, vascular malformations, intracranial bleeding

   e. Ventricles, obstructive hydrocephalus

C. Loss of consciousness

Ask directly about any previous episodes of loss of consciousness: head injury, fainting or blackout spells, epileptic seizures, meningitis, or encephalitis. Although you may elect to do a full mental status examination at this point, usually it is better to investigate the mental status near the end of the ROS when you will have a better idea of what and how to do it (see Chapter 9).

D. Next, visualize each special sense.

1. After asking about headache or other head pains, ask about each special sense. Mentally dissect out the special sensory organs of the head by visualizing the face into transverse planes that separate the eyes, ears, nose, and mouth (Fig. 7–1D).

2. If the patient responds positively to an open question about a part, such as "Do you have any trouble with your vision?" ask for a description. Then add closed questions:

   a. "Do you wear glasses?"

   b. "Do you have eye pain?" Consider photophobia, glaucoma, temporal arteritis, and iritis.

   c. "Do you have dimness or blurring of vision?"

   d. "Can you read newsprint?"

   e. "Do you have double vision?"

   f. "Do you have trouble seeing at night?"

   g. "Do you see spots before your eyes?"

   h. Finally, for selected patients who may be mentally ill, you may ask, "Do you see unusual images or visions?" or "Do you see visions or images that other people do not see?"

   i. If the patient has a visual symptom, ask whether it affects one or both eyes or follows a quadranopic or hemianopic pattern.

3. Then, visualize the middle transverse plane and nose and ask about smell and taste. Ask about nasal discharge and nosebleeds.

4. Then, in the same middle transverse plane, visualize the ears and nerve VIII with its auditory and vestibular divisions (Fig. 7–1D).

   a. Ask about earaches and discharge from the ear.

   b. Auditory screening:

      (1) "How is your hearing?"

      (2) "Do you experience buzzing, popping, or ringing in your ears?"

(3) "Do you have trouble locating the source of sounds?"

(4) As with vision, you may need to ask selected patients about auditory hallucinations: "Do you hear voices when no one is present?"

   c. Vestibular screening:

(1) "Do you feel dizzy, like being on a merry-go-round?"

(2) "Do you feel unsteady when you are walking?"

(3) "Do you feel unsteady or dizzy when you change position, stand up, or turn over?"

5. Visualize the third or lower transverse plane of Figure 7–1D and ask about taste. Lack of smell (*anosmia*) and lack of taste (*dysgeusia*) often run together.

6. Alternatively, you can run through the cranial nerves for the special senses in serial order: I, smell; II, vision; VII, taste; and VIII, hearing and equilibrium.

7. If the history suggests neurologic disease, think through the levels of the brainstem, the midbrain, pons, and medulla (Fig. 7–1B), and ask about sensory and motor dysfunctions characteristic of each level (DeMyer, 2004). For the localization or exclusion of a neurologic lesion, you need to know what functions the disease has spared, as well as those affected.

  E. General somatic sensation

After finishing the inquiries for the special senses, visualize the trigeminal nerve, spinal cord, nerve roots, plexuses, and peripheral nerves in rostrocaudal order (Fig. 7–1E). For the open question, ask "Do you have numbness, tingling, or pain in the face, arms, or legs?"

IV. Visualize the Muscular System (Fig. 7–1F)

  A. Start by visualizing facial and oropharyngeal movements

1. Open question: "Do you have any trouble with face movements, speaking chewing, or swallowing?"

2. Then ask directly about the following:

   a. Involuntary facial movements, particularly eyelid twitching (*blepharospasm*) or drooping of eyelids (*ptosis*)

   b. Vocal or oropharyngeal tics

   c. Facial weakness or paralysis

3. Then, although often evident during the history, ask directly about the five *dys's*.

       a. *Dysphonia*: hoarseness or difficulty producing the voice

       b. *Dysarthria*: poor articulation or pronunciation of words

       c. *Dysphagia*: gagging or difficulty swallowing

       d. *Dysprosody*: stuttering, pauses, and hesitations or poor inflections or intonation

       e. *Dysphasia*: difficulty finding and expressing the right words

B. Next, visualize the muscles of the limbs and trunk (Fig. 7–1F)

    1. Open question: "Do you have trouble with your muscles or movements?"

    2. Then ask directly about the following:

       a. Stumbling or falling

       b. Weakness, fatigability, or endurance. If the patient reports weakness, determine its distribution: unilateral, bilateral, symmetrical, asymmetrical, and proximal or distal.

       c. Involuntary movements, tremors, or twitching of muscles (fasciculations or myoclonic jerks)

       d. Cramps, stiffness, or exercise intolerance

       e. Ask whether an elderly patient can climb stairs and get up from a chair or whether a child can run normally and hop, skip, and jump.

V. Next, Visualize the Skeletal System (Fig. 7–1G)

A. Open question: "Do you have any problems with your bones or joints?"

B. Then ask directly about the following:

    1. Pain in the neck and back

    2. Pain, redness, swelling, or stiffness in the joints of the shoulders, arms, fingers, hips, knees, and feet. Notice how you apply anatomic principles by starting rostrally and proximally at the neck and vertebral column and then systematically working caudally and distally from the hip and shoulder girdles to the digits of the hands and feet.

    3. Bone pain

    4. Fractures, sprains, and dislocations

VI. Next, Visualize the Bone Marrow (Fig. 7–1H)

A. Open question: "Have you had any blood disorders or abnormal bleeding?"

B. Then ask directly about the following:
1. Anemia or pallor
2. Unusual bruising or bleeding from nose, gums, or rectum
3. Unexplained fever and malaise
4. Blood transfusions or receipt of other blood products such as platelets or γ-globulin
5. You may choose to ask about the lymphoid system now or later (Fig. 7–1O, P).

VII. **Next, Visualize the Chest and Its Contents and Start with the Respiratory System (Fig. 7–1I, J)**
A. Open question: "Do you have problems breathing?"
B. Then ask directly about the following:
1. Chest pain (see next section on the cardiovascular system)
2. Shortness of breath (*dyspnea*), hyperventilation, wheezing. Find out whether the dyspneic patient has asthma, exertional dyspnea, or orthopnea.
3. Snoring or sleep apnea
4. Cough and sputum production and character—thin/thick, copious/scanty, clear/purulent, rusty, or frankly bloody (*hemoptysis*)
5. Smoking
6. If the patient has respiratory symptoms, ask about exposure to allergens, tuberculosis, birds (psittacosis), and previous respiratory infections

VIII. **Next, Visualize the Cardiovascular System (see Fig. 7–1J)**
A. Open question: "Do you have any heart problems?"
B. Then ask directly about the following:
1. Chest pain (angina pectoris) or pleuritic (a sharp catch of pain on attempting to breathe) retrosternal pain, left arm pain
   a. Spontaneous pain
   b. Exertional pain (angina pectoris)
   c. Feelings of tightness or aching in chest or upper abdomen
   d. Deep chest pain arises in several intrathoracic structures, the heart, lungs, and esophagus, innervated by thoracic dermatomes 1–6, so-called 6-dermatomal pain (Castell, 1992), that includes

myocardial ischemia, esophageal irritation/rupture, pericarditis, pulmonary embolism/infarction, pneumothorax, dissecting aortic aneurysm, subphrenic disease, and hiatal hernia. Table 7–1 contrasts the history to distinguish anginal pain from heartburn or gastroesophageal reflux disease (GERD), two fairly common conditions.

   e. Just as in adults, GERD in infants may cause irritability, anorexia, aspiration, and wheezing.

2. Blood pressure: hypertension or hypotension
3. Palpitations, cardiac arrhythmias (pulse irregularities), and any accompanying symptoms of dizziness, anxiety, nausea, sweating, and fear of dying. Ask about any triggering events such as caffeine ingestion or exercise.
   a. Tachycardias (tachyarrhythmias: supraventricular, atrial fibrillation, atrial flutter, infraventricular)
   b. Bradycardias (bradyarrhythmias) and asystole
4. Cyanosis, blanching or redness of face or extremities (Raynaud phenomenon)
5. Varicosities
6. Intermittent claudication
7. Swelling of feet (pedal edema)
8. Congestive heart failure syndrome: fatigue, cough, shortness of breath, orthopnea, palpitations, anorexia, and nocturia. Physical signs that complete the diagnosis are jugular vein distension, hepatosplenomegaly, and pedal edema.

Table 7–1. Differences in Angina Pectoris and Heartburn, Disclosed by the History

Characteristic	Angina Pectoris	Heartburn
Trigger factors	Exercise but sometimes when reclining, feeling emotion, and eating	After eating or when reclining
Quality of pain	Feeling of tightness or pressure; accompanied by fear, apprehension, nausea, and perspiration	Burning in the chest and often regurgitation of gastric contents into the throat
Localization	Radiates to the jaw, left shoulder or arm, and sometimes the back	In the middle of the chest
Duration	1–10 minutes	Longer
Drug response	Responds to nitroglycerine but not antacids	Responds to antacids or maybe to nitroglycerine

IX. **Next, Visualize the Gastrointestinal System (Fig. 7–1K)**
   A. Open questions: "How is your appetite? Do you have any problems with your stomach, digestion, or bowel movements?" Ask the patient to describe eating habits (bulimia or anorexia, weight/diet/food intolerances).
   B. Then ask directly about the following:
      1. If not asked previously, ask about chewing and swallowing and continue through the gastrointestinal tract in rostrocaudal order, starting at the mouth.
      2. Heartburn, abdominal discomfort, pain, and relation to meals. In the analysis of acute abdominal pain in the emergency room patient, the history and physical, augmented by nonenhanced computed tomography, had a sensitivity of 92% and a specificity of 90% for the cause (Gerhardt et al., 2005).
      3. Nausea and vomiting of food (projectile or moderate, spontaneous or induced by eating), blood (hematemesis), or bile. Large bowel obstruction can cause vomiting of feces.
      4. Gas, belching, and flatus
      5. Previous liver disease: hepatitis, liver failure, or jaundice
      6. Bowel habits: "Do you have any trouble with bowel movements?"
         a. Changes in bowel habits, frequency of stools, straining, constipation, diarrhea, or fecal incontinence
         b. Character of bowel movements: volume, consistency, mucus, rectal bleeding, and stool color (pallid, clay-colored, or black, "tarry" stools). If the stools are dark or black, ask about ingestion of iron, bismuth, licorice, or charcoal; otherwise, suspect blood.
         c. Enemas, laxatives, or antacids
         d. Rectal pain, bleeding, piles, or itching (pruritis ani)

X. **Next, Visualize the Renal System (Fig. 7–1L, M)**
   A. Open question: "Do you have any problems urinating?"
   B. Then ask directly about the following:
      1. Incontinence and dribbling
      2. Bed-wetting
      3. Inability to start and stop the stream
      4. Frequency and amount of urination (polyuria is more than 2500 ml/day and oliguria is less than 500 ml/day)

   5. Dysuria, burning on urination
   6. Ability to feel full bladder
   7. Urine color, clear or cloudy, pus or blood in the urine. Dark urine may signify concentration or myoglobinuria, hemoglobinuria, porphyria, drugs, or dietary intake.
   8. Flank pain
   9. Previous episodes of cystitis or nephritis, kidney failure, or uremia
  10. Urinary odor

XI. Next, Visualize the Reproductive System (Figs. 7–1L, M)
  A. When to take the sexual history
   1. One appropriate time arises in the ROS because you arrive at the reproductive system in the natural rostrocaudal progression of questions. A second appropriate time arises during the psychosocial history, in asking about marital adjustment and interpersonal relationships. If you tend to take copious notes, lay your pen aside during the sexual history.
   2. Some timid physicians may omit this part of the history or try to complete it during the physical examination. With the woman racked up in stirrups for the pelvic examination or the man or woman in a flimsy robe in front of you, these are the times that try patients' souls, not for probing sexuality. The patient feels too exposed and too vulnerable. Moreover, you must focus full attention on the technique and findings of the physical examination and not meander off into the history. Wait until the patient has redressed and regrouped if you need to extend the sexual history.
   3. In discussing sexuality, avoid technical terms like "mons," "perineum," "cervix," or "glans" but also avoid slang or vulgarities. Acceptable terms include "penis," "vagina," "intercourse," "orgasm," "climax," "foreplay," "masturbation," and "sexually transmitted diseases" ("STDs"). Encourage the patient to ask for clarification of any terms misunderstood. Use the same tone of voice as for any other part of the history. Many physicians will have to overcome personal embarrassment to question teenaged patients or patients of the opposite sex. Avoid jokes or double entendres. For details of a complete sexual

history, see Jones and Barton (2004), Pomeroy (1982), and Ross et al. (2000).

B. Open question: "Do you have any questions or worries about sex or reproduction?"

C. Questions for both males and females
  1. Sexually active? Marital status/cohabitation, single or multiple partners?
  2. Satisfactions or dissatisfactions of the patient and partner?
  3. Sexual orientation?
  4. Interest in sex, foreplay, arousal, coitus, orgasm?
  5. Masturbation?
  6. Vaginal, oral, or anal sex?
  7. Contraception: rhythm method/condom/hormonal/or surgical (i.e., vasectomy for males or tubal ligation/hysterectomy for females)?
  8. Venereal disease?
      a. Half or more of the new infections with venereal diseases occur in the 15–24 year age range.
      b. Ask about risk factors for STDs. Review the sex of the sex partners, unprotected anal sex, intravenous drug use, and blood transfusion.
      c. Sores on the genitalia: herpes or chancre
      d. If the patient or the patient's partner has multiple partners, suspect particularly gonorrhea, HIV, human papillomavirus, chlamydia, trichomoniasis, and genital herpes.
      e. Chlamydia usually causes symptomatic urethritis in males, but many females lack symptoms.
      f. Immunization against human papillomavirus protects females from cervical cancer.

D. Males only, ask about the following:
  1. Erectile dysfunction and premature ejaculation
  2. Penile discharge or overt sores
  3. Fertility/number of children
  4. Testicular masses

E. Females only, ask about the following:
  1. Breast pain, nipple discharge, lumps, frequency and technique of self-examination, and radiographic screening
  2. Pelvic and genital pain
  3. Vaginal discharge, itching, or infections, particularly yeast and herpes

143

    4. Vaginal dryness/dyspareunia/vaginismus

    5. Douching

    6. Menstruation

      a. Menarche and periods: frequency and quantity of menstrual flow, clots, interperiod bleeding, and discomfort

      b. Cyclic changes such as edema and emotionality

      c. Menopause-related symptoms: irregularity of flow, cessation of flow, hot flashes, fatigability, irritability, and cardiac irregularities. Encourage the patient to discuss her feelings about menopause.

    7. Reproduction: previous pregnancies and outcome, contraception, number of children, and any pregnancy-related or birth-related maternal illnesses. Spontaneous miscarriages or induced abortions. (See sections II and III of Chapter 10 for the complete pregnancy history as related to the health of the fetus.) Kaplan (2006) describes special characteristics of neurologic disease in women.

F. Paraphilias and gender concerns

The foregoing standard questions may provide clues for further investigation of the patient's sexual fantasies or practices.

    1. Child molestation, with patient as victim or pedophile

    2. Incest

    3. Sadomasochism

    4. Fetishism

    5. Transvestitism

    6. Exhibitionism

    7. Voyeurism

    8. Necrophilia

    9. Bestiality

G. Rape

    1. Ask about forced sexual encounters or abuse (Diaz et al., 2004).

    2. Temper the history from a victim of rape with the utmost sensitivity to the patient's anguish.

    3. In interviewing an acute rape victim, utilize a coordinated multidisciplinary team integrated with law enforcement (Hampton, 1995).

XII. Next, Visualize the Endocrine System (Fig. 7–1N)

   A. Open question: "Have you had any glandular or hormonal troubles?"

   B. Then, visualize the endocrine glands in rostrocaudal order, starting with the pituitary and ask about symptoms of hormonal dysfunction

   1. Visualize the adenohypophysis and neurohypophysis and their hormones.

   a. Ask about the onset of puberty. Menstrual and reproductive disorders were covered previously in the ROS.

   b. Observe the patient for dwarfism or gigantism or any abnormalities of fat distribution or of body habitus (adiposogenital dystrophy, acromegaly, etc.)

   c. Ask about excessive thirst (*polydipsia*) and food intake (*polyphagia*) that may indicate diabetes mellitus (pancreatic dysfunction) or diabetes insipidus (neurohypophyseal dysfunction). Appetite disturbances may also include anorexia, hyperphagia, and bingeing.

   d. Ask about hair distribution, hair texture, hair loss, and, for males, the frequency of shaving.

   e. Masculinization/feminization

   2. Heat or cold intolerance (hyper- or hypothyroidism)

   3. Bronzing of skin and salt craving (adrenal insufficiency, Addison disease)

XIII. Next, Visualize the Immune and Lymphatic Systems

   A. Open question: "Do you have allergies, intolerances, or sensitivities?"

   B. Then, ask directly about the following:

   1. Infections

   a. Frequency and type of infections

   b. Infectious disease exposures

   c. Unexplained fevers, chills, and night sweats

   2. Immunizations. Record dates and agents protected against: tetanus, poliomyelitis, diphtheria, rubella, measles, mumps, pertussis, influenza.

   3. Allergies and sensitivities

   a. Sneezing, wheezing, hay fever, and asthma

   b. Hives

      c. Food intolerances
      d. Medication sensitivities
      e. Anaphylactic reactions
        (1) Bee or hornet stings
        (2) Snake venoms
        (3) Insect bites
    4. Enlarged lymphoid tissue
      a. Lymphadenopathy: cervical, axillary, and inguinal
      b. Tonsillitis
      c. Nocturnal snoring: enlarged adenoids and tonsils

XIV. Finally, Visualize the Skin
    A. Open question: "Do you have any skin problems?"
    B. Then, ask directly about the following:
      1. Eruptions, redness, rashes, itching, or wheals
      2. Infections: tinea crura or pedis, folliculitis, or acne
      3. Dryness
      4. Excessive sweating (*hyperhidrosis*) or loss of sweating
        (*anhidrosis*)
      5. Cold-induced acrocyanosis and pain (Raynaud
        phenomenon)
      6. Ulcerations of skin or mucous membranes
      7. Vascular lesions: hemangiomas or spider nevi
      8. Changes in pigmentation: light spots (vitiligo) or
        brown spots (café au lait spots, moles, or freckles).
        Recording the actual diameter of some skin lesions
        provides a baseline for future evaluation.
      9. Warts, growths, or cancer
    10. Sun exposure and tanning
    11. Nails: infections, brittleness
    12. Edema or puffiness of the skin, such as periorbital, or of
        lips, arms, legs, or abdomen
    13. Scars: location, operative or accidental
    14. Tattoos

XV. Environmental/Toxic Exposure History
    A history exploring environmental and toxic exposures is
    especially important when the patient has an otherwise
    puzzling disorder (see Chapter 11). Ask about exposure at
    home or in the workplace to chemicals, such as carbon
    monoxide, lead, arsenic, pesticides, and organic solvents.
    Check on water supply and air pollution. Physical hazards

include radiation, noise, vibration, and other unusual mechanical stresses at work or during hobbies. Ask the patient whether other persons in the same environment or workplace have had similar symptoms. (Access the Agency for Toxic Substances and Disease Registry, www.atsdr.cdc.gov/, to download a detailed form for taking a toxic exposure history.)

XVI. **Supplementing the Standard History and ROS with Inventories, Rating Scales, and Structured Interviews**
    A. Checklists
        Efforts have been made to shorten the history and ROS by checklists, such as the Cornell Medical Inventory or a list of questions to screen for alcoholism (see Table 9–5). Why not just give the patient a checklist that covers everything? A checklist is too mechanical and too impersonal. It does not promote the knowing and trust that the history should produce. Hypochondriacs will check off too many symptoms, while stoics will check off too few. A checklist or computerized form can never substitute for the mutual knowing and trust produced by a face-to-face interview.
    B. Structured interviews and rating scales
        Sometimes the history offers tantalizing clues but leaves the diagnosis in question. Further help may come from a structured interview or rating scale or tests that have a diagnostic scoring system. While generally designed as research protocols, these scales may prove of value in selected patients (Herndon, 2006; Hersen, 2004).

XVII. **Efficiency in the ROS: The Long and Short of It**
    A. The short of it
        1. Given an intelligent, medically knowledgeable, previously healthy patient, you may be tempted to limit the ROS to "Do you have any other health concerns that we should discuss?" But that is not quite enough.
        2. If you curtail the questioning too much or fire questions too rapidly, with obvious intent to save time, you may discourage patients from revealing important symptoms. For a minimum acceptable ROS, ask at least one open question to screen each body system, in essence working sequentially through Figure 7–1.
           a. "Do you have headaches?"
           b. "Do you have any blackout or dizzy spells?"

   c. "Do you have any problems with your vision, hearing, taste, or smell?"

   d. "Do you have any pain, numbness, or tingling in your face, hands, or feet?"

   e. "Do you have any problems speaking or swallowing?"

   f. "Do you have any trouble walking, tremors, or excessive movements?"

   g. "Do you feel weak, fatigued, or worn out?"

   h. "Do you have pain in your neck or back or pain or swelling of your joints?"

   i. "Do you have any trouble breathing, shortness of breath, persistent cough, or chest pain?"

   j. "Have you ever had anything wrong with your heart, pulse rate, or blood pressure? Do you have chest pain on exertion?"

   k. "How is your appetite, digestion, diet, and bowel movement. Is your weight staying the same?"

   l. "Do you have nausea, vomiting, discomfort, or pain in your abdomen?"

   m. "Do you have any trouble with urination or bowel movements? Do you have any incontinence of bowel or bladder or any blood in the urine or stool?"

   n. "Do you have any problems with reproduction, pregnancy, menstruation, or sexuality?"

   o. "Do you have any allergies? Recurrent infections? Are you immunized?"

   p. "Do you have heat or cold intolerance?"

   q. "Do you have any skin problems, itching, or infections?"

   r. Mental status: "How is life going for you in general? Have you been feeling blue or down in the dumps?" Do you have any particular worries or concerns that you want to discuss?" Then do the mental status screening history, as outlined in Table 9–2. Decide whether further tests for organic brain disease such as the Mini-Mental State Exam or more extensive neuropsychiatric testing are required (Chapter 9).

B. The long of it

The physician could extend the ROS to a book-length list of questions that no one would attempt at one sitting.

Fortunately, you do not have to ask every possible question of every patient, just as you do not have to do every possible maneuver on the physical examination or every possible laboratory test. You always have to balance doing too much against doing too little. Instead, tailor the questions to the particular patient. Insure that the patient understands the meaning and intent of the questions asked and feels invited to discuss any unmentioned concerns.

C. Coping with adverse circumstances that prolong the history and ROS
Hostile, depressed, passive–aggressive, hypochondriacal, overly talkative, or inarticulate patients can make even a brief ROS tedious. Chapter 12 discusses the techniques for these situations.

D. Leaven the ROS by some gaps in the drone of questions
Do not just pound through the ROS always in hot pursuit of symptoms. Impressionable patients may begin to imagine more symptoms than actually exist and report them to "please the doctor." Detour now and then to learn about the patient as a person. If the patient reports spraining an ankle while playing tennis, take the opportunity to learn something about the patient's level of skill, interest in the game, and what the activity means to the patient. This technique will improve the quality of the ROS and the interest for both parties, as well as often actually shortening the ROS as contrasted to a relentless barrage of questions. For example, if the patient can play three consecutive sets of tennis without discomfort, you don't have to ask about exertional dyspnea, anginal pain, intermittent claudication, or physical fitness.

> If all you listen to are symptoms, then all you will hear from your patient are symptoms. If you can listen to a variety of subjects, then fewer and fewer of your patients will have symptoms.
>
> —Clifton K. Meador
> (see Meador, 1992, rule 123)

XVIII. Summary

A. The past clinical history
After completing the present illness, the physician asks about the past clinical history, which includes previous illnesses, hospitalizations, operations, medical workups,

and treatment. Obtain actual copies of previous medical documents.

B. The ROS

1. The physician asks an organized series of questions to assay the functions of the various organ systems. This process identifies any other health problems not covered in the present illness and past clinical history.

2. To insure inclusion of every system, visualize the body systems anatomically, starting with the head and nervous system and working rostrocaudally through the chest and abdomen to the anogenital region (Fig. 7–1).

3. The physician first asks an open question pertaining to the system under review and then, as needed, a series of direct or closed questions that will disclose the symptoms arising from dysfunction of the organs. The extent of the ROS, beyond a minimum questioning about each organ system, depends on the previous health, intelligence, and knowledge of the patient.

4. Consider whether the patient may have an environmental/toxic cause for the illness.

5. Do not riddle the patient with question after question. Learn about the person answering the question.

6. Close the ROS by asking the patient "Do you have any other worries about your health."

References

DeMyer WE. Technique of the Neurologic Examination, 5th ed. New York: McGraw-Hill, 2004.

Castell DO, ed. Chest pain of undetermined origin: proceedings of a symposium. Am J Med 1992;(Suppl 5):1–129.

Diaz A, Edwards S, Neal WP, et al. Obtaining a history of sexual victimization from adolescent females seeking routine health care. Mt Sinai J Med 2004;71:170–173.

Gerhardt RT, Nelson BK, Keenan S, et al. Derivation of a clinical guideline for the assessment of nonspecific abdominal pain: the Guideline for Abdominal Pain in the ED Setting (GAPEDS) Phase 1 Study. Am J Emerg Med 2005;23:709–717.

Hampton HL. Care of the woman who has been raped. N Engl J Med 1995;332:234–237.

Herndon RM, ed. Handbook of Neurologic Rating Scales, 2nd ed. New York: Demos Medical, 2006.

Hersen M, ed. Comprehensive Handbook of Psychological Assessment. Hoboken, NJ: John Wiley & Sons, 2004.

Jones R, Barton S. Introduction to history taking and principles of sexual health. Postgrad Med J 2004;80:444–446.

Kaplan PW, ed. Neurologic Disease in Women, 2nd ed. New York: Demos Medical, 2006.

Meador CK. A Little Book of Doctors' Rules. Philadelphia: Hanley & Belfus, 1992, rule 123

Newman LS. Occupational illness. N Engl J Med 1995;333:1128–1134.

Pomeroy W. Taking a Sex History: Interviewing and Recording. Old Tappan, NJ: Free Press, 1982.

Ross MW, Channon-Little LD, Simon Rosser BR. Sexual Health Concerns: Interviewing and History Taking for Health Practitioners. Philadelphia: FA Davis, 2000.

The Family History

8

I. Transition to the Family History

A. Perspectives on the family history

The family history discloses specific risks for many patients, such as for breast cancer and diabetes. The technological advances of genomic medicine, in fact, make the time-honored family history more important and indispensable than ever because it provides the basis for genetic testing, genetic counseling (Harper, 2004), and preventive medicine (Guttmacher et al., 2004; King et al., 2002; Rimoin et al., 2001; Yoon et al., 2003). Although not a routine part of the family history, an *ecomap* (relationships between the family, stressors, and environment) and genogram may be added to the standard pedigree described here (McGuinness et al., 2005; also access online Wikipedia/genogram or ecomap).

B. Receptivity of the patient to the family history

The primary-care physician should always elicit a family history (Bennett, 2004; Berry and Shooner, 2004; Rich et al., 2004). Most patients will answer questions about the family history directly but may deny familial illness, particularly neurologic and mental illnesses. Some patients resist because of guilt or shame. Patients also fear that acknowledging a familial disease may reduce their chances of getting health insurance or employment—another example of third-party intrusion into the patient–physician relationship. When eliciting a family history from a reluctant patient, make every effort to assure confidentiality.

C. Transitional statements to open the family history

After ending the ROS, say to the patient "Let's see about the health of other family members." Introduce the family history by asking about the health of other family members, rather than asking "Do any diseases run in your family?" That question may make the patient defensive. If the patient has already articulated a chief concern and present illness that may be genetic in origin, an excellent transition question to the family history is "Does anyone else in your family have a disorder like yours?" Later, ask a series of closed questions about common disorders such as hypertension, diabetes, and cancer.

II. Drawing up the Pedigree

A. Review the pedigree symbols in Figure 8–1.

B. Construct a pedigree

1. When asking the opening question, produce a blank sheet of paper and actually diagram the pedigree, in sight of the patient, while the patient narrates the information. Later, insert the sheet in the patient's medical record.

2. For step A, Figure 8–2, start by drawing the patient as a square (male) or a circle (female), about halfway down the page. Indicate by an arrow that the patient is the index case (propositus or proband), around whom the pedigree is constructed.

3. Step B, Figure 8–2: Add the patient's siblings in order of age. Connect the top of the squares or circles with a straight line to indicate a sibship.

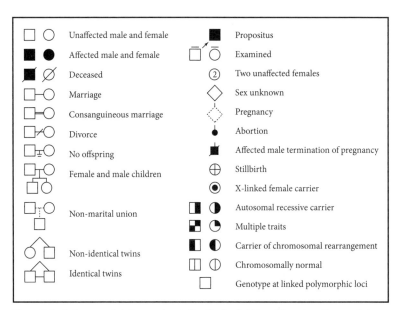

Figure 8–1. Pedigree symbols to use when taking the family history. (Reproduced by permission from Rimoin DL, Conner JM, Pyeritz RE. Emery and Rimoin's Principles and Practice of Medical Genetics, 5th ed. New York: Churchill Livingstone, 2007, Fig 25–3.)

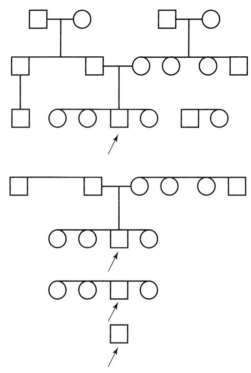

Figure 8–2. Progressogram to illustrate how to draw up a pedigree. The examiner draws up the pedigree while the patient watches and includes the finished page in the patient's record. See the text for explanation.

4. Step C, Figure 8–2: Add the parents. Draw a horizontal line from the midpoint of the symbols for the parents to indicate parentage, and draw a vertical line to connect the parents to the propositus and siblings. Add the brothers and sisters (siblings) of the parents and their ages. As you proceed, the informant quickly understands how you want to organize the information. Upon adding each person's symbol, inquire about that person's health and record any diseases reported or the cause of death. Unless you do a person-by-person review in this manner, the patient may not remember or may fail to report significant genetic information.

5. Step D, Figure 8–2: Add the children of the aunts and uncles. Inquire about the health and development of each one.

6. Step E, Figure 8–2: Add the patient's grandparents. Continue with the pedigree as long as the process produces useful information (Wattendorf and Hadley, 2005).

7. After you complete steps 1–6, draw up the pedigree of your own family, using yourself as the index patient.

8. Several electronic sources provide detailed instructions for compiling pedigrees (the National Society of Genetic Counselors, http://www.nsgc.org/, and the U.S. Surgeon General, www.hhs.gov/familyhistory).

C. Closed questions for the family history

1. Having learned whether disorders resembling the patient's occur in the family, inquire about common diseases. Again, start with the head and headaches and work caudally as a mnemonic, as described in Chapter 7.

2. Ask particularly about neuropsychiatric disorders, such as mental retardation, dementia, seizures, and movement disorders. Ask about depression, suicides, schizophrenia, and treatments or hospitalizations for mental illness.

3. Ask about personality traits in the family, education, employment, and ethnic and geographic origin, if pertinent to the patient's problem.

4. Then, proceed through the other systems, asking about heart disease and hypertension, stroke, lung disease, kidney disease, cancer, arthritis, allergies, blood disorders, hormonal disorders, skin spots or disorders, and exposures to infectious diseases such as tuberculosis.

5. If the patient reports a significant illness in a family member, learn how the diagnosis was made and whether it was objectively confirmed, as by biopsy or autopsy. Arrange to get any medical records pertinent to the patient's health.

6. Record the cause of death of any close relatives and observe the patient's reaction to the deaths and terminal management.

7. If the patient has no apparent genetic illness and none of the near relatives has an evident developmental or genetic disorder, end the family history.

8. Frequently, the initial family history will disclose gaps in the patient's knowledge or mistaken memories. From your questions, the patient will have learned how to investigate the family. Encourage the patient to actively ask family

members, particularly grandparents, about familial
disorders. Reopen the questioning on a follow-up
visit.

D. Utilize the family history to discover management-relevant
attitudes of the patient

1. Clues may come from the patient's tone of voice and word
choice as to how threatened the patient feels by a familial
illness or deaths of close members of the family.

2. By encouraging the patient to talk about the cause of
death of relatives and the terminal management, you will
discover the patient's attitude toward life, terminal illness,
and death. This process discloses the patient's attitude
toward terminal care as a natural evolution of the patient–
physician relationship, not in the totally artificial
circumstance of drawing up a "living will" in a lawyer's
office. The lawyer has no training or incentive to inquire
into the causes of the patient's attitudes, to educate the
patient, or to even understand what care physicians and
genetic consultants can offer.

III. **Special Problems in the Family History of Pediatric Patients**

A. The question of biological parenthood

1. When a couple brings in a child for medical care, make no
assumptions as to the identity of the biological parents.
Today's families may include children of five origins:

a. *Their* children by the present union

b. *His* children by a previous union

c. *Her* children by a previous union

d. An *adopted* child

e. A *foster* child

2. The informants may not offer that information
spontaneously, particularly if you have made the error of
taking the history in the presence of the children.
Generally, the correct information about paternity comes
from interviewing the woman alone, without either the
accompanying male or the children present. Ask directly
whether the mother is the biological mother and whether
the male is the biological father, and determine his status
as husband or live-in boyfriend. Start on the pedigree of a
pediatric patient only after identifying the biological
parents (Fig. 8–3)!

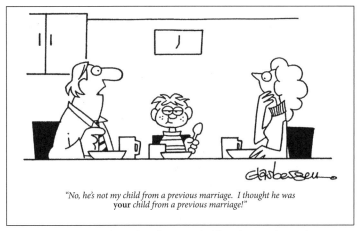

*"No, he's not my child from a previous marriage. I thought he was
your child from a previous marriage!"*

Figure 8–3. Whose child is it? (Reproduced by permission from the *Saturday Evening Post,* 1983.)

    3. In asking about parentage, use the term "union," which
avoids asking about marital status. You should ask "Your
first union produced a boy and a girl, and your second a
boy?" not "Your first *marriage* produced a boy and a girl
and your second a boy?" One or more of the children may
not have come from a marriage, but all came from a
"union."

    4. If the patient is adopted, respect the patient's wishes about
the wisdom of searching previous records or trying to
contact the biological parents.

B. Specific questions when the pedigree indicates a
developmental or genetic neurologic disorder

    1. Ask specifically about the usual birth weight of infants in
the family and their usual age at first walking and
talking.

    2. Ask specifically about seizures, cerebral palsy, mental
retardation, and learning disabilities or whether any
children have required institutional care or hospitalization.
Chapter 10 details the developmental history.

    3. When doubt exists or the information seems incomplete,
call in one of the family elders, preferably a grandparent.

    4. Finally, reopen the family history on a subsequent visit. The
parents will have inquired around or remembered a piece of
information missing on the initial interview, after having

discovered from the physician's questions what to ask about. patients may resist disclosing pedigree information until they understand its medical significance and trust how the physician will use it.

5. The disclosure or admission, as it were, of a genetic disorder in the family of one of the parents may result in feelings of guilt and anxiety by that parent. Be aware of this possibility and deal with it compassionately. Sometimes the reluctance of one parent to give genetic information may signal this problem. Leaven the impact of passing on a hereditary disease by pointing out that we all pass on undesirable traits: hypertension in one family, diabetes in another, cancer, and so on. Point out that reproduction always involves the risk of transmitting a hereditary disorder or a harmful spontaneous mutation.

6. Sometimes reluctance of the patient to answer questions about the family history stems from embarrassment about consanguinity or interracial unions.

C. Examination of the family to resolve physical findings of uncertain significance

1. Ask whether any of the family members have any of the unusual mental or physical characteristics found in the patient, such as breath-holding spells, toe walking, or a large head. If an infant's face or somatotype looks at all dysmorphic or a little unusual, ask whether the infant resembles other members of the family or the paternal or maternal side. Don't comment that the child looks a little odd. Merely ask if others have the trait (e.g., a very small jaw). Ask for photographs or videos of other family members for comparison. Ask about head size, narrow-set or wide-set eyes, or delayed walking or talking.

2. If a patient has a borderline finding, such as occipitofrontal head circumference (OFC) or height or weight, always measure the parents and other available family members. If the family consists of people about five feet tall who have slender somatotypes, the child who has an OFC and height and weight in the 5th percentile may merely reflect genetic background, not a disease.

3. In addition to resolving borderline dysmorphic features, examination of the parents or siblings often resolves other questions.

a. The presence of hypertension in other family members may establish the cause as a genetic predisposition, rather than an acquired disease.

b. The presence of pseudopapilledema in other family members means that the patient with headaches and blurred optic disk margins in all likelihood does not have true papilledema from increased intracranial pressure.

c. Identification of neurocutaneous stigmata in other family members, particularly café au lait spots and depigmented, ash leaf spots, confirms neurofibromatosis and tuberous sclerosis, respectively, as inherited rather than new mutations in the child. Subsequent children of the affected parent will have a 50:50 chance of inheriting the disease, whereas if a new mutation has caused the patient's disease, the reproductive risk if the parents have another child about equals the risk for the population at large.

D. Establish a working relationship with a genetic counselor
The complexities of a genetic workup and genetic counseling mean that the practicing physician, particularly one who sees children, will need a working relationship with a trained genetic consultant.

IV. **Summary**

A. The family history clarifies whether the patient may have a hereditary disorder as the basis for the presenting illness or whether the patient may be at risk for some hereditary disorder unrelated to the present illness that may require further investigation.

B. Patients sometimes conceal familial illnesses because of fear, guilt, or the possibility that they cannot get insurance or employment.

C. Using standard pedigree symbols, the physician should draw up a pedigree in sight of the patient and inquire about the health of each person represented.

D. Using a brief review of systems approach (see Chapter 7), inquire about the health of close relatives.

E. The physician can gain insight into the attitudes of patients to life, death, and terminal medical management by listening to how patients describe the illnesses, final days, and deaths of family members.

F. With a pediatric patient, always ask directly, but discretely, about the paternity and origin of the child—whether the child is his, hers, theirs, adopted, or fostered.

G. By history and by physical examination of available family members, the physician should ascertain whether mental traits, dysmorphic stigmata, or physical findings, such as small stature, occur genetically in the family or come from an acquired illness.

References

Bennett RL. The family clinical history. Prim Care 2004;31:479–495.

Berry T, Shooner KA. Family history: the first genetic screen. Nurse Pract 2004;29:14–25.

Guttmacher AE, Collins FS, Carmona RH. The family history—more important than ever. N Engl J Med 2004;351:2333–2336.

Harper PS. Practical Genetic Counseling. New York: Oxford University Press, 2004.

King RA, Rotter JI, Motulsky AG, eds. The Genetic Basis of Common Diseases. New York: Oxford University Press, 2002.

McGuinness TM, Noonan P, Dyer JG. Family history as a tool for psychiatric nurses. Arch Psychiatric Nursing 2005;19:116–124.

Rich EC, Burke W, Heaton CJ, et al. Reconsidering the family history in primary care. J Gen Intern Med 2004;19:273–280.

Rimoin DL, Conner JM, Pyeritz RE. Emery and Rimoin's Principles and Practice of Medical Genetics, 4th ed. New York: Churchill Livingstone, 2001.

Rimoin DL, Conner JM, Pyeritz RE. Emery and Rimoin's Principles and Practice of Medical Genetics, 5th ed. New York: Churchill Livingstone, 2007, Fig 25–3.

Wattendorf DJ, Hadley DW. Family history: the three-generation pedigree. Am Fam Physician 2005;72:441–448.

Yoon PW, Scheuner MT, Khoury MJ. Research priorities for evaluating family history in the prevention of common diseases. Am J Prev Med 2003;24:128–135.

The Mental Status and Psychosocial History

9

I. Introduction to the Mental Status Examination

> Generally speaking, if the whole thing is a matter of mental disturbance, this is more easily recognized by the method of questioning than by any other.
>
> —Rufus of Ephesus, 1st century
> (reproduced in Brock, 1929, p 114)

A. Definition of the mental status examination
  1. The mental status examination consists of a series of inquiries and observations that evaluate the patient's mental state in regard to the following:
    a. Overall life adjustment
    b. Symptoms of mental illness
    c. Cognitive abilities: normal, retarded, or demented
    d. Emotionality
    e. Sensorium
  2. Many of the inquiries consist of test questions with specified, objective end points, such as knowing the day and date, whereas in the history per se the patient simply relates what has previously occurred or has previously been experienced. Nevertheless, the techniques for exploring the mental status are the same as those for eliciting the history.
B. The medical model and the concept of mental health and mental illness
  1. Just as we can envision a physically normal person in regard to body dimensions and functions, such as blood pressure, height, and weight, we can envision a mentally normal person (Table 9–1).
  2. Of course, no sharp line separates mental health from mental illness, but patients who depart significantly from the criteria in Table 9–1 generally display mental characteristics that impair their pursuit of life, liberty, and happiness.
C. Conduct the mental status examination as an integral part of the history and review of systems (ROS).

Table 9–1. Some Criteria for a Mentally Normal Person

1. Displays an intact mental status, perceives reality correctly, thinks more or less rationally, has adequate overall intelligence, and has common sense (as technically defined in section IV, D)
2. Suffers no crippling addictions, compulsions, obsessions, phobias, mood swings, illusions, delusions, or hallucinations
3. Loves other persons, relates to them for long-term give-and-take relationships, and mourns over their death
4. Respects the rights and needs of other persons
5. Observes rules of propriety and personal and public hygiene
6. Obtains an education, works, and retires at appropriate times in the life cycle
7. Shows an appropriate balance between social compliance and rebellion or aggression
8. Has an appropriate self-image
9. Plays and has sources of recreation and enjoyment
10. Feels that life is precious and interesting, has an overall sense of reward and satisfaction, and strongly desires to live

1. Physicians tend to shirk the mental status examination. They think it takes too much time, lack confidence in their abilities, and misperceive it as requiring special rites outside of the ordinary course of inquiry.

2. Properly done, the mental status examination emerges naturally from the moment-to-moment interchanges of the clinical history so that the clinical history, mental status examination, and psychosocial history merge seamlessly. If you conduct it as a formal inquisition or as a separate thing unto itself, some patients will perceive you as snooping for mental illness and will react adversely.

II. **Quick (but Effective) Questions to Screen the Patient's Mental and Psychosocial Status**

A. Transition to the formal mental status questions and psychosocial history

1. After the interview has matured to an appropriate point, generally after the ROS, and you have shown your willingness to listen, start to review the patient's mental status by asking a very broad, open question: "How is life going for you?" or "Do you have any particular worries or life problems that you want to discuss?" or "Is there something about your life that you feel needs to change?"

2. These open, nonthreatening questions afford the patient a chance to adjust to the new line of inquiry. You can then screen the average patient quickly, yet very effectively, for mental illness by asking a few questions about each of the

Table 9–2. To Screen the Patient Quickly for Mental Illness, Ask at Least One Open Question About Each of the Nine Categories

Children	Adults
I. Mood and satisfactions/dissatisfactions	I. Mood and satisfactions/dissatisfactions
II. Family interactions: with siblings and parents	II. Family interactions: with children, spouse, and other relatives
III. Peer relations: playmates	III. Peer relations: friends
IV. School performance	IV. Work performance
V. Play activities and hobbies	V. Recreation, hobbies, exercise, and fitness
VI. Personal habits (adolescents or teens): tobacco, alcohol, and other drugs	VI. Personal habits: tobacco, alcohol, other drugs, gambling, and lifestyle
VII. Sleep	VII. Sleep
VIII. Legal problems: truancy and delinquency	VIII. Legal problems: arrests, convictions, bankruptcy, divorce, and lawsuits
IX. Sexuality: orientation, precocity	IX. Sexuality: orientation—satisfactions and dissatisfactions

highly significant interpersonal relations and life activities listed in Table 9–2.

3. Most mentally ill patients will function poorly in one or more of these categories, whether they have a so-called functional or an organic mental disorder. The self-sufficient patient who functions well in each of the areas listed probably does not have a severe mental illness.

4. If the patient gives a faint, noncommittal, or disturbing answer to any of the inquiries, explore that area further. Conversely, perk up your ears if the patient quickly dismisses all of your inquiries with "Everything's just fine."

B. Three tables guide the mental status examination (Tables 9–2 to 9–4)

1. If the history otherwise indicates or answers to Table 9–2 suggest mental illness, explore the mental status in depth, using headings III–VI in Table 9–3 (DeMyer, 2004; Trzepacz and Baker, 1993). You may then ask further specific questions to identify criteria for the suspected psychiatric syndrome or disease (*Diagnostic and Statistical Manual of Mental Disorders* [DSM-IV], 2000).

2. If the inquiries suggest that the patient might have organic brain disease, explore the sensorium by the detailed inquiries listed in Table 9–4. (See the discussion of the sensorium in section IV of this chapter.) You may also complete a bedside neuropsychological screening battery

Table 9–3. Formal Outline of the Mental Status Examination

I. General behavior and appearance: Is the patient normal, hyperactive, or agitated? Is the patient neat or slovenly? Are the demeanor and clothes in accordance with the patient's age, peers, sex, and background?

II. Stream of talk: Does the patient converse normally? Is the speech rapid, incessant, or under great pressure? Or is it slow and lacking in amount or spontaneity? Is the patient evasive, discursive, or tangential and unable to reach conversational goals?

III. Mood and affective responses: Is the patient euphoric, agitated, inappropriately gay and giggling, or silent, weeping, or angry? Does the patient's mood swing in a direction appropriate to the subject matter of the conversation? Is the patient emotionally labile, histrionic, expansive, or overtly depressed?

IV. Content of thought: Does the patient correctly perceive reality or have obsessions, illusions, hallucinations, or phobias? Does the patient have delusions of persecution, maltreatment, or thought control by malicious forces? Is the patient preoccupied with bodily complaints or fears of cancer, heart disease, or other phobias?

V. Intellectual capacity: Is the patient bright, average, dull, or apparently demented or mentally retarded?

VI. Sensorium:
    A. Consciousness
    B. Orientation for time, place, and person
    C. Memory: recent and remote
    D. Attention span
    E. Calculation
    F. Fund of information
    G. Insight, judgment, and planning

Adapted by permission from DeMyer, W. Technique of the Neurologic Examination, 5th ed. New York: McGraw-Hill, 2004.

such as the Halstead-Reitan (DeMyer, 2004; Cipolotti and Warrington, 1995; Reitan 1984; Reitan and Wolfson, 1993; Weinberg et al., 1995) or the Mini-Mental State Examination (Grigoletto et al., 1999).

3. These screening tests will help determine whether the patient needs an extensive, formal neuropsychological battery. (See section III, E of this chapter.)

4. For all patients, especially women (Woods and Heitkemper, 2004), the physician should seek insight into the self-image and view of their role in life. Addressing the patient's self-doubts may provide valuable clues to the cause of obscure symptoms and for optimal management.

C. General mood and satisfactions/dissatisfactions
The mentally ill patient often has a mood disorder, manifested by hostility, anger, mania, or depression. At some point, ask directly about the patient's mood: "How has your mood been?" or "Have you been feeling down or blue?" If the reply suggests

Table 9–4. Sample Questions to Screen the Patient's Sensorium

Area of Sensorium Tested	Sample Questions
Orientation for time, place, and person; recent and remote memory	What is your name? What is the time of day/date/month/year? Where are you? How old are you? When is your birthday? What is your address? What kind of work do you do? Do you have a spouse/children? What are their names/ages/occupations/addresses?
Recent memory	What is the season/weather? Have you waited long to see me? What did you do this morning/yesterday? How has your memory been? Does it worry you? Give the patient a name, address, and color to remember; at the end of the interview, ask "Can you name the three items?"
Calculation, attention span	Can you subtract 7 from 100 and continue subtracting? Spell the word "world" backward. Can you spell the word "world" by the alphabetical sequence of the letters?
Fund of information, attention span, memory	What's been happening in the news? What do you think of (mention a recent news event)? Can you name the last several presidents?
Insight, judgment, and planning	What are your plans for the future? What have you come to see me about? Do you feel any need for medical help? How long do you expect to be off work?
Recent memory	Ask the patient to repeat the three items mentioned above.

Adapted by permission from DeMyer, W. Technique of the Neurologic Examination, 5th ed. New York: McGraw-Hill, 2004.

a mood disorder, proceed with more detailed questions. (See section III, C for an exploration of mood disorders.)

D. Family interactions

    1. The mentally ill patient usually relates poorly to one or more family members. Open this topic by asking about the patient's living arrangements and the number of persons in the household. Then ask "How do things go for you at home?" Then ask about relations to each individual in the household (spouse, live-in mate, and children).

        a. Excellent questions are "How are your relations to your partner?" and "What do you like best about your partner?" and "What do you dislike the most?"

        b. At some point, take a sexual history (see Chapter 7, section XI, A) (Jones and Barton, 2004).

    2. If the patient is a child, ask the child and the parents how the child gets along with the siblings and with each of the parents.

3. At some point in the history, ask specifically about domestic violence involving partners or spouses (Jaffee et al., 2005; Minsky-Kelly et al., 2005), children (Giardino and Finkel, 2005; Horner, 2005) including children with disabilities (Hibbard and Desch, 2007), pregnant women (Chambliss, 2007; see also the website for the American College of Obstetricians and Gynecologists, http://www.acog.org/departments), and the elderly (Gorbien, 2005; Kurrie, 2005). You should be aware of the local laws regarding investigation and reporting of intrafamilial sexual and physical abuse. Also learn whether family members have previously been arrested or imprisoned.

4. Take a child abuse history if concerns about a battered child arise in questioning the adults involved. Clues are unexplained bruises and injuries, multiple visits to emergency rooms for the child, and a living arrangement where the mother works and an unemployed male, often not the actual father, stays home to attend to the child (Flaherty and Sege, 2005; Matthews, 2004).

E. Peer relationships (Table 9–2, III)

1. The mentally ill patient usually relates poorly to peers. For children, ask parents about overall activity level and temperament. Ask how a child gets along with other children, whether the child can share toys, tries to dominate other children, is too aggressive, and always has to be first. Particularly ask whether the playmates tease or bully the patient and whether other children spontaneously seek out the child as a playmate. Anderson et al. (1999) give a checklist to screen for mental disorders in children, and Greenspan and Greenspan (2003) give sample interviews.

2. For adult patients, ask about social activities and friendships.

F. School or work (Table 9–2, IV)

1. The mentally ill patient usually functions poorly in school or at work. Ask whether the child likes school. As an index of the child's feelings about school, ask whether the child willingly gets ready in the mornings to go to school or balks. Ask about current grades, grade placement (regular classes or special), attendance, attitude toward teacher, and behavior evaluation by the teacher. Ask about performance on achievement tests.

2. Ask adults what kind of work they do and how things go at work in regard to job performance, promotions, and relations to coworkers.

G. Play/hobbies/recreation (Table 9–2, V)

1. The mentally ill patient often lacks interest in play or recreation, whereas the mentally normal person usually has hobbies and interests. Ask parents and the child about the child's play activities, interests, and talents (Cepeda, 2000). A revealing question often is "What does the child do if left alone?" Ask about fascination with weapons, fire-setting, cruelty to animals, and persistent lying or stealing— predictors of a highly disturbed child.

2. Ask adults about hobbies, interests, and physical fitness activities. Recall the importance of a flower garden for patient 1 (see Chapter 3, section II, B and C).

H. Personal habits (Table 9–2, VI)

1. Drug addiction: Ask specifically about use of tobacco, alcohol, and sleeping pills. Then ask about "street drugs" and list them by name: marijuana, cocaine, speed, LSD, heroin, and any other "uppers or downers."

a. Frequently, the patient can more readily admit drug use if the physician asks about past rather than present use: "Have you used (such and such a drug) in the past?" The physician can then creep up to the present by asking "In the past year? Month? Days?" It's always easier to admit past sins than current ones.

b. If the adult patient uses alcohol or other drugs, you need to find out how much. Remember, however, that one of the diagnostic features of addiction is denial, especially with alcoholism. The alcoholic invariably minimizes the amount of alcohol ingested: "Only a few drinks now and then" or "Only a few beers." Discovering the true amount may require later visits or questioning family members. The patient's work record and number of days off may prove helpful in assessing the degree of alcoholism. Patients often deny or minimize the use of other self-medications, such as laxatives, sleeping pills, and stimulants. Obese patients understate the amount of food ingested, whereas anorexics claim they eat too much.

Table 9–5. Sample Questions for Taking a History of Alcoholism

1. Do you drink alcoholic beverages?
2. Describe your drinking habits.
3. Do you drink daily? Describe alcohol use on a routine workday or weekend.
4. Do you regularly go to bars, drink with friends, or mostly drink alone?
5. Do you get drunk? Never? Infrequently? Frequently?
6. Do you worry about excess use of alcohol?
7. Do you feel a need to curtail or stop drinking?
8. Have you ever sworn completely off?
9. Do your family/spouse/friends think you should cut down on drinking?
10. Do you keep bottles of liquor stashed away at home or work?
11. How does alcohol affect your mood?
12. Do you get belligerent when drinking?
13. Have you missed days at work/school because of alcohol?
14. Have you experienced any "lost weekends" or any period of lost memory from drinking?
15. Have you had the "shakes" from drinking?
16. Have you ever been hospitalized or treated for alcohol problems?
17. Have you been arrested for drunken driving?

    c. Table 9–5 lists sample questions to use in taking an alcoholism history.

    d. The CAGE mnemonic summarizes these questions

> "Have you ever felt that you should Cut down in alcohol use?"
>
> "Does criticism of drinking Annoy you?"
>
> "Have you felt Guilt about drinking?"
>
> "Do you take a morning Eye-opener?"

    e. The Michigan Alcoholism Screening Test (MAST) is a full twenty-five-question, scored battery (Selzer, 1971).

2. Specific history from all addicted patients: Most of the questions about alcoholism in Table 9–5 also apply to all addictive substances.

    a. Agents used

    b. Age at first use, duration (most recent use), frequency and amount: daily, weekly, binges

    c. Adverse reactions

    d. Route of administration: oral, nasal, inhalation, injection

    e. Previous efforts at withdrawal

    f. Impact on family and work

    g. Amount of money spent

    h. Conflict with the law

3. Gambling and other obsessions or compulsions, if not covered elsewhere in the ROS

I. Psychosocial summary

At this point you will have attained a fairly broad perspective of the possible role of psychosocial factors as the background for the patient's state of health. You may need to ask more about employment, life satisfactions, and living circumstances (Carlat, 2005; White, 2005).

J. Sleep disorders (Table 9–2, VII)

1. Ask about the bedroom and circumstances for sleeping, the presleep routine, time of retiring and arising, daytime napping, ability to fall asleep and time required, nocturnal awakenings, frightening dreams, bed-wetting, sleepwalking, and restorative effect of sleep. Things that interfere with sleep may cause irritability and malaise the next day.

2. Ask the patient to describe the transition from sleep to wakefulness in the mornings.

3. Also ask about snoring, sleep apnea, jerks (sleep myoclonus), and specifically leg cramps and restless legs. A patient with restless legs syndrome has unpleasant feelings in the legs. Ask "Do you have restless feelings in your legs that require you to move them (or even get up and walk) for comfort?" Simple leg cramps differ in being relieved by stretching of the involved muscle.

4. Ask whether the patient has hypersomnolence, insomnia, or a parasomnia and the time of night the disturbance appears (relation to rapid eye movement [REM] periods). This information often best comes from a partner or parent who has observed the patient during sleep.

5. Find out whether the patient arouses habitually at night to urinate or drink water.

6. Ask about medications, including caffeine and alcohol, which could affect sleep and the use of sleeping pills.

7. A nosology of sleep disorders again serves as a reminder of the range of disorders to consider during the sleep history (Table 9–6). As with seizures and headache, you may need a full structured interview in selected patients (Schramm et al., 1993). As in video monitoring of seizure disorders, an overnight polysomnogram that includes an electroencephalogram (EEG) may help to substantiate the diagnosis. The American Sleep Disorders Association (1997, p 15–17) and Chokroverty (1994) give the diagnostic criteria for the various sleep disorders listed in Table 9–6.

Table 9–6. International Classification of Sleep Disorders

I. Dyssomnias (disorders of initiating and maintaining sleep and disorders of excessive sleepiness)
  A. Intrinsic sleep disorders
    1. Psychophysiological insomnia
    2. Sleep state misperception
    3. Idiopathic insomnia
    4. Narcolepsy
    5. Recurrent hypersomnia
    6. Idiopathic hypersomnia
    7. Posttraumatic hypersomnia
    8. Obstructive sleep apnea syndrome
    9. Central sleep apnea syndrome
    10. Central alveolar hypoventilation syndrome
    11. Periodic limb movement disorder
    12. Restless legs syndrome
    13. Intrinsic sleep disorder NOS
  B. Extrinsic sleep disorders
    1. Inadequate sleep hygiene
    2. Environmental sleep disorder
    3. Altitude insomnia
    4. Adjustment sleep disorder
    5. Insufficient sleep syndrome
    6. Limit-setting sleep disorder
    7. Sleep-onset association disorder
    8. Food allergy insomnia
    9. Nocturnal eating (drinking) syndrome
    10. Hypnotic-dependent sleep disorder
    11. Stimulant-dependent sleep disorder
    12. Alcohol-dependent sleep disorder
    13. Toxin-induced sleep disorder
    14. Extrinsic sleep disorder NOS
  C. Circadian rhythm sleep disorders
    1. Time zone change (jet lag) syndrome
    2. Shift work sleep disorder
    3. Irregular sleep–wake pattern
    4. Delayed sleep phase syndrome
    5. Advanced sleep phase syndrome
    6. Non-24 hour sleep–wake disorder
    7. Circadian rhythm sleep disorder NOS
II. Parasomnias (disorders that primarily do not cause a complaint of insomnia or excessive sleepiness)
  A. Arousal disorders
    1. Confusional arousals
    2. Sleepwalking
    3. Sleep terrors
  B. Sleep–wake transition disorders
    1. Rhythmic movement disorder
    2. Sleep starts
    3. Sleep talking
    4. Nocturnal leg cramps
  C. Parasomnias usually associated with rapid eye movement (REM) sleep
    1. Nightmares
    2. Sleep paralysis
    3. Impaired sleep-related penile erections
    4. Sleep-related painful erections
    5. REM sleep–related sinus arrest
    6. REM sleep behavior disorder
  D. Other parasomnias
    1. Sleep bruxism
    2. Sleep enuresis
    3. Sleep-related abnormal swallowing syndrome
    4. Nocturnal paroxysmal dystonia
    5. Sudden unexplained nocturnal death syndrome
    6. Primary snoring
    7. Infant sleep apnea
    8. Congenital central hypoventilation syndrome
    9. Sudden infant death syndrome
    10. Benign neonatal sleep myoclonus
    11. Other parasomnias NOS

8. For children, ask about position during sleep, nightmares and night terrors, "things that go bump in the night," sleep phobias, and enuresis. Ask specifically about snoring. Snoring is abnormal in a child and generally requires investigation by an overnight polysomnogram. Tonsillectomy and adenoidectomy often correct the problem.

Table 9–6. *(continued)*

III. Sleep disorders associated with medical/ psychiatric disorders	4. Sleep-related asthma
A. Associated with mental disorders	5. Sleep-related gastroesophageal reflux
1. Psychoses	6. Peptic ulcer disease
2. Mood disorders	7. Fibrositis syndrome
3. Anxiety disorders	IV. Proposed sleep disorders: These are disorders
4. Panic disorder	for which insufficient information is available
5. Alcoholism	to confirm their acceptance as definitive sleep
B. Associated with neurologic disorders	disorders.
1. Cerebral degenerative disorders	1. Short sleeper
2. Dementia	2. Long sleeper
3. Parkinsonism	3. Subwakefulness syndrome
4. Fatal familial insomnia	4. Fragmentary myoclonus
5. Sleep-related epilepsy	5. Sleep hyperhidrosis
6. Electrical status epilepticus of sleep	6. Menstruation-associated sleep disorder
7. Sleep-related headaches	7. Pregnancy-associated sleep disorder
C. Associated with other medical disorders	8. Terrifying hypnagogic hallucinations
1. Sleeping sickness	9. Sleep-related neurogenic tachypnea
2. Nocturnal cardiac ischemia	10. Sleep-related laryngospasm
3. Chronic obstructive pulmonary disease	11. Sleep choking syndrome

American Sleep Disorders Association. International classification of sleep disorders, revised: Diagnostic and coding manual. Rochester, Minnesota: American Sleep Disorders Association, 1997.

    K. Legal problems/criminal record/delinquency (Table 9–2, VIII)
       1. For a child, ask the parent about truancy, gang membership, and juvenile delinquency.
       2. Ask an adult "Have you had any legal problems? Arrests? Convictions?"
       3. In some discrete fashion you need to learn whether the patient is involved in a lawsuit over any medical problems, particularly related to the present illness.
       4. The ascertainment in retrospect by physicians of the patient's state of mind during a crime is fraught with uncertainty and highly subjective, as in judging mental competence in making out a will. In such circumstances, the history narrated by the patient may fail (Simon and Shuman, 2002).
    L. Sexuality
      Inquire about sexuality by questions appropriate to the age of the patient (see Chapter 7, section XI, A–F).

III. Detailed Inquiries into the Patient's Mental Status
    A. Format for a detailed mental status examination

If the presenting problem of the patient or the screening of the mental status items in Table 9–2 suggests mental or neurological illness, proceed with a detailed formal mental status examination by inquiring into the categories outlined in Tables 9–3 and 9–4. Again, you do not need to pursue each item in the order outlined when taking the history but should assemble the information in sequence in the write-up.

B. General behavior, appearance, and stream of talk
Items I and II of Table 9–3 are self-explanatory and depend essentially on observations during the history and physical examination. The mentally ill patient may produce too much speech, showing pressure of speech, or remain nearly silent or completely mute. Some children who talk normally at home may display elective mutism and say little or nothing in the physician's office or at school.

C. Mood and affective responses (Table 9–3, III)
1. Kinds of affective responses
To evaluate the patient's mood, observe the quality of the patient's emotional responses during the interview: appropriate, blunted, or excessive. The patient may show too little affect, a condition called a *blunted affect*, or too much, a condition called *excessive affect*, or may rapidly shift from one affective state to another, a condition called *labile affect*. The patient may also show an inappropriate affect, that is, no emotional responses or giggling or smiling when discussing the death of a family member.

2. Asking about depression
a. Since both mental and physical illnesses commonly cause depression, always ask specifically "Have you been feeling blue or sad?" It is often best to avoid the word "depression" because it connotes a finalized clinical diagnosis rather than inviting patients to talk about their feelings. Getting too "psychiatric" too soon may alienate some patients.

b. Observe the patient's facial expression for clues to depression. Most depressed patients have a slack face and slumped posture, speak slowly and softly, and move slowly; but patients with agitated depression may pace and wring their hands.

c. Some depressed patients will produce an automatic, wan smile in response to every question asked, the "automatic smiler" syndrome, which usually masks hostility that the patient cannot express overtly. Thus, the smiling behavior is separated from the usual emotion it should express.

(1) The automatic smiler syndrome has in itself a differential diagnosis. Some passive–aggressive patients also display automatic smiling, although to a different purpose from the depressed patient. (The automatic smiler syndrome also afflicts politicians and diplomats, who smile inappropriately no matter what the gravity of the topic of discussion.)

(2) Diffuse brain impairment, particularly bilateral interruption of the corticobulbar tracts, causes a syndrome called "pseudobulbar palsy." The patient displays affective lability, shifting rapidly from crying to laughter or laughter to crying, and has dysphagia and dysarthria (DeMyer, 2004). A pseudobulbar (labile) affect may also occur in cerebral palsied children, but some children, usually severely retarded, may automatically smile to almost any stimulus, whereas others may automatically fret or cry.

d. For the overtly depressed patient, the physician may be more direct: "It seems you have been feeling blue" or "I wonder whether you have been feeling blue. Would you want to talk about it?" Such inquiries often result in a diagnostic response: a sad look, a sagging of the shoulders, a sigh, or even overt tears.

e. Ask about mood changes, sleep disturbances, loss of interest in usual activities, *anhedonia* (loss of ability to enjoy life), and lack of energy. Table 9–7 lists the diagnostic features of major depression that the history will disclose (Simon and Hales, 2006).

f. You can convert the DSM-IV criteria of Table 9–7 into questions or use the patient Health Questionnaire (PHQ-9), a nine-item depression questionnaire (access by Google, "PHQ-9").

g. During this phase of the history you should ask directly about suicidal thoughts (Barber et al., 1998; Shea, 1999), particularly in the presence of risk factors (Table 9–8). Around 30,000 deaths per year are attributed to suicide in the United States.

Table 9–7. Symptoms of Major Depression and Dysthymia (Based on DSM-IV-TR, 2000)

1. Depressed mood most of the day, nearly every day
2. Extreme disinterest and loss of pleasure in all or almost all activities
3. Extreme weight loss or gain or decrease or increase in appetite
4. Insomnia or hypersomnia nearly every day
5. Psychomotor agitation or retardation nearly every day
6. Fatigue or loss of energy nearly every day
7. Feelings of worthlessness or excessive or inappropriate guilt
8. Diminished ability to think or concentrate or indecisiveness
9. Recurrent thoughts of death or suicidal ideation or attempt
10. Feelings of hopelessness

Major depression *is defined as the presence of symptom 1 or 2 (or both) plus enough of symptoms 3–9 to make a total of five or more symptoms with a minimum duration of 2 weeks.* Dysthymia *is defined as chronic (persisting for at least 2 years) depressed mood plus at least two of symptoms 3, 4, 6–8, and 10.*

h. Use questions such as "Have you felt like doing away with yourself?" and "Do you wish you weren't here?" and "How does the future look to you?" Active inquiry is necessary because patients do not often bring up suicide attempts spontaneously (Hirschfeld and Russel, 1997). Ask the patient what problems suicide would solve and how the suicide might affect family members. Suicide often reflects profound hostility toward the family. Such a message of hostility and revenge stands out unmistakably when someone shoots her- or himself under circumstances that insure that a family member, usually a

Table 9–8. Risk Factors for Suicide

1. Previous suicide attempts
2. History of mental disorders, particularly depression and schizophrenia
3. History of alcohol and substance abuse
4. Family history of suicide
5. Family history of child abuse
6. Feelings of hopelessness
7. Loss (relational, social, work, or financial)
8. Feelings of isolation or being cut off from other people
9. Impulsive or aggressive tendencies
10. Easy access to lethal agents, particularly guns
11. Financial barriers to mental health treatment
12. Resistance to seek help because of mental illness stigma
13. Cultural and religious beliefs
14. Local epidemics of suicide
15. Physical illness

(Based on www.cdc.gov/ncipc)

spouse, will walk in and unexpectedly discover the blood-soaked corpse, with half of its head blown off. The corpse speaks more eloquently than the person while alive: "Look! You made my life so bad that I had to kill myself. See what you made me do! You'll be sorry now."

    i. If the patient has had recurrent thoughts of suicide or has made overt attempts, the physician generally should "hand-carry" the patient to a psychiatrist.

  3. The manic–depressive or bipolar patient
The manic patient acts just the opposite to a depressed patient when questioned about mood or how life is going. Ask directly about cycles of excessive thoughts and behaviors. The manic expansively describes how great everything is and declaims numerous imagined financial and personal triumphs and grandiose but unrealistic schemes. Because of impaired judgment during the mania, the patient may have spent himself or herself into bankruptcy and made personal commitments and promises that are impossible to fulfill.

D. Content of thought (Table 9–3, IV)

  1. Preoccupations or obsessions generally come to light as the patient returns to them time and again during the history or betrays them with strong emotional responses.

  2. Illusions, delusions, and hallucinations are technically defined (DeMyer, 2004).

    a. *Illusions* are false sensory perceptions based on natural stimulation of a sensory receptor, for example, the illusion of water shimmering on the highway on a hot summer's day or misinterpreting a shadow or a pile of leaves as a cat.

    b. *Hallucinations* are false sensory perceptions not based on natural or normal stimulation of a sensory pathway, for example, the experience of seeing faces peering through the window or hearing voices, although no one is actually there. Hallucinations take many forms—visual, auditory, visceral, and somatic—depending on the sensory avenue involved. They may arise from specific brain lesions or from thought disorders such as schizophrenia.

    c. *Delusions* are false beliefs which neither reason nor the patient's own reality testing can dispel, for example, believing that radio waves are controlling the patient's thoughts or interpreting the normal daily irritations of living as a plot deliberately designed by malicious persons or forces to harass the patient.

3. The timing of questions about the content of thought
   a. Obviously, you have to choose the patient and the optimal time during the interview to ask questions about preoccupations, phobias, illusions, hallucinations, or delusions. To ask in an inappropriate context "Do you hear voices and see visions?" will displease a normal person to some degree, but it may lead a mentally ill patient to react very adversely.
   b. Yet, when the patient relays some unusual mental phenomenon, a question such as "Have you experienced voices although no one was present?" may encourage the patient to report a very distressing auditory hallucination, such as a voice that repeatedly commands the patient to drown her baby.

E. Intellectual capacity (Table 9–3, V)
   1. The physician needs an estimate of the patient's intellect and education for diagnosis as well as to judge the patient's capability to make decisions. Is the patient frankly mentally retarded or overtly demented? Is the patient of low, normal, average, or superior intelligence?
   2. Middle-class English and grammar, normal conceptualization, and a bona fide high school diploma suggest at least adequate intelligence, whereas a college degree generally requires average to above average intelligence. However, absence of these criteria does not identify a patient of inferior intellect.
   3. If the clinical problem requires exploration of the patient's intellect, IQ, or educational achievement, order full, formal neuropsychological batteries. Do not rely simply on clinical intuition, particularly with a patient from a different socioeconomic stratum, race, language, or culture or if motor deficits preclude expression of the intellect, as in cerebral palsied children. Neuropsychological batteries give a standardized appraisal of the patient's mental strengths and deficits, whether psychiatric or organic.

      a. For adults, see Cippoloti and Warrington, l995; Heilman and Valenstein, 2003; Jarvis and Barth, 1984; Reitan and Wolfson, 1993; Strauss et al., 2006.

      b. For children, as in evaluating for learning disability, see Cordoni, 1995; Fennell, l995; and Weinberg et al., 1995. (See Chapter 10 for developmental milestones for clinical evaluation of retardation.)

IV. The Sensorium or Sensorium Commune: Common Sense and Its Testing

A. What is the sensorium?

  1. Intuition tells us that somewhere within the body resides a mechanism, a sensorium, which receives and monitors all of our incoming external and internal sensations and integrates them with our needs, desires, and memories. This surveillance produces a stream of consciousness that makes us aware of ourselves and our environment. This awareness leads to appropriate behaviors to survive the contingencies of our daily lives.

  2. The sensorium consists of neural circuitry that functions in three ways:

      a. To receive and monitor ongoing events, as detected by sensory receptors and conducted as nerve impulses to the brain by sensory pathways

      b. To integrate this ongoing sensory information with memories, desires, and emotions

      c. To respond with forecasts and plans that lead to behaviors that promote one's purposes and one's survival

  3. In the fewest words, the sensorium is the neural mechanism that

      a. Perceives what's going on

      b. Processes it

      c. Responds with appropriate behavior (Fig. 9–1)

  4. Since sensorial functions are highly susceptible to organic disorders of the brain, their testing is essential in the mental status examination. To test them, physicians ask a series of questions that have specified, objective answers. These answers demonstrate whether the patient's perceptions and responses match those of the standard normal person and that the patient shares the senses

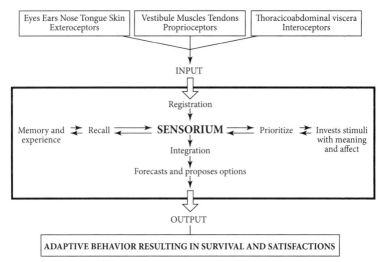

| Eyes Ears Nose Tongue Skin
Exteroceptors | Vestibule Muscles Tendons
Proprioceptors | Thoracicoabdominal viscera
Interoceptors |

INPUT

Registration

Memory and ⇄ Recall ⇄ **SENSORIUM** ⇄ Prioritize ⇄ Invests stimuli
experience   Integration   with meaning
                         and affect

Forecasts and proposes options

OUTPUT

ADAPTIVE BEHAVIOR RESULTING IN SURVIVAL AND SATISFACTIONS

Figure 9–1. Diagram of the sensorium as an input–output system. (Reproduced by permission from DeMyer, W. Technique of the Neurologic Examination, 5th ed. New York, McGraw-Hill, 2004.)

common to us all. In other words, the sensorium of one person with a normal brain and normal life experiences closely matches everyone else's. We all recognize what time of day it is, whether it's raining outside, whether it's noisy or quiet, and so on. We all retreat from a blazing fire or tread cautiously at the edge of a precipice. This phenomenon of humans having common perceptions and responses when facing like circumstances we call "common sense," the *sensorium commune* of the ancient philosophers.

  B. What is common sense?

    1. Common sense means that confronted with the same events or choices everyone whose mental status is normal will perceive the events more or less the same and will choose to respond to them more or less the same.

    2. Uncommon sense is what we differ about: Does God exist? Are abortion and euthanasia murder? Should we prohibit guns? Is capital punishment justified? Obviously, we do not share a common sense about these questions. To evaluate the sensorium, physicians avoid such questions because they

elicit unquantifiable argumentation, not objective, definable end points such as "What is the date today?"

C. Where is the sensorium?

1. Aristotle (384–322 BCE) located the sensorium—sensation, emotion, and consciousness—in the heart. Certainly, all of these functions stop when the heart stops but only because blood flow to the brain also stops.

2. Some contemporaries and successors of Aristotle, such as Theophrastus (371–287 BCE), Herophilus (about 335–280 BCE), and Erasistratus (304–250 BCE), advocated the brain as the site of the sensorium; but Galen's work (130–200 CE), as much as anyone's, firmly established the brain as the correct organ. Decisive modern proof comes from heart transplantation, which does not change the recipient's sensorium.

3. We now know that the sensorium resides in the circuits of the rostral brainstem reticular formation, diencephalon, and cerebrum. In spite of the fact that the sensorium resides in the head, we retain the notion that emotions arise in the heart. We still say that a person with no sympathy "has no heart," one who is generous is "full of heart," and one who is brave is "lion-hearted." An "affair of the heart" and even the heart-shaped images of Valentine's Day derive from the outmoded Aristotelian notions. We still dichotomize "head" and "heart" as if reason, which arises in the head, struggles against emotion, which was erroneously believed to arise in the heart.

D. Common sense as a clinically testable aspect of the patient's history and mental status

1. Because of our common perceptions, each of us agrees as to who we and who others are and as to our respective roles, as to where we are, as to what day and time of day it is, as to what season it is, as to what's going on, and as to how to behave appropriately to survive. Our common sense tells us all to avoid the edge of cliffs and not to run on ice. In brief, "Does the person have the common sense to come in out of the rain?" (But an exuberant few will romp in the rain and enjoy it.)

2. To test the integrity of the sensorial circuitry, the physician simply asks *who, when, where, what,* and *how* questions,

each question posing a definable end point that assesses
processing by the sensorium (Table 9–4).

E. Taking a prompt history for screening a patient's sensorium in
an emergency

1. *Pt 12:* A 21-year-old football player was knocked
momentarily unconscious. The team physician runs onto
the field and must quickly but effectively screen the player's
sensorium. The physician first asks the athlete for his own
name and then to identify the physician by name (*who*
questions); to name the day, date, and time (*when*
questions); to state the location of the game (*where*
questions); to name the opponent and the score of the
contest (*what's happening* questions). These questions test
whether the patient's sensorium perceives the current
circumstances, in effect knows what's happening in
common with other persons. In fact, the single best question
to test for the return of the athlete's sensorium to normal is
to ask the athlete "What is the score of the game?" We even
intuitively ask that question when we greet someone by
saying "What's the score?" Thus, these simple *who, where,
when*, and *what* questions enable the physician's
consciousness to evaluate the patient's consciousness by
testing for the mental state that everyone should hold in
common, that is, appropriate perceptions and responses to
current circumstances, a simple matching of two persons'
perceptions.

2. Automatic testing of the sensorium in everyday life
By habit, we intuitively test and monitor the sensorium of
everyone we meet. That is exactly our agenda when we greet
anyone: "Hello, how are you?" or, in street talk, "Hey, what's
happening?" or "What's coming down?" or "What's the
score, man?" These ploys invite the other person to display
his or her perceptions and intents for you to sample and
compare with your own. You have to ask yourself
immediately "Does this person display common sense?" or
"Is this a madman? Had I better get out of here?" or "OK,
this one seems safe enough" (matches well against yourself)
or "Hey, this one's all right—simpatico—I'll foster this one."
It's like two stray dogs warily eyeing, nuzzling, sniffing, and
licking each other, that is, each maximizing its sensory
input, by vision, touch, smell, taste and body language—one

organism strutting and titrating its perceptions and projected actions against another. This process is basically a stimulus–response paradigm that amounts to testing for the species norm of common sense. Each individual asks "What are the possibilities and what is appropriate here?" "What do I do or not do?" We return to a basic principle of the medical examination: Match the findings for the patient against a norm, in this case the norm of common sense. Thus, the *who, where, when,* and *what* questions formally require the other person to display his or her sensorium for evaluation by your own.

F. How not to ask questions to test the patient's sensorium
   1. In emergencies to screen immediately for the return of consciousness, as in the previous patient, ask several simplistic questions in a row; but you should not elicit the mental status history from the usual patient in that way. The inexperienced physician often tests the patient's sensorium and mental status (and forbearance) with a barrage of direct but disconnected questions, fired machine gun-style:
     a. "Who are you?"
     b. "Do you hear voices talking to you?"
     c. "Do you see snakes on the wall?"
     d. "What is this place?"
     e. "Who am I?"
     f. "Who is the president?"
     g. "What is 100 minus 7?"
     h. "What is the date today?"
   2. While circumstances may justify each of these inquiries, their unnatural order and obvious purpose will annoy many patients, particularly patients who are worried about their mental status or paranoid.
     a. The reticent or normal patient, embarrassed, responds to the amateurish, machine-gun technique with a forbearing smile.
     b. The touchy patient, irked, replies with a not-so-amused "Do you think I'm crazy, Doc?" Again, the "Doc" puts the patient down a little as the patient expresses veiled resentment.
     c. The paranoid patient will lapse into silence and glare at you.

     d. Remember that such adverse responses usually result from a breach of technique in asking questions.

  G. How to ask the questions and gather the information required to evaluate the sensorium

    1. To diagnose the patient's mental status requires all of the data outlined in Table 9–3, but you do not need to follow the sequence of the table in asking the questions that elicit the information.

    2. Subtle, unobtrusive introduction of the mental status questions produces much more information than rapid-fire questioning because it does not alienate the patient. Develop the mental status data by bits and pieces as the subjects naturally and appropriately arise during the entire interview.

  H. Techniques to evaluate the sensorium

    1. Evaluating consciousness and attention span

      a. Evaluate consciousness by determining how the patient responds to ordinary conversational approaches and attends to ordinary environmental stimuli. Judge attention span by the length of time the patient can focus on the subject at hand.

      b. Full evaluation of partially conscious patients requires physical examination techniques (DeMyer, 2004) beyond the usual clinical history.

    2. Evaluating orientation to time, person, and place

      a. Determine the patient's orientation to time, person, and place during the initial chitchat and initial stages of the interview by noting how the patient can relate the dates of the symptoms and during the ROS.

      b. The patient with temporal disorientation will have trouble dating *when* and *what happened* questions: "When were you last well?" "What happened next?"

    3. Testing for temporal disorientation and loss of memory (amnesia)

      a. Entree questions

        (1) If the patient appears confused about temporal orientation and memory, the physician may appropriately ask "It seems you are having some problem keeping track of time. Could you tell me the date today?" In such a context, when you express appropriate interest and concern, the patient accepts

the inquiry readily. You then may also ask about time of day and day of the week and the year without insulting the patient.

(2) If you suspect temporal disorientation, ask "Have you noticed any trouble with your memory?" Then pose questions to test remote memory, recent memory, and recall. Questions such as "Who has come to visit you today?" and "When did you get up today?" provide natural, subtle ways to test recent memory, without offending the patient.

  b. Standard recent memory test

(1) If faulty answers to the foregoing questions suggest a memory deficit, introduce a standard test for recent memory. Ask the patient to remember three unrelated items, as follows: "Let's see how your memory is working. I'll give you three things to remember, and I will ask for them at the end of the examination today. The first is an address, 5327 Broadway. The second is an item, a table. The third is a color, orange."

(2) Then say, "Now repeat those three things to be sure you have them."

(3) Then require the patient to repeat the three items at the end of the history or physical examination. Normal individuals remember all three items accurately.

  c. Remote memory test: Ask about distant dates such as birthdays or graduation dates. Organic brain disease impairs recent memory more than remote.

4. Testing for inability to calculate (*dyscalculia*)

  a. To test arithmetic ability, ask "Have you noticed any trouble making change?" or "Do you balance your checkbook?"

  b. Follow up by asking "If you gave a cashier a dollar for a seven-cent item, how much change should you get?" Ask the patient to continue to subtract sevens serially from the previous answer: "What is ninety-three minus seven?" then, "What is eighty-six minus seven," etc.

5. Testing the patient's fund of information
Mentally healthy persons know what's going on in the city, state, nation, and world. The introductory chitchat will

disclose much about the patient's fund of information. If not, at some appropriate point, ask about some general newsworthy event to test the patient's awareness. Ask the patient "Do you read the newspapers every day? What's happening that particularly interests you?" If the patient flounders, ask questions such as "What is the president trying to do?" or, more bluntly, "Who is the president?" or to name previous presidents or recent events that everyone should know about.

6. Testing for lack of insight, judgment, and planning
   a. If the sensorium is working properly, the patient's insight, judgment, and planning will match the real circumstances. Simply ask for the patient's future plans. Ask what the patient intends to do for the next several hours or for the next several days, months, or years.
   b. From the answers, you can judge whether the patient has the insight to recognize the presence of the illness, to understand the need for medical care, and to realize how the illness affects future plans. Judge whether the patient appreciates the effect of the illness on life activities, such as walking, returning to work, or driving. Judge whether the patient's plans realistically match the patient's mental or physical capabilities and prognosis.
   c. Formal tests of judgment include asking how the patient would handle commonplace events: "What would you do if you found a letter on the sidewalk?" or "What would you do if you discovered a fire in a crowded theater?"

V. **An Ethics, Values, and Spiritual History**
Management decisions need to take into account the patient's general philosophy, values, and spiritual beliefs. Although you should learn about the patient's beliefs, you should listen to them nonjudgmentally, avoiding debate or proselytizing (see Chapter 14, section VI, D).

VI. **Special Features of the History in Suspected Dementia**
A. Changes reported by the patient's family

1. Usually, the family brings in an elderly person whom they suspect of declining mentality because "Grandpa just doesn't act like himself anymore."
2. The history will disclose that the patient has become forgetful, socially inappropriate, negativistic, childish, unable to make judgments, and irritable or apathetic (Albert and Knofel, 1994; Christensen, 2004; DeMyer, 2004; Lesser et al., 2005). The patient typically is worse at night than during the day.
3. Frequently, the family will note that the patient has "aged" rapidly over the last few months. Ask about physical changes, such as lack of facial expression, small steps, loss of balance, tremor, dysarthria, word searching, poverty of thought, and recent changes in habits (Christensen, 2004).
4. Remember, too, when questioning family members that they will have become perplexed or dramatically saddened by the transformation of the vibrant person they once knew into a demented stranger.

> The mother I knew has died and I do not know the woman who has taken her place.
>
> —Marc Agronin (see Agronin, 2007)

B. Scoring the patient's mental status
   1. If the history suggests brain disease, the physician may complete a formal screening test, such as the Mini-Mental State Examination (Dick et al., 1984; Folstein et al., 1975; Grigoletto et al., 1999). A somewhat longer test is the Halstead-Reitan test for cerebral dysfunction (DeMyer, 2004; Jarvis and Barth, 1984; Reitan and Wolfson, 1993).
   2. After the mental status history and the screening tests provide a preliminary appraisal at the bedside, you have to decide whether the patient requires an extensive neuropsychological battery (see section III, E of this chapter). For an extensive compilation of rating scales and measures for psychiatric illness, see Rush et al. (2008).

VII. A Historical Tutorial with Rufus of Ephesus
Now that you understand the mental status and psychosocial history, I urge you to take the time to read the treatise by Rufus of Ephesus, entitled "Interrogation of the patient" (reproduced

in Brock, 1929). It deals with many of the principles that we use today and will give you a marvelous feeling of the continuity of yourself and the founders of our profession, which nothing else can duplicate. It will give you one of the best experiences of your whole medical education.

VIII. **Summary**

A. The mental status examination is not a special rite but emerges naturally by weaving in the required questions at opportune moments during the regular clinical history. Follow all of the rules: maintain privacy and confidentiality, ask all questions nonjudgmentally, introduce each area to be examined by an open question followed by direct questions as indicated. Don't insult the patient by a barrage of disconnected questions that have simplistic answers. If the patient truly has organic defects and realizes them, the machine-gun approach riddles the patient's dignity as bullet after bullet strikes the target. The patient may feel obliged to apologize or may even break into tears.

B. You can screen the patient's overall mental health quickly and efficiently by asking about several psychosocial items (Table 9–2). Explore the possibility of depression by asking directly about the patient's mood and general feeling about life. If the screening questions suggest a mental disorder, continue with more detailed inquiries according to Tables 9–3 to 9–8 and formal neuropsychological tests.

C. Much of the information to evaluate the patient's sensorium (e.g., orientation to time, place, and person; memory and judgment; and insight and planning) emerges incidentally during the ordinary questioning of the clinical history. If the physician uses the correct technique of questioning, the patient experiences the whole process as an ordinary conversation, not an inquisition. In an emergency, however, the physician can screen the patient's sensorium by a series of simple *who, where, when,* and *what's happening* questions (Table 9–4).

> Rule 1 for the mental status examination: Technique and timing are all important.

> Rule 2: If not an emergency, do not press to learn too much too fast.

References

Albert ML, Knofel JE. Clinical Neurology of Aging, 2nd ed. New York: Oxford University Press, 1994.

Agronin ME. Roots. CNS news topics in geriatrics, August 2007 (http://www.cnsnewsonline.com).

American Sleep Disorders Association. International Classification of Sleep Disorders, revised. Diagnostic and coding manual. Rochester, MN: ASDA, 1997, p 15–17.

Anderson DL, Spratt EG, Macias MM, et al. Use of the pediatric symptom checklist in the pediatric neurology population. Pediatr Neurol 1999; 20:116–120.

Barber ME, Marzuk PM, Leon AC, et al. Aborted suicide attempts: a new classification of suicidal behavior. Am J Psychiatry 1998;155:385–389.

Brock AJ, ed. Appendix I: On the interrogation of the patient in Greek Medicine: Being Extracts Illustrative of Medical Writers from Hippocrates to Galen. London: JM Dent & Sons, 1929, p 114.

Carlat DJ. The Psychiatric Interview: A Practical Guide, 2nd ed. Philadelphia: Lippincott Williams & Wilkins, 2005.

Cepeda C. Concise Guide to the Psychiatric Interview of Children and Adolescents. Washington DC: American Psychiatric Publishing, 2000.

Chambliss LR. Letter to the editor. N Engl J Med 2007;357:2310.

Chokroverty S. Sleep Disorders Medicine: Basic Science, Technical Considerations, and Clinical Aspects. Boston: Butterworth-Heinemann, 1994.

Christensen RC. Assessing new-onset mental status changes in patients with dementia. Am J Emerg Med 2004;22:228–229.

Cipolotti L, Warrington EK. Neuropsychological assessment. J Neurol Neurosurg Psychiatry 1995;(Suppl):655–664.

Cordoni B. Psychoeducational assessment for learning disabilities. J Child Neurol l995;(Suppl):31–35.

DeMyer WE. Technique of the Neurologic Examination, 5th ed. New York: McGraw-Hill, 2004.

Diagnostic and Statistical Manual of Mental Disorders, 4th ed. Washington DC: American Psychiatric Association, 2000.

Dick JPR, Guiloff RJ, Stewart A, et al. Mini-Mental State Examination in neurological patients. J Neurol Neurosurg Psychiatry 1984;47:496–499.

Fennell EB. The role of neuropsychological assessment in learning disabilities. J Child Neurol 1995;(Suppl):36–41.

Flaherty EG, Sege R. Barriers to physician identification and reporting of child abuse. Pediatr Ann 2005;34:349–356.

Folstein MF, Folstein SE, McHugh PR. "Mini-Mental State": a practical method for grading the cognitive state of patients for the clinician. J Psychiatr Res 1975;12:189–198.

Giardino AP, Finkel MA. Evaluating child sexual abuse. Pediatr Ann 2005; 34:382–394.

Gorbien MF, ed. Elder Abuse and Neglect. Clinics in Geriatric Medicine. Philadelphia: WB Saunders, 2005.

Greenspan SI, Greenspan NT. The Clinical Interview of the Child, 3rd ed. Washington DC: American Psychiatric Publishing, 2003.

Grigoletto F, Zappalà G, Anderson D. Norms for the Mini Mental State Examination in a healthy population. Neurology 1999;53:315–320.

Heilman KM, Valenstein D. Clinical Neuropsychology, 4th ed. New York: Oxford University Press, 2003.

Hibbard R, Desch LW. Maltreatment of children with disabilities. Pediatrics 2007;119:1018–1025.

Hirschfeld MA, Russell JM. Assessment and treatment of suicidal patients. N Engl J Med 1997;337:910–915.

Horner G. Physical abuse: recognition and reporting. J Pediatr Health Care 2005;19:4–11.

Jaffee KD, Epling JW, Grant W, et al. Physician-identified barriers to intimate partner violence screening. J Women's Health 2005;14:713–729.

Jarvis PE, Barth JT. Halstead-Reitan Test Battery: An Interpretive Guide. Odessa, FL: Psychological Assessment Resources, 1984.

Jones R, Barton S. Introduction to history taking and principles of sexual health. Postgrad Med J 2004;80:444–446.

Kurrie S. Abuse of the elderly. Aust Fam Physician 1992;21:1742–1748.

Lesser JM, Hughes SV, Jemelka JR, et al. Compiling a complete clinical history in the elderly: challenges and strategies for taking a comprehensive history in the elderly. Geriatrics 2005;60:22–25.

Mathews DD, ed. Child Abuse Sourcebook. Detroit: Omnigraphics, 2004.

Minsky-Kelly D, Hamberger LK, Pape DA, et al. We've had training, now what? Qualitative analysis of barriers to domestic violence screening and referral in a health care setting. J Interpers Violence 2005;20: 1288–1309.

Reitan RM. Aphasia and Sensory-Perceptual Deficits in Adults. Tucson: Reitan Neuropsychology Laboratories, 1984.

Reitan RM, Wolfson D. The Halstead-Reitan Neuropsychological Test Battery: Theory and Clinical Interpretation, 2nd ed. Tucson: Neuropsychology Press, 1993.

Rush AJ Jr, First MB, Blacker D. Handbook of Psychiatric Measures, 2nd ed. Washington DC: American Psychiatric Publishing, 2008.

Schramm E, Hohagen F, Grasshoff U, et al. Test–retest reliability and validity of the structured interview for sleep disorders according to DSM-III-R. Am J Psychiatry 1993;150:867–872.

Selzer ML. The Michigan alcoholism screening test. Am J Psychiatry 1971;127:1653.

Shea SC. The Practical Art of Suicide Assessment: A Guide for Mental Health Professionals and Substance Abuse Counselors. New York: John Wiley, 1999.

Simon RI, Hales RE, eds. The American Psychiatric Publishing Textbook of Suicide Assessment and Management. Washington DC: American Psychiatric Publishing, 2006.

Simon RI, Shuman DW. Retrospective Assessment of Mental States in Litigation. Washington DC: American Psychiatric Publishing, 2002.

Strauss E, Sherman EMS, Spreen O. A Compendium of Neuropsychological Tests. Administration, Norms, and Commentary, 3rd ed. New York: Oxford University Press, 2006.

Trzepacz PT, Baker RW. The Psychiatric Mental Status Examination. New York: Oxford University Press, 1993.

Weinberg WA, Harper CR, Brumback RA. Use of symbol language and communication battery in the physician's office for assessment of higher brain functions. J Child Neurol 1995;10(Suppl 1):S23–S31.

White P, ed. Biopsychosocial Medicine: An Integrated Approach to Understanding Illness. New York: Oxford University Press, 2005.

Woods NF, Heitkemper M, eds. Woman's Health. Philadelphia: WB Saunders, 2004.

The Pregnancy and Developmental History (for Pediatric Patients)

10

I. Introduction to the Developmental History

A. Threefold goals of the developmental history

1. To disclose risk factors for the infant's brain by reviewing the pedigree, pregnancy, perinatal events, and postnatal illnesses of the infant or child

2. To disclose whether the infant or child's psychomotor development matches or lags behind the normal timetable

3. To disclose any parental worries or concerns about the infant's development and to learn about the child-rearing practices and expectations of the parents

B. Glossary of developmental stages (Table 10–1)

Table 10–1. Definitions and Durations of Developmental Stages

I. Developmental stages and duration
   A. Conceptus: all derivatives of a fertilized ovum from time of conception to birth, including the membranes
   B. Embryo: conception to 8 weeks
   C. Fetus: 8 weeks to birth (whether full term or not)
   D. Neonate: birth (whether premature or not) to 4 weeks
   E. Infant: 4 weeks to 2 years
   F. Toddler: stage of walking with short steps, broad based gait, and semi-flexed arms, during the second year of life
   G. Child: 2 years to puberty

II. Definition of stages of maturity as estimated by birth weight
   A. Immature: 500–999 g (12 oz to 2.2 lb)
   B. Premature: 1000–2499 g (2.2–5.5 lb)
   C. Mature: >2500 g (5.5 lb or more)

III. Definition of time of birth in relation to normal term of 41 weeks
   A. Preterm: born before completion of week 37 (259 days of gestation)
   B. Term: born between the beginning of week 38 of gestation and the end of week 41 (260–287 days)
   C. Postterm: born any time after the beginning of week 42 (after 288 days of gestation)

IV. Definition of gestational, chronologic, and developmental (maturational) ages
   A. Gestational age: age of the embryo or fetus as dated from the time of conception or the last menstrual period
   B. Chronological age: age of an individual as dated from the time of birth, irrespective of gestational age at birth
   C. Developmental age: functional age of the patient as determined by formal testing of abilities and comparison with normal infants

Table 10–2. Outline of the Developmental History

I. Fertility and health history of the mother before and during pregnancy
II. Ultrasound examinations and quickening
III. Labor and delivery
IV. Neonatal history: spontaneous breathing and feeding, Apgar scores
V. Developmental timetable, ages birth to 5 years
    A. Motor
    B. Sensory
    C. Mental/social (psychosocial)
VI. Scholastic timetable, ages 5–18 years
VII. Puberty

C. Outline of the developmental history (Table 10–2)
D. Setting for the pregnancy and developmental history
    1. Insure privacy during this part of the history because you probe the mother's reproductive and sexual past for risk factors that may have harmed the infant or child (Table 10–3).
    2. The mother may not want to disclose this information in the presence of her male partner or children old enough to understand. The mother knows much more about the infant than the father and can relay it more freely in private. Of course, you must also question the father at some point, either with or without the mother present; usually you will discuss the management with both parents present.
    3. Insure that you ask questions and accept the responses nonjudgmentally. Questions about the pregnancy, reproduction, and health of the baby can easily translate into accusations that invoke feelings of guilt and resistance.
        a. Ask "Have you been pregnant before? What was the outcome?" not "Have you had any abortions?"
        b. Ask "Was the baby planned?" not "Was the pregnancy an accident?"
        c. Ask "Have you had sex with other partners?" not "Have you been sexually promiscuous?"
    4. Topics to ask about in the routine pregnancy and developmental history
        a. Previous pregnancies and their outcome, including miscarriages, spontaneous or induced abortions, or stillbirths. The mother's responses will disclose much about her general attitude toward children and in particular about whether she wanted and has accepted

Table 10–3. Factors that Cause or Statistically Correlate with Increased Risk of Brain Dysfunction in Infants and Children

---

I. Prenatal factors which cause or statistically correlate with risk of brain dysfunction
  A. Family history of consanguinity, hereditary degenerative or metabolic neurologic disorders, previous sibs with cerebral palsy or mental retardation, or parental mental retardation
  B. History of pregnancy wastage or prolonged infertility
  C. Male sex
  D. Maternal age less than 20 or over 29 years if white and less than 30 or over 39 years if black, menarche after 14 years (Broman et al., 1975)
  E. Small maternal stature
  F. Maternal systemic illness: anemia, malnutrition, and diabetes
  G. Maternal history of smoking, street drugs, or alcoholism
  H. Maternal ingestion of anticonvulsant drugs and other prescription drugs (see www. nvp-volumes.org/p2_4.htm)
  I. Extreme maternal obesity or malnutrition
  J. Eclampsia or HELLP syndrome
  K. Multiple fetuses
  L. Chromosomal aberrations: excesses of genetic material, translocations, and deletions
  M. Aminoacidurias, organic acidurias
  N. Large family
  O. Low socioeconomic class
  P. Severe psychosocial and emotional stress (Lou et al., 1994) or child abuse
II. Perinatal factors which cause or statistically correlate with risk of brain dysfunction
  A. Prematurity, premature rupture of membranes, or postmaturity
  B. Bleeding or prolonged labor
  C. Breech presentation
  D. Birth injury, skull fracture, subdural hematoma, and intracranial hemorrhage
  E. Low birth weight for gestational age or excessive birth weight for gestational age
  F. Persistently low Apgar score
  G. Respiratory distress, hypoxia, cyanosis
  H. Convulsions, persistent tremor, or extreme irritability
  I. Hyperbilirubinemia
  J. Congenital infections: toxoplasmosis, cytomegalovirus, herpes, syphilis, and AIDS
  K. Prolonged hypoglycemia or hypothermia
  L. Poor sucking or inability to feed
  M. Extreme hypotonia
  N. Craniofacial or multiple extracephalic malformations
III. Postnatal factors which cause or statistically correlate with risk of brain dysfunction
  A. Social and emotional deprivation (developmental timetable of young infants is mainly biological rather than environmental)
  B. Inattentive, unreactive baby who never makes demands and is "too good" or is the opposite, implacably irritable
  C. Battered child or other head trauma, particularly if it caused loss of consciousness
  D. Myoclonic seizures and other forms of epilepsy
  E. Delayed developmental milestones
  F. Delayed or poor vocalizations or speech
  G. Disordered sleep pattern and appetite
  H. Failure to thrive
  I. Malnutrition
  J. Repeated hospitalizations, especially three or more
  K. Meningitis/encephalitis
  L. Lead intoxication

Based in part on, but updated from, Broman et al. (1975).

the new baby. The presence of another person will inhibit the free expression of these feelings.

   b. Postpartum depression with previous births

   c. Use of prescription or street drugs and alcohol during the pregnancy

   d. Previous exposure to venereal disease, particularly syphilis, AIDS, and herpes, which might infect the neonate

   e. Ask whether the putative father is the biological father of the child. You must know that before charting the family pedigree (see Chapter 8).

   f. Ask about abuse of the mother herself or the child by the male partner (see Chapter 9, section II, D; also see American College of Obstetricians and Gynecologists, 2008).

5. Equally important as a reason for privacy, the mother may harbor feelings about her baby that she cannot disclose to anyone other than her physician. The most powerful abreaction I have encountered in over 50 years of practice evolved this way:

Pt 13: The mother came to me for another opinion about her infant's diagnosis and prognosis. The infant, a 23-month-old male, born prematurely at 32 weeks of gestation, had suffered severe neonatal hypoxia, convulsions, and intraventricular hemorrhage. He had made essentially no developmental progress and showed no social interactions. He had daily convulsions in spite of all medications. He had a tracheostomy and was fed by gastrostomy. He had microcephaly and spastic quadriparesis. Magnetic resonance imaging (MRI) showed severe polycystic porencephaly involving the entire cerebrum. He could not fixate or follow with his eyes; could not sit, stand, or speak; and made no movements that could be considered voluntary. He would startle to sound and withdrew his extremities reflexly from a noxious stimulus. He responded with fretful, high-pitched cries to touch or movement. He had no potential for any development, and the mother, after struggling with the problems daily for 2 years, realized the hopeless outlook.

I interviewed the mother, a 22-year-old single woman, in private. I asked her sister, who accompanied her, to remain in the waiting area with the infant because I knew that the fretful infant and even the sister would be a distraction during the history. Since his birth, the mother had devoted almost every waking moment to the patient, denying herself any other life or activities, like many grief- or guilt-stricken mothers. The history proceeded uneventfully until near the end, when I asked about previous pregnancies. She replied, "Yes. One other time, I was pregnant when I was 17." I asked, "What was the outcome?" She said almost matter-of-factly, "I had an abortion." She then paused and blanched. Her composure evaporated as an abreaction overwhelmed her. She then painfully whispered, "I . . . I . . . th . . . think, maybe, I think maybe I k . . . k . . . killed the wrong one." And then, fully realizing the implications of that judgment, she lapsed into a catatonic state of silent grief, too profound for tears. Finally, she began to sob, immense voiceless sobs, too profound for sound, thus experiencing the catharsis. forecast by Hawthorne in the *Scarlet Letter* (1919, p 127) when "...the soul of the sufferer [will] be dissolved and flow forth in a dark but transparent stream." I held her hands, in silence, for several minutes, until she regained enough composure to speak again.

The conflict between her image of herself as a nurturing mother, her feelings of rejection of the severely impaired infant, and the thought that the aborted baby might have been normal overwhelmed her. I arranged for her sister to spend the rest of the day and the night with her. I made an appointment for her to return the next day, to learn how she was faring and to complete the medical aspects of her visit.

The catharsis marked a turning point in her life. She ultimately began to cope with her feelings, obtained day care for her boy in a nursing home, and started school to learn a career. In the privacy of the consulting room, free from attending to the moment-to-moment demands of the infant and from censuring her thoughts because of a third party in the room, she attended to her real feelings and needs. She had given expression to the most profound feelings of her life and crossed a beneficent bridge to her physician.

Suppose I had conducted my interview with the sister present or anyone who might not have known of the mother's previous pregnancy, or suppose she had had to attend constantly to the fretful baby during the interview, giving only half of her mind to her own feelings and needs.

A second example of the revelation of true feelings during a private interview was another mother who said in despair about her retarded hyperactive, oppositional, hyperaggressive 3-year-old child, "I think they gave me the wrong one when I left the hospital after he was born." Then, the mother quickly flushed as she added, "You didn't hear me say that," realizing the depth of her rejection of the child. I will reiterate a previous statement: Unless you conduct private interviews, you will never understand their importance and you will never know what you have missed.

E. The battered or sexually abused child

The private interview with the mother becomes especially important to pursue suspicions about physical or sexual abuse of children or herself (American College of Obstetricians and Gynecologists, 2008). Recognition of either physical or sexual abuse requires particular attention as to how and whom to interview and when to notify law enforcement. Conduct private interviews with each adult involved and determine the state of the couple's relationship to each other and to the child. Remember that the mother may be in denial or unable to face the realities. (For a general discussion and references on intrafamily abuses, see Chapter 9, section II, D.)

II. Reproductive History

A. Fertility history

1. Open question: "Did you have any problem getting pregnant?"
2. Closed questions:
   a. Menarche and regularity of periods
   b. Assisted fertilization or implantation
   c. Previous pregnancies and outcomes: miscarriages, stillbirths, or premature births
   d. Contraceptive methods

B. Screening the pregnancy history when the patient is a seemingly normal infant or young child

If the infant seems developmentally normal, ask the mother several screening questions about the pregnancy, delivery, and neonatal period.

1. Open question: "How was your health during the pregnancy?"
2. Closed questions:

     a. Prenatal care

     b. Diet, weight gain, and morning sickness

     c. Spotting or vaginal bleeding

     d. Uterine cramping/premature labor

     e. Systemic illnesses: diabetes mellitus, thyroid disease, hypertension

     f. Use of prescription or street drugs, tobacco, or alcohol

     g. Work history/toxic exposure

     h. Radiation exposure

     i. Onset of quickening and its persistence

     j. Mental status during pregnancy and attitude toward the new baby

     k. Outcome of previous pregnancies

C. Extended pregnancy history when the physician suspects a brain disorder of prenatal or perinatal origin

  1. The concept of risk factors for the infant's brain

     a. If a brain disorder is suspected, the physician has to consider a range of risk factors that can act during intrauterine development or perinatally. The mother and the developing embryo and fetus constitute a delicate ecological system. The nervous system has countless types of neurons, each with its own particular structure, metabolic requirements, and schedule of development. In contrast, muscle, liver, and other organs have at most a few types of parenchymal cells. Each population of neurons goes through critical metabolic stages, a determination period, that make those particular neurons susceptible to given teratogens; hence, numerous agents can impair brain development (Broman et al., 1975; Carey and Bamshad, 2003; Diav-Citrin and Koren, 2000; Koren, 1990; Lou et al., 1994) (see Table 10–3).

     b. Many factors in Table 10–3 directly impair the developing brain, while others statistically correlate with impaired function but do not necessarily directly cause it. For example, alcohol can cause direct fetal brain damage by its pharmacological effect. Thus, it acts as a proximate cause that justifies defining fetal alcohol effects as a syndrome or disease (see the definitions of "disease" and "syndrome" in Chapter 2). Contrarily, low socioeconomic class statistically correlates with a lower intellectual performance on the average but per se does not constitute a proximate cause of overt brain damage. Correlation is not necessarily causation.

c. We lack comprehensive data on the effect of teratogens on sperm, but agents that may alter germ cells of either sex may cause a defective brain.

2. Identification of risk factors—genetic, endogenous, or exogenous—provides the basis for preventive counseling. If the risk factor is not preventable, the parents can at least decide, on the basis of informed consent, whether to risk having other children. Use Table 10–3 to extend the history to search for causes of early brain impairment.

III. **Labor and Delivery History**

A. Open question: "Tell me about the birth of [Denise]." Remember the three P's that influence the outcome at delivery: the Powers, the Passageway, and the Passenger. The *powers* are the uterine and abdominal contractions, the *passageway* means the pelvic outlet, and the *passenger* refers to the characteristics of the infant. Malformed or grossly defective infants are more likely than normal infants to present abnormally and to have difficult deliveries. Brain damage then may be falsely attributed to the difficult delivery rather than correctly to a defective fetus.

B. Closed questions

1. Duration of the pregnancy: Was the baby immature, premature, mature (term), postmature? The normal duration of pregnancy is 38–42 weeks (Table 10–1).

2. Spontaneous or induced delivery, vaginal, or C-section

3. Duration of labor: time from onset of labor to delivery

4. Presentation: cephalic, breech, or transverse

5. Presence of quickening movements of the fetus

6. Some common complications of labor:

a. Premature rupture of membranes. Ask "When did your water break?"

b. Placenta previa

c. Fetal distress, slowing of the fetal pulse

d. Meconium staining

e. Arrest of labor and failure of progression

7. Question the mother about previous pregnancies and their outcome.

IV. Neonatal History

A. Open question: "How did [Denise] do immediately after birth?"

Then ask specifically whether the baby breathed and fed spontaneously or required any special efforts to breathe and feed.

B. Closed questions:

1. Neonatal distress

a. Ask whether the infant required support to breathe or feed, whether hospitalization in a neonatal intensive care unit was required and what had to be done and for how long, whether the neonate required only oxygen supplementation or intubation.

b. Meconium staining of amniotic fluid

c. Apgar score

d. Seizures

e. Jaundice

f. Meningitis or encephalitis

g. Duration of time in special care nursery or hospital

2. Find out whether the birth weight and birth occipitofrontal circumference (OFC) were small, appropriate, or large for gestational age.

a. The OFC is the single most important dimension of the infant at any age (DeMyer, 1999, 2007), and body weight is the second most important.

b. Prematurity and low birth weight from any cause are common risk factors for brain impairment. The effect of prematurity may range from overt developmental retardation, seizures, and cerebral palsy to minimal behavioral or learning disabilities. Prematurity carries the risk of anoxia, intraventricular hemorrhage, periventricular leukomalacia, sepsis and meningitis, feeding and breathing difficulties, retinopathy of prematurity (and its extreme form, retrolental fibroplasia), metabolic imbalance, and nutritional deficiencies.

c. The overweight neonate with its larger body and head also has a greater risk for brain impairment than the normal–birth weight infant (DeMyer, 1999; Babson et al., 1969).

3. Ask about feeding, appetite, and weight gain.

V. **Classification of Infant Behaviors for Judging the Neurodevelopmental History and the Neurodevelopmental Examination**
  A. Four types of infant behavior
    For this discussion, I define *behavior* as any observable change produced by nerve impulses acting on an effector (a gland or a muscle). Thus, crying is a behavior, as is the pupillary reaction to light. Various behaviors appear or disappear according to a definite timetable (Gesell and Amatruda, 1965). They should not appear before or persist after their genetically and environmentally programmed times. The four types of behaviors based on time of appearance are as follows:
    1. Inborn behaviors that should be present at birth and that should persist
    2. Inborn behaviors present at birth and that should disappear
    3. Inborn behaviors not present at birth and that should appear
    4. Volitional and learned behaviors that should appear, dependent on environmental exposures, such as language, toilet training, social graces, and reading
  B. Inborn behaviors present at birth and that should persist
    Some inborn behaviors, such as breathing, pupillary light reflexes, and muscle stretch reflexes, should persist during the person's entire life. They do not depend on psychosocial development or intelligence. A baby with gross defects in the cerebrum, such as anencephaly or hydranencephaly, may display these behaviors.
  C. Inborn behaviors present at birth and that should disappear (Table 10–4)
    Behaviors that persist after they should have disappeared indicate developmental impairment. For example, the grasp reflex of the newborn should decrease during the first several weeks. Persistent fisting and a persistently strong grasp reflex imply deficiency of the corticofugal tracts. Similarly, the Moro reflex and the asymmetric tonic neck reflex should disappear by around 6 months. Persistence of these primitive reflexes predicts poor motor control.
  D. Inborn behaviors not present at birth and that should appear
    Delay in the inborn behaviors that should appear is always ominous. For example, the pursuit of moving objects by the

199

Table 10–4. Timetable (gestational age) for Appearance and Disappearance of Automatisms and Reflexes in Normal Infants

Reflex or Automatism	Appearance	Disappearance
Sucking	2–3 fetal months	Several months
Rooting	2–3 fetal months	3–4 months
Pupillary	6–7 fetal months	Persists
Doll's eye movements	6–7 fetal months	1 month
Tonic neck	6–7 fetal months	6–7 months
Neck righting	7–8.5 fetal months	9–12 months
Moro	7 fetal months	4–6 months
Traction	8–9 fetal months	4–6 months
Palmar grasp	4–6 months	5–6 months
Plantar grasp	4–6 fetal months	9–12 months
Crossed extension	5–6 fetal months	Persists
Positive supporting	8–9 fetal months	2–3 months
Automatic stepping	8–9 fetal months	3–4 months
Placing	8–9 fetal months	up to 1 year

baby's eyes, eye–hand coordination, head and trunk supporting responses, and the parachute response should appear at specific times (Table 10–5).

E. Volitional and learned behaviors that should appear
Most important for assaying development are the volitional behaviors that should appear according to the developmental timetable, such as sitting, imitative babbling, walking, and

Table 10–5. Timetable for Behaviors that Should Appear After Birth in Normal Infants

Behavior	Time of appearance
Breathing, sucking, swallowing	Present by birth
Smiling	4–6 weeks
Supports head in upright position	6 weeks
Fixation plus pursuit by the eyes	6 weeks
No head lag when pulled upright	4 months
Hands together in the midline	4 months
Transfers hand to hand	6–7 months
Sitting unsupported, at least briefly	6–7 month
Pulls up to standing	9 months
Parachute response	9–10 months
Cruising (walking holding on)	10–11 months
Walking	12 months
Talking (single words)	12 months
Pincer grasp	12 months
Running (stiff legged, toddler gait)	16–18 months
Runs well	24 months

talking. Developmentally abnormal infants will fail in some degree to achieve the new behaviors, reflex and volitional, that should develop after birth and will tend to retain those inborn behaviors that should disappear.

VI. **Attending to the Mother's Concern About Her Infant's Development**
   A. The transition question
      1. Start the developmental history by asking the mother the most important question of all: "Do you think [Denise] is developing normally?" or "Is there anything about [Denise's] development that worries you?" Use the baby's name instead of referring to it as "the baby" or "it" (review Chapter 6, Section III, B, if you have forgotten the vignette).
      2. This question demonstrates to the mother that you value her opinions and observations, making her a peer of the physician in a developmental watching team. Most mothers, even if mentally ill, have a fair idea of the developmental level of their infant because they have read the "baby book" and have compared their infant to their previous children or the children of friends. On the other hand, you must learn whether the mother holds unrealistic opinions about her baby's development.
      3. Most mothers remember and can readily answer most of the standard questions about their child's development, even years later. If the mother cannot answer the main questions, such as when the infant walked and talked, consider whether she is emotionally detached from the infant or depressed.
   B. Responses to avoid in the developmental history
      1. The commonest complaint by mothers of retarded babies about the history is that they repeatedly mentioned their concerns but the physician either paid no attention or offered some platitude: "Oh the baby's just lazy" or "You just wait on him too much" or "Not all babies do things at the same time" or, the ultimate putdown, "Oh, you just worry too much." A comparable situation occurs when the physician states to an adult patient "There is nothing wrong with you. It's all in your mind." Consign those statements to the category of things never to be said.

After all, discovering parental worries about the child is one of the major goals of the developmental history. Of course, the mother expresses concern, curiosity, and even anxiety about her baby's development. It is a focal point of her whole life. The most important rule in the pediatric history is this: Listen to what the mother says and respond to her concerns.

2. Particularly with a stable, experienced mother who has raised several infants, you dismiss the problem as an "overanxious mother" at your peril. Most mothers are well versed in child development and accurate in their appraisal (Harris, 1994).

3. If the mother has unrealistic anxieties that persist, extending the history will generally disclose an underlying emotional problem, a frank mental illness, or a bad marriage. Consider the possibility of an abused mother or other domestic problems, and encourage the mother to express such problems to you or to a counselor.

VII. **The Developmental History for Infants from Birth to 2 Years of Age**
 A. Adjusting for prematurity
   To judge developmental progress during the baby's first year requires adjusting for prematurity. Do not judge the infant prematurely born at 34 weeks of gestational age as a 6-week-old when examined 6 weeks postnatally. Judge that infant as if it were a term infant (40–41 weeks). Premature delivery does not speed up development. Quite the contrary, the factors that cause prematurity may also impair the brain and thus retard development.
 B. Determine the current developmental level
   Having asked the mother an open question, "Do you feel that [Denise] is developing normally?" proceed to the specific questions that disclose the infant's motor, vocal, and social progression. After learning the baby's gestational and chronological age, determine whether the baby matches the norms listed in Tables 10–5 to 10–11 or in standard developmental texts (Bower, 1977).
 C. Motor timetable
  1. Table 10–5 and Figure 10–1 review the major motor milestones from birth to 1 year. Ask particularly about

hand use: opening of the fingers versus persistent fisting, hand-to-mouth actions, grasping, eye–hand coordination in reaching for objects, midline transfer of objects, and the pincer grasp.

2. Ask whether the infant uses both hands equally. The normal infant may show some preference for the future dominant hand, but consistent use of one hand and neglect of the other hand often indicates a "hemisyndrome," such as infantile hemiplegia. By turning over, sitting, and standing, the infant demonstrates normal trunk control (Table 10–5 and Fig. 10–1).

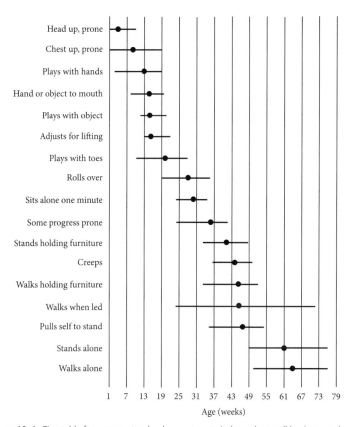

Figure 10–1. Timetable for gross motor development up to independent walking in normal infants. (Reproduced by permission from Bower TGR. A Primer of Infant Development. San Francisco: Freeman, 1977, fig. 6–1.)

Table 10–6. Timetable for Visual Development in Normal Infants

Visual function	Time
Brief fixation, crude OKN	Term birth
Fixation and pursuit	6 weeks
Plays with own fingers held in front of face	12 weeks
Eye–hand coordination: reaches for and holds toy	16 weeks
Recognizes strangers and cries if picked up	6 months+
Visual attention to more and more distant objects	6–12 months

D. Visual timetable
   Determine whether the infant's visual performance matches the timetable (Table 10–6).
E. Vocalization timetable
   1. At birth the infant can only cry. Ask the mother whether the infant's cry sounds normal in quantity and quality. Brain-impaired infants often have a scratchy, high-pitched, irritating cry. Various other disorders from hypothyroidism to *cri du chat*, or cat's cry, syndrome (chromosome 5 deletion) cause characteristic alterations in crying. Persistent inconsolable crying suggests a colicky baby and requires a detailed inquiry into the feeding practices, diet, and examination for gastroesophageal reflux. In the latter case, the infant cries after feeding.
   2. Ask whether the infant's vocalizations follow the normal sequence: crying at birth, then throaty sounds and cooing, followed by automatic babbling, then imitative babbling, and finally single-word speech that emerges at 1 year of age. Phrases and sentences appear by 18–24 months. Any failure to produce imitative babbling or delayed language development always requires investigation, first of all an evaluation of the infant's hearing (Table 10–7).
F. Hearing timetable
   1. Ask the mother "Does [Denise] react to ordinary sounds? Does she turn to your voice?" (see Table 10–8).
   2. Until 6 months of age, a deaf infant vocalizes much like a hearing one because the early vocalizations are inborn rather than learned behaviors.
   3. If the history suggests a hearing disorder, ask about risk factors (Table 10–9) and refer the infant for audiometry.
G. Feeding Timetable

Table 10–7. Timetable for Sequences of Vocalization and Expressive Language in Normal Infants

Vocalization	Age at appearance
Audible cry	32 weeks of gestational age
Organized crescendo–decrescendo cry	Term birth
Vocal grunts and small throaty sounds	1–6 weeks
Cooing sounds ("pleasure vocalizations")	6–16 weeks
Automatic babbling	3–6 months: "Goo-goo, "Ugh-Ugh," and "Ba-ba" sounds, consisting of consonants or consonant–vowel combinations
Imitative babbling (echolalia)	6 months: infant begins to imitate or feed back certain sounds made by parents
Prosody	6–12 months: infant jabbers with prosody (inflections, rhythms, and intonations), although without actual words
Combines syllables: "baba," "mama," etc.	8 months
Simple single words	12 months (8–13 months): uses "Mama" and "Dada" appropriately
Numerous single words and some word combinations	15–18 months
Simple sentences	24 months: uses meaningful sentences that reflect grammatical rules

Table 10–8. Timetable for Auditory Responses in Normal Infants

Auditopalpebral reflex	Neonatal period
Arrest of movement in response to sound	6 weeks and after
Turns to lateralized sound	16–24 weeks
Imitative babbling (*prima facie* evidence of hearing)	6 months and after
Single words (*prima facie* evidence of hearing)	12 months
Hands over toys on request or follows other simple requests	14 months

Table 10–9. Risk Factors for Impaired Hearing in Normal Infants and Children

Family history of deafness
Birth weight <1500 g
Congenital or perinatal infection: rubella, cytomegalovirus, herpes simplex, toxoplasmosis or syphilis
Bacterial meningitis/antibiotic therapy
Recurrent middle ear infections
Antibiotics
Hyperbilirubinemia
Severe asphyxia
Ear, jaw, and palatal malformations

Find out whether the mother breast-feeds, her attitude toward breast-feeding, and her understanding of the nutritional needs of infants. Breast-feeding generally extends through the first 5–6 months of life. Then, the mother introduces pureed food and cereals. Match the child's feeding history against Table 10–10.

H. Toileting timetable

1. Bowel control precedes bladder control. Bowel training becomes feasible at 18–24 months for some infants. By 30 months about 90% of girls and 75% of boys will defecate in a toilet. By 4 years of age 95% of normal children have achieved bowel training.

2. The frequency of bowel movements in normal children varies from several per day to one every 2 or 3 days.

3. Children achieve bladder control during the daytime prior to continence at night. About 50% of children have daytime control by 2 years and 95% by 5 years. About 66% of children achieve urinary continence at night by 3 years and 90% by 8–9 years.

I. Psychosocial timetable

1. Match the infant's socialization against Table 10–11.

Table 10–10. Timetable for Feeding Behavior in Normal Infants

Age (months)	Feeding behaviors	Food
0–2	Automatic sucking, rooting and swallowing, and tongue extension	Breast milk/formula per bottle
4–6	Head and neck balance improving, tongue more mobile	Single-grain cereal, usually rice, fortified with iron, mixed with milk
5–7	Biting and sucking reflexes fading, opens mouth to accept spoon or turns head to indicate preferences or satiety	Strained or pureed vegetables and then fruits
6–9	Grasps finger foods and gets hand to mouth, rotary chewing, teeth erupt	Continues strained or pureed fruits, vegetables, meats, and beans; will accept small pieces of food like cheese and meat
9–12	Sticks out tongue, spits, drinks from cup; wean from bottle or breast	Accepts range of table foods, meats, vegetables, starches, and raw peeled fruit
12–24	Expresses food preferences, can name some foods, begins to handle cup and utensils	Eats most of normal diet but may have temporary strong preferences

Table 10–11. Timetable for Psychosocial Responses in Normal Infants

Response	Time of Response
Crying	Neonatal period
Smiles (automatic at first, then social)	4–6 weeks
Laughing	3 months
Smiles at mirror	5 months
Expresses pleasure and displeasure and shows food preferences	6 months
Displeased if picked up by strangers	6 months and after
Responds to "No"	8 months
Plays patty-cake, peek-a boo, and bye-bye	8 months
Understands names of objects	12 months
Requests by pointing	15 months
Obeys several commands	18 months

2. Ask about the child-care arrangement and whether the father participates in the child's daily care.

3. Ask how the family members, especially siblings, react to the baby.

4. Sometimes the mother describes the baby as "too good," by which she means the baby lies passively for prolonged periods of time, interacting but little with caregivers or environmental stimuli. This history always raises the question of mental retardation or ultimately autism. Normal babies are interactive and clamorous and will fuss up a storm at times.

J. Response to handling

1. One of the most basic operations of parenting is to pick up the infant in order to cuddle, comfort, feed, and talk to him or her. In addition to other psychosocial responses, ask about the infant's response to handling: "How does [Denise] respond to being picked up?" Determine whether the baby is
   a. Cuddly, conformable, consolable
   b. Irritable and inconsolable
   c. Loose, floppy
   d. Stiff or fails to conform, particularly whether the head arches back (opisthotonic arching). The infant should also accept the supine position for diapering and bathing.

2. The brachial support response to vertical suspension
   a. When a person inserts hands in the infant's armpits to pick her or him up, the infant should reciprocate by tensing its upper arms for support.

b. Most babies will accept being picked up by anyone, including strangers, until about 6 months of age. After that they show an aversion to strangers.
3. Ask about smiling. Smiling is automatic at first, but reactive smiling should appear by 4 weeks. The often blank, seemingly nonsmiling face of the neonate provides no reinforcing feedback for mothering and can contribute to postpartum depression of the mother.

VIII. **The Developmental History for Children More Than 2 Years of Age**
A. Inquire about the major milestones for the first 2 years. The child of 2 years should feed itself, walk, run, respond socially, and speak in phrases and sentences. Concentrate more on these current developmental attainments rather than on precise details of earlier developmental milestones. The Capute scales cover the age range from birth to 3 years (Accardo and Capute, 2005). The Denver Developmental Screening Test II (Swaiman, 2006) assays the current developmental level of children from birth to 6 years of age, as does the Child Development Inventory to 5 years (Ireton and Glascow, 1995). These tests depend on parent reporting.
B. Screening questions to ask about the development of children 2–6 years of age
1. "Is the child's overall behavior within acceptable limits?"
2. "Does the child more or less easily follow the routines of the household and the limits you set?"
3. "How does the child respond to discipline? What kind of discipline do you use?"
4. "Does the child behave much differently with the two parents together, one parent, the grandparents, or at school?"
5. "Is the child hyperactive or laid back?"
6. "Does the child have a short attention span?"
7. "Does the child recognize and avoid danger?"
8. "Can the child play with other children and share toys?"
9. "Does the child have unusual fears or phobias?"
C. Psychosocial screening questions for mothers of school-age children

    1. Ask most of the foregoing questions and ask about nursery school, kindergarten, grade level, and whether any formal scholastic test scores are available.

    2. Has the child repeated grades or required special education?

    3. Is the mother satisfied with the school and the child's acceptance of the school?

    4. How does the teacher appraise the child's behavior on the report card?

    5. If school problems exist, ask the mother's permission to contact school authorities and to review school records.

    6. Does the child respond to discipline and reward?

    7. Does the child consistently lie and deny the obvious or blame others for transgressions?

    8. Ask whether the child is a fire-setter, is enuretic, is cruel to animals, or has an undue obsession for guns, knives, and violence. These characteristics predict a grim prognosis. A psychosocial screening checklist will assist in identifying aberrant psychosocial characteristics (Anderson et al., 1999).

D. Immunization history

Record the dates of immunizations, check on currency of immunizations, and make appointments for future immunizations for all infants and children. (For references to immunization schedules, see Chapter 11, section II, B.)

E. Extending the developmental history by quantitative determination of the child's developmental level

Rapin (1995) succinctly summarizes the tests and investigations to quantify the child's developmental level.

IX. Discussing Developmental Retardation with Parents

A. Avoid pejorative terms when taking the history

    1. When the history and physical examination disclose developmental retardation, generally avoid using the term "mentally retarded," which parents resent. Always ask the parents how they think the patient is developing. Ask how the infant's development compares with that of siblings or other children of the same age. The wise physician reviews the age-appropriate attainments and thus leads the parents to make their own judgments—in other words, offers the parents the opportunity to judge the evidence,

rather than declaiming an unfavorable diagnosis and prognosis. Then, the physician merely has to agree with the (astute) conclusions of the parents, rather than getting shot as the messenger who brings bad news.

2. The parent will often offer as an explanation that the infant doesn't walk because "We always carried him" or doesn't talk because "We always waited on him and anticipated everything he needed." Often, the parents have reversed cause and effect. They carried the infant all of the time because of his or her inability to walk, and they waited on the infant because of his or her inability to do things for him- or herself or express his or her wants verbally.

B. Gentle ways to speak about mental retardation

1. When the clinical workup discloses a brain condition that will cause retardation, I generally advise the parents "It appears that [Denise] has a brain problem that may affect her ability to develop," and then I go on to review the evidence for that concern from the history, physical findings, and laboratory workup. I often will show the parents the infant's MRI scan along with a normal one. The physician should keep all statements conditional, "It appears that . . ." or "I suspect that . . .," rather than dogmatic.

2. I point out to the parents that we have to be cautious about predicting the developmental potential for any infant and that the younger the child at the time of the examination, the less accurate the prediction. No matter how retarded the infant, one of the worst things the physician can do is to pronounce that the child is a hopeless vegetable and belongs in a nursing home because of no potential for development. Remember, with humility and grace, that prognosis is the most difficult of all of the arts of medicine. Even when the dire predictions are true, the parents need some time to discover the outcome for themselves. In the meantime, the physician provides support by saying, "Each time you bring [Denise] in for a routine visit we will carefully check on her developmental status." This statement allies the physician with the parent in observing what the infant actually will achieve.

3. Since the term "mental retardation" generates anxiety, clinicians try to soften it by using terms like "developmental

lag" and "developmental delay." Parents may misunderstand these terms because they suggest that, given time, the infant will catch up, whereas in fact the child my fall further and further behind. Indeed, often parents ask just that question, "When will [Denise] catch up?" I try to say things such as "[Denise] is somewhat behind the usual timetable" and then wait to see what terms the parents use as they come to realize that their child is retarded. A compassionate history that elicits the parents' attitudes is the best guide for the vocabulary the physician should use.

4. The physician may automatically assume that the parents devalue an overtly retarded or grossly deformed child. The physician may unwisely tend to speak of the child pejoratively, but the mother may have as strong a feeling of attachment for the defective child as for a normal one. In fact, she may become pathologically bonded to the child.

5. Address the child by name, gently, as a person because the mother will view her child, retarded or not, as a person.

6. Realize also that when conveying bad news, such as a severe heart or brain malformation or informing adults that they have cancer, the emotional turmoil may prevent patients from hearing much of what you are trying to say. patients' knowledge and understanding of what you have said and their grasp of the real circumstances need to be reviewed by gentle questioning as you go along and at subsequent visits.

7. Some patients request a tape recording of your discussion. I generally say, "Let's discuss the situation first, and then I will make a summary for you." This often produces better communication than recording a lengthy conversation verbatim.

X. Summary

A. The developmental history has three major goals:

1. To learn whether the infant or child has been exposed to any risk factors for the brain (Table 10–3)

2. To determine whether the infant is developing normally

3. To disclose any parental worries or concerns about the infant's development and the overall parental attitudes toward the infant

B. Precautions in the developmental history
The physician should insure privacy for questioning the mother about her reproductive and sexual history, infectious disease exposures (particularly venereal diseases), pregnancy loss, family history, and personal habits such as drug and alcohol use. Because of the profound emotional impact of many of these topics, the physician should phrase the questions circumspectly and respond nonjudgmentally.

C. Behavioral timetables
The behaviors of the fetus and infant should progress according to timetables. The physician must know which behaviors are present at birth and normally persist or disappear and which ones appear after birth and may persist or disappear. Tables 10–4 to 10–11 list the normal behavioral sequences, which the physician should review at each visit.

D. Always ask the mother how she thinks her infant is developing
Listen carefully to any concerns she may express. The first rule of the pediatric history is to listen to the mother. Never dismiss the mother's developmental concerns by a patronizing admonition such as "You worry too much" or "He will grow out of it." Address her concerns respectfully.

E. Avoid overtly pejorative terms like "mentally retarded" or "vegetable"
Adopt the terms the parents use as they come to realize that their child is retarded. The parents will soon enough discover where their child stands on the developmental scale. Do not adopt an adversarial position by declaiming a hopeless or abysmal prognosis. Instead, join with the parents to carefully watch and measure whatever development the child may actually show.

References

Accardo PJ, Capute, AJ. The Capute Scales: Cognitive Adaptive Test/Clinical/ Linguistic & Auditory Milestone Scale. Baltimore: Brooks, 2005.

American College of Obstetricians and Gynecologists. Violence against women, 2008 (http://www.acog.org/departments).

Anderson DL, Spratt EG, Macias MM, et al. Use of the Pediatric Symptom Checklist in the pediatric neurology population. Pediatr Neurol 1999; 20:116–120.

Babson SG, Henderson N, Clark WM. The preschool intelligence of over-sized newborns. Pediatrics 1969;44:536–538.

Bower TGR. A Primer of Infant Development. San Francisco: Freeman, 1977.

Broman SH, Nichols PL, Kennedy WA. Preschool IQ. Prenatal and Developmental Correlates. New York: John Wiley and Sons, 1975.

Carey C, Bamshad MJ. Clinical genetics and dysmorphology. In: Rudolph C, Rudolph AM (eds), Rudolph's Pediatrics, 21st ed. New York: McGraw-Hill, 2003.

DeMyer WE. Microcephaly, micrencephaly, megalocephaly, and megalencephaly. In: Swaiman K, Ashwal S (eds), Pediatric Neurology, 3rd ed. St. Louis: Mosby-Year Book, 1999.

DeMyer WE. Small, large, and abnormally shaped head. In: Maria BL (ed), Current Management in Child Neurology, 3rd ed. London: BC Decker, 2007.

Diav-Citin O, Koren G. Human teratogens: a critical evaluation. In: Koren G, Bishai R (eds), Nausea and Vomiting of Pregnancy: State of the Art 2000. Toronto: Motherisk, 2000 (www.nvp-volumes.org/p2_4.htm).

Gesell A, CS Amatruda. Developmental Diagnosis: Normal and Abnormal Child Development, 2nd ed. New York: Hoeber Medical Division, Harper & Row, 1965.

Harris SR. Parents' and caregivers' perceptions of their children's development. Dev Med Child Neurol 1994;36:918–923.

Hawthorne N. The Scarlet Letter. New York: Charles Scribner's Sons, 1919, p 127.

Ireton H, Glascow FP. Assessing children's development using parents' reports. The Child Development Inventory. Clin Pediatr 1995;343:248–255.

Koren G. Maternal–Fetal Toxicology. A Clinician's Guide. New York: Marcel Dekker, 1990.

Lou HC, Hansen D, Nordentoft M, et al. Prenatal stressors of human life affect fetal brain development. Dev Med Child Neurol 1994;36:826–832.

Rapin I. Physician's testing of children with developmental disabilities. J Child Neurol 1995;10(Suppl 1):S11–S15.

Swaiman K. General aspects of the patient's neurologic history. In: Swaiman KF, Ashwal S, Ferriero DM (eds), Pediatric Neurology: Principles and Practice. Philadelphia: Mosby Elsevier, 2006.

The Preventive History and Wellness

I. Importance of the Preventive History

A. Why the patient comes to the physician

Patients usually visit physicians because of an emergency, because of an overt feeling of illness, or to get a routine medical checkup, rather than specifically to anticipate and prevent future health problems (Baker, 1993; Kottke et al., 1993; Masterson, 1998; Wender and Nevin, 2002). Although third-party payers offer little incentive for it, prevention, as part of the overall management plan, constitutes one of the cornerstones of the medical model (see Fig. 4–1). Patients welcome inquiries into their overall functioning and well-being (Schor et al., 1995).

B. Components of a prevention plan

1. The regular history provides much of the information for a preventive program. Sox (1994) argues that preventive measures against disease should not depend primarily on exhaustive histories and head-to-toe physical examination. Instead, the physician should focus on selective screening for frequent or high-risk diseases. However, the person with a rare disease has as much right to a diagnosis and treatment as one with a common disease. Utilization of population statistics need not diminish the traditional emphasis on maximal benefit for each individual and the respect for each individual's health. When ill, none of us wants to be regarded as a population statistic. Unfortunately, even the early discovery of some serious illness may not lead to effective intervention (Welch, 1996).

2. A cornerstone of any prevention and wellness program for patients of any age is regularly scheduled visits to the physician. These visits cement the knowing relationship that serves the patient best and enables the physician to review the changing health needs at various ages and to incorporate other professionals such as dentists and audiologists in the overall health program.

II. Preventive History and Preventive Programs for Infants and Children

A. Monitor developmental progress

1. Check the developmental progress of the infant during regular "well baby" appointments. Chapter 10 reviews the developmental milestones to ask about.

2. Chart the height, weight, and occipitofrontal circumference regularly for infants and children.

3. If questions of physical or sexual abuse arise, see Chapter 9, section II, D.

B. Monitor immunization

Ask parents about immunizations and check against a standard schedule (Harrison, 2008; Heisler and Richmond, 1994; Rudolph and Rudolph, 2003; Centers for Disease Control and Prevention, 2008). The American Academy of Pediatrics keeps updated immunization schedules for infants and children as well as discussions of parental misconceptions about immunizations. (www.cispimmunize.org)·

C. Readiness for learning and school

1. Do regular physical examinations and formal screening tests for vision and hearing in infancy and in the preschool period.

2. Order formal tests for developmental delays and learning disability if the history suggests the need, in order to plan an appropriate educational program (see Chapter 10).

3. Ask about the ability of the child to separate from the mother and to engage in peer play.

4. Determine whether the infant needs a "First Steps" program or referral for occupational, physical, or speech therapy.

D. Environmental exposures

1. Question the parents about exposure to lead in toys or the environment. Simply knowing the patient's address, in an old neighborhood where lead paints have been used, is one clue.

2. Check on access of child to toxins and medications.

III. Preventive History and Preventive Programs for Adolescents and Teens

A. Major shifts in health risks arise during the teen years. Automobile accidents, sexually transmitted diseases, unwanted pregnancy, suicide, alcohol and drug use, and alienation from parents and school become major concerns (Borkowski and Weaver, 2006; Montalto, 2008, pp 10–22). Montalto (2008) lists twenty-four recommendations for preventive services for adolescents. The history and selected tests should probe for these factors. Again, privacy is often of critical importance in taking the history from teenagers (see Chapter 5, section I, E).

B. A relatively recent addition to the immunization schedule, recommended by the Centers for Disease Control and Prevention, now includes multiple injections beginning in females 11–12 years old to protect against the human papillomavirus and its threat of cervical cancer.

C. Ask whether the parents wish the physician to participate in teaching the child about safety practices such as seat belts and bicycle helmets and later about menstruation, reproduction, and drug use.

IV. Preventive History and Preventive Programs for Adults

A. Routine health care

1. Review plans for routine physicals; laboratory tests that screen for cardiovascular disease, diabetes, and cancer; as well as mammograms, chest radiographs, Pap smears, prostate and rectal examinations, colonoscopies, and infectious disease prevention (Lyons, 2008 pp 22–33). Table 11–1 summarizes the minimal routine preventive measures for adults, even though the history discloses no known risk factors (Sox, 1994). Beyond the routine measures, the extent of the investigation depends on the identification of risk factors by a careful history, including the family history.

2. Formal lists of preventive measures for particular categories of patients also prove useful (Dexter et al., 2001). For special preventive programs for females, see Rosenfeld (2001). The U.S. Department of Health and Human Services maintains updated recommendations for screening tests and immunizations (Centers for Disease Control and Prevention, 2008).

3. Routinely inquire about mood, depression, and suicidal ideation.

Table 11–1. Minimal Preventive and Wellness Measures for Adults (Particularly Those Past 40 Years of Age)

I. Men and women
  A. Periodic history and physical examination, including rectal examination/colonoscopy; review of diet, use of alcohol and other drugs, and smoking; and mental health review
  B. Blood pressure measurement
  C. Lipoprotein profile: total cholesterol, low-density lipoproteins, high-density lipoproteins, and triglycerides
  D. Diabetic screening
  E. Intraocular pressure measurements for glaucoma after the age of 40 years
  F. Immunizations: See updated recommendations of the American Academy of Pediatrics (www.cispimmunize.org) and the Centers for Disease Control (2008): pneumococcal pneumonia, influenza, hepatitis B, tetanus, diphtheria, rubella, and measles. Further immunizations tailored to foreign travel.
  G. Yearly dental examinations
  H. Aerobic fitness program
II. Women
  A. Breast examination, self to age 40 years and by physician after age 40
  B. Annual mammography after 50 years of age (age range still debatable)
  C. Cervical cytological screening (Pap smear), unnecessary after age 65 years
III. Men
  A. Rectal examination/prostrate cancer screening

B. Review diet and physical fitness programs
   Ask about fad diets and adequate calcium intake for women, and ask all patients about regular aerobic exercise.
C. Occupational disease prevention
   1. Survey the patient's work history and regularity of employment.
   2. Ask about occupational hazards and industrial exposures: air quality, organic solvents, lead, mercury, noise, and other physical hazards in the workplace and physical stresses on the body (Newman, 1995).
   3. Ask selected patients to describe a typical day at work.
D. Home hazard prevention
   1. Many of the questions that explore occupational disease prevention apply to home hazards in respect to possible toxic chemicals and pesticides.
   2. Fire alarm and fire prevention
   3. Firearm storage
   4. Quality of housing, heating, and water supply
E. Infectious disease prevention
   1. Determine whether measures such as antibiotic prophylaxis for bladder and ear infections, bacterial endocarditis, and rheumatic fever are indicated.

2. The elderly require immunization programs, as do younger individuals. A vaccine can prevent pneumococcal pneumonia, the third leading cause of death in individuals over 65 years of age, exceeded only by heart disease and cancer. The elderly also may need ad hoc flu vaccination.

3. Review the patient's knowledge of the transmission of venereal disease. If the patient has a venereal disease, the issue of partner notification arises as part of the management of treatment and prevention. To treat one partner for gonorrhea and not the other insures its recurrence. In notifying the patient's partners, the physician has to follow public-health laws and circumspection. North and Rothenberg (1993) point out the threat of violence to women whose partners learn that they have HIV/AIDS.

4. Counsel homosexuals about risks for infectious diseases and anogenital cancer (Makadon, 2006).

F. Accident prevention: seat belts for everyone, gun safety, helmets for bicycle or motorcycle riding, soccer, and football

G. Heredofamilial disease prevention

1. Prevention starts with a family history that searches for familial disorders. Newborn screening, which is mandatory in most states, detects a number of inborn disorders that, if identified, permit treatment (Khoury et al., 2003).

2. If the patient has a heredofamilial disease, offer to examine other family members and to provide genetic counseling, which may require referral to a geneticist (Rosenberg and Iannaccone, 1995). Physical examination may disclose signs of heredofamilial diseases, such as café au lait spots indicative of neurofibromatosis, or chemical or genetic tests may identify many other heredofamilial diseases.

3. The role of anticipatory genomic screening raises ethical questions as to their value and the effect on the individual. If one of your parents has Huntington chorea (an autosomal dominant disorder of adult onset), do you want to be tested at 20 years of age and learn that at 37 years you will start to twitch and become progressively demented, as you have already seen in one of your parents and the relatives of that parent? (See also Chapter 14, section II, G.)

H. Birth defect prevention

Ask whether prospective mothers and fathers realize that they should avoid ingestion of medications, street drugs, tobacco, and alcohol during the conception and pregnancy (Koren, 1990). Take an extended dietary history. Routine folic acid supplementation reduces neural tube defects (Czeizel and Dudas, 1992). Insure that the prospective mother understands the importance of prenatal care. Ask prospective mothers, before pregnancy, whether they have had immunizations against flu and rubella and have been tested for diabetes.

I. Disease prevention in the elderly

1. A person 65 or more years old qualifies as elderly, but physiological age and chronological age differ. A truism is that if you look 80 years old at 70, you probably won't reach 80.

2. Include in the history questions about inevitable difficulties in balance, gait, stair climbing, getting in and out of a bathtub, or simply flexing the thigh to put on a sock and shoe. Reduction in flexibility of the neck impairs the ability to look right and left at street intersections or to look backward. Rising after a fall becomes difficult.

3. Ask specifically about falling. Every elderly person falls at some time, making serious injury, a hip fracture or brain injury, an ever present threat, along with the other ever present threats of heart disease, stroke, cancer, and dementia (Richardson, 2008, pp 33–37). The elderly also realize that life is shutting down. If the history indicates one fall, others are likely. Balance and gait can be tested during free walking and by using a formal test: Get-Up-and-Go Test, Timed Get-Up-and-Go Test, and the Tinetti mobility scale. These tests can be accessed through Google. One simple predictor of a falling tendency or gait defect is to count how many times the patient has to try to elevate to a standing position from a sitting position on a chair or toilet stool by extending the thighs and legs. If the patient requires more than one trial to rise, a gait and balance disorder is highly probable; and two or more trials is a distinct warning.

4. Asking the elderly about these problems will establish immediate rapport: "Thank goodness, this doctor understands what I'm facing."

5. See www.preventiveservices@ahrq.gov for a ranking of evidence-based preventive measures. The principles are the same as for younger individuals, but the specific details differ in respect to immunization, types of cancer, disease

susceptibility, mental health, exercise, injury prevention, response to medications, and the likelihood of comorbidities.

6. Screening guidelines for cancer. The common cancers associated with, but not limited to, older individuals are breast, cervical, uterine, ovarian, prostate, and colorectal. Especially important is periodic colonoscopy screening for colorectal cancer, starting annually at 50 years and in increasing intervals thereafter. Colorectal cancer affects one in 18 persons over a lifetime. The American Cancer Society maintains updated guidelines for screening for all cancers (www.cancer.org).

J. Disease prevention in international travelers

1. Provide appropriate immunization and risk warnings to patients planning international travel. Focus the preventive practices for immigrants on the major diseases found in their land of origin.

2. Discuss jet lag prevention (Revell and Eastman, 2005). Workers who change from day to night also can learn how to more effectively shift their circadian rhythms. Effective management has safety and performance implications for the individual as well as the public.

3. For children adopted from abroad, insure routine screening tests for diseases such as tuberculosis, syphilis, cytomegalovirus, hepatitis B, HIV, and intestinal parasites (Elder et al., 2008 pp 38-45; Ericsson et al., 2004; Hostetter et al., 1991; Keystone et al., 2004).

K. Mental illness prevention

1. The psychosocial history and mental status examination (see Chapter 9) will provide the information to decide whether the patient needs mental health treatment. Explore any possible suicidal tendencies in depressed patients, troubled teenagers, drug users, and alcoholics.

2. Review possible use of alcohol, tobacco, analgesics, laxatives, sleeping pills, street drugs, prescription drugs, and dousing with herbs and vitamins.

3. Question the patient about environmental and occupational exposures that can impair mental as well as physical health (Lundberg, 1998).

4. At some point in the history, ask "What kind of things do you enjoy doing?" as a way to explore the patient's overall adjustment to life and its rewards and satisfactions.

L. Prevention beyond the individual patient
As an aphorism, one might say "I can be disease-free only when you are disease-free." It applies to such diseases as malaria, tuberculosis, and many other parasitic, infectious, and transmissible environmental pathogens that we possess the knowledge to eradicate but for which we lack the political commitment required to mount prevention programs. Sachs (2008) outlines ten practical programs that would save the lives of millions upon millions of adults and children worldwide, at essentially negligible costs to developed nations.

V. The Positive Promotion of Wellness

A. The issue of promoting wellness

> Hollywood and Madison Avenue tell us we should be energy-packed, physically perfect, and pain-free. There is an unspoken belief that if we think right, feel right, eat right, and breathe right, we will never be afflicted by a terrible disease.
>
> —Edward Campion
> (Campion, 1993, p 382)

1. Physicians today focus more on diagnosing, treating, and preventing specific diseases, rather than positively promoting health and wellness. In years past, patients consulted a physician only after getting ill. One fault of this approach is that children and mentally ill individuals lack the capacity to decide when they need medical help, and other people wait too long out of fear, ignorance, or inability to pay. If the physician wants to shift from treating disease to actively purveying wellness, the history must reflect this new goal.

2. Before enshrining programs that add the positive promotion of health, as contrasted to disease prophylaxis, consider first the worst possible situation. Worst of all would be a formal definition of physical and mental health composed by a Wellness, Correct thinking and Health Committee, codified by law and regulation, and enforced by the Bureau of Health Police or third-party carriers. That should not replace the decision of responsible individuals as to when they need professional consultation about their health and lifestyle. External coercion would remove the incentive, reward, and personal growth that come from making our own decisions and learning from our own

errors (Fitzgerald, 1994; Illich, 1974). However, this is not an advocacy of the "right to die insane." It only emphasizes the difficulty in trying to separate wellness from the extremes of normal behavior (Lane, 2007).

B. Wellness and *primum non nocere*

1. Some institutions and authors publish newsletters or legitimate books on wellness (Rippe, 1999), but of course the paramedical fringe, sundry fitness gurus and trainers, and the ubiquitous diet industry tout themselves as wellness advisors. The commercialization of wellness poses a danger as one vendor tries to outadvertise, outclaim, and outmarket the other. The public has no way of adjudicating these extravagant claims (Angell and Kassirer, 1994), and the science of wellness needs comprehensive, evidence-based data.

2. Any new wellness programs require an even more cautious advocacy than prevention programs. Since the physician in a sense meddles with a healthy person, each proposed intervention must meet the *primum non nocere* rule by rigorous scientific tests for safety and efficacy to justify adoption.

C. Wellness promotion and the clinical history

> How much happiness is gained, and how much misery escaped, by frequent and violent agitation of the body.
> —Samuel Johnson (1709–1784)
> (Johnson, 1888, p 96)

1. The traditional clinical history focuses on what makes patients feel ill rather than what makes them feel well. Scientific studies have clearly proven the value of exercise in preventing disease and promoting health, but before embarking on an exercise program or any other health program, a person still needs the standard history and physical. Valid practices to promote wellness and make patients feel well must come from accurate clinical appraisal. I find it curious, or perhaps droll, that in all of the agitation about wellness, the time-honored clinical history, with the patient and physician sequestered in the consulting room, still holds its indispensable place in patient management whether we want to detect disease or promote wellness.

2. Finally, an obsession with health can become in itself a disease, a tyranny of health (Barsky, 1988). Health includes the ability to cope with pain, sickness, disappointment, and death as integral parts of life, rather than medicalizing all adversities in the disease prevention model (Barsky, 1988; Fitzgerald, 1994).

VI. Summary

A. The standard history provides much information about preventive needs, but further questioning may be necessary before proposing a formal preventive and wellness program (see Fig. 4–1).

B. How to incorporate wellness questions into the traditional history, which focuses on disease recognition, remains an issue. We cannot leave the matter of health and wellness to the gurus who now pose as experts. The basic principles of the medical model should guide the adoption of any wellness programs. Because of the *primum non nocere* ethic, we should not meddle in the lives of ostensibly healthy people without solid scientific proof of the safety and efficacy of wellness programs. To learn what promotes wellness, just as to learn what causes disease, we still have to start with the clinical history.

References

Angell M, Kassirer JP. Clinical research—what should the public believe? N Engl J Med 1994;331:189–190.

Baker H. Health care challenge. Mayo Clin Proc 1993;68:792–793.

Barsky AJ. Worried Sick: Our Worried Quest for Wellness. Boston: Little Brown, 1988.

Borkowski JF, Weaver CM. Prevention: The Science and Art of Promoting Healthy Child and Adolescent Development. Baltimore: Brooks, 2006.

Campion EW. Why unconventional medicine? N Engl J Med 1993;328: 382–383, p 382.

Centers for Disease Control and Prevention. 2008 Child & Adolescent Immunization Schedules, 2008 (www.cdc.gov/nip/recs/child-schedule. htm).

Czeizel AE, Dudas I. Prevention of the first occurrence of neural-tube defects by periconceptional vitamin supplementation. N Engl J Med 1992;327:1832–1835.

Dexter PR, Perkins S, Overhage JM, et al. A computerized reminder system to increase the use of preventive care for hospitalized patients. N Engl J Med 2001;345:965–969.

Elder NC, Schlaudecker JD, Peters M, et al. Health care for the international traveler. In: Paulman PM, Paulman AA, Harrison JD (eds), Taylor's Manual of Family Medicine. Philadelphia: Wolters Kluwer/Lippincott Williams & Wilkins, 2008, pp 38–45.

Ericsson CD, DuPont HL, Steffen R. Travelers' Diarrhea. Hamilton: BC Decker, 2004.

Fitzgerald FT. The tyranny of health. N Engl J Med 1994;331:196–198.

Harrison R. Health maintenance for infants and children. In: Paulman PM, Paulman AA, Harrison JD (eds), Taylor's Manual of Family Medicine. Philadelphia: Wolters Kluwer/Lippincott Williams & Wilkins, 2008, pp 1–10.

Heisler MB, Richmond JB. Lessons from Finland's successful immunization program. N Engl J Med 1994;331:1446–1447.

Hostetter MK, Iverson S, Thomas W, et al. Medical evaluation of internationally adopted children. N Engl J Med 1991;325:479–485.

Illich I. Medical nemesis. Lancet 1974;1:918–921.

Johnson Samuel. Wit and Wisdon of Samuel Johnson, compiled by Birkbeck G, Hill N, Clarendon press, 1888, p. 96.

Keystone JS, Kozarsky PE, Freedman DO, et al. Travel Medicine. Philadelphia: Mosby, 2004.

Khoury MJ, McCabe LL, McCabe ERB. Population screening in the age of genomic medicine. N Engl J Med 2003;348:50–58.

Koren G. Maternal–Fetal Toxicology. A Clinician's Guide. New York: Marcel Dekker, 1990.

Kottke T, Brekke M, Solberg L. Making „time" for preventive services. Mayo Clin Proc 1993;68:785–791.

Lane C. Shyness: How Normal Behavior Became a Sickness. New Haven: Yale University Press, 2007.

Lundberg A. The Environment and Mental Health: A Guide for Clinicians. Mahwah, NJ: Lawrence Erlbaum, 1998.

Lyons PE, Health maintenance for adult patients. In: Paulman PM, Paulman AA, Harrison JD (eds), Taylor's Manual of Family Medicine. Philadelphia: Wolters Kluwer/Lippincott Williams & Wilkins, 2008, pp 22–33.

Makadon HJ. Improving health care for the lesbian and gay communities. N Engl J Med 2006;354:895–897.

Masterson TM, ed. A Pocketful of Prevention: Preventive Care Guidelines Adapted from the United States Preventive Services Task Force. McLean, VA: International Medical Publishing, 1998.

Montalto N. Health maintenance for adolescents. In: Paulman PM, Paulman AA, Harrison JD (eds), Taylor's Manual of Family Medicine. Philadelphia: Wolters Kluwer/Lippincott Williams & Wilkins, 2008, pp 10–22.

Newman LS. Occupational illness. N Engl J Med 1995;333:1128–1134.

North RL, Rothenberg KH. Partner notification and the threat of domestic violence against women with HIV. N Engl J Med 1993;329: 1194–1196.

Revell VL, Eastman CI. How to trick mother nature into letting you fly around or stay up all night. J Biol Rhythms 2005;20:353–365.

Richardson JP. Health maintenance in older adults. In: Paulman PM, Paulman AA, Harrison JD (eds), Taylor's Manual of Family Medicine. Philadelphia: Wolters Kluwer/Lippincott Williams & Wilkins, 2008, pp 33–37.

Rippe JM, ed. Life Style Medicine. Malden MA: Blackwell Science, 1999.

Rosenberg RN, Iannaccone ST. The prevention of neurogenetic disease. Arch Neurol 1995;52:356–362.

Rosenfeld JA, ed. Handbook of Women's Health: An Evidence-Based Approach. New York: Cambridge University Press, 2001.

Rudolph CD, Rudolph AM, eds. Rudolph's Pediatrics, 21st ed. New York: McGraw-Hill, 2003.

Sachs JD. Primary health for all: ten resolutions could globally ensure a basic human right at almost unnoticeable cost. Sci Am 2008;297: 35–36.

Schor EL, Werner DJ, Malspeis S. Physicians' assessment of functional health status and well-being. Arch Intern Med 1995;155:309–314.

Sox HC. Preventive health services in adults. N Engl J Med 1994;330: 1589–1595.

Welch HG. Questions about the value of early intervention. N Engl J Med 1996;334:1472–1473.

Wender RC, Nevin JE, eds. Preventive Medicine. Philadelphia: WB Saunders, 2002.

Succeeding with the Difficult History

12

I. **The Good and the Poor Historian**
   A. What determines the quality of the history?
      1. When reciting histories to me, medical students often apologize by stating that their patient gave a "poor" history. Students often consider as a poor historian any patient whose vocabulary, diction, education, and logic differ from theirs, while a "good" historian usually matches the student in these attributes.
      2. Given any patient with adequate intelligence, the quality of the history depends much more on the physician than the patient because the experienced physician adapts to extract what the patient knows. The better your technique of interviewing, the less often will you label patients as "poor" historians. Make a "good" history a matter of professional pride.
   B. The novelty of being a patient
      Why expect the average person to provide a free-flowing, "good" history when facing a stranger who asks intimate questions? The patient has not thought through the disease process in logical cause-and-effect sequence, has no training to know which life events relate to the disease, and may not have practiced the degree of introspection and self-observation required for insightful answers. When reflecting on the questions and struggling to give answers, the patient may appear indecisive or evasive. These difficulties of normal persons tend to irritate the physician, who just wants to push on.
   C. Consider the difficult history as a problem of differential diagnosis
      When the history is difficult, the issue becomes *why*. Instead of reacting impatiently, think clinically, in terms of an interesting puzzle in differential diagnosis. Often, symptoms of frank mental illness intrude in lesser but still recognizable form to impede the history. The physician who responds analytically and nonjudgmentally by asking "What factors are making this

history difficult?" will recognize the reason for the difficulty and cope with it.

D. Organic symptoms in psychiatric patients
Symptoms of organic diseases are often difficult to separate as such from mental illness. Is a visual hallucination a symptom of schizophrenia or an occipital lobe lesion? Is the symptom or sign a medication effect? The possibility of one disease camouflaging another is ever present.

II. Causes for Difficult Histories and Their Differential Diagnosis

A. Factors in the patient that cause a difficult history. The text discusses these factors in the order listed in Table 12–1.

1. The patient with an unexpressed or unrecognized agenda
Even a skilled interviewer may not uncover the patient's chief concern or agenda readily. The reasons for the visit may remain hidden because of embarrassment, fear, or unconscious motivation. If the opening questions disclose no special reason or a vague reason for the visit, defer the search for a single chief concern or a single stated medical problem until after the physical examination or until a later appointment.

Table 12–1. Differential Diagnosis of Causes for the Difficult Clinical History, Based on Factors Intrinsic to the Patient

Patient with an unvoiced or unrecognized agenda
Passive–aggressive patient
Depressed patient
Pure paranoid patient
Manic patient
Schizophrenic patient
Demented or retarded patient
Nonstop talker or logorrheic patient
Obsessive–compulsive patient
Hysterical patient (conversion reaction)
Hypochondriacal patient (somatization disorder)
Psychophysiological overreactor
Hostile patient or informant
Chronic pain patient (somatiform pain disorder)
Malingering/Munchausen syndrome patient
Deaf patient or one who speaks only a foreign language
Mute patient
Cross-cultural patient
Comatose patient
Acute severe pain patient

2. The passive–aggressive patient
   a. Passive–aggressive patients respond with noninformative or evasive answers. They habitually express interpersonal hostility by obstructing the proceedings. If you ask "When did your pain begin?" the patient replies, often with a dainty or sly smile, "Oh, I'll have to check my calendar," although knowing full well the answer. Then deliberately, as it were, wasting time, the patient rummages through a purse or bag for the calendar, which she or he can never find. If you ask "Where is the pain?" the patient replies, "Well, sometimes I can't tell," and so it goes, as the physician strives to extract usable information. In such patients, the response pattern provides the significant diagnostic information rather than the specific content of the responses.
   b. The passive–aggressiveness, driven by unconscious motivations, victimizes the patient by interfering with her or his whole life. The way the patient relates to you mirrors the way the patient will relate to others. The disorder prevents the patient from completing simple, everyday interactions, but the patient blames events and others for problems and feels that others do not appreciate her or his valiant efforts to "cooperate." Passive–aggressive personality disorder may in fact underlie the bellyache, headache, or fatigability that brought the patient in. Far from a "poor" historian, the patient has offered you the diagnosis on a platter. The perceived impediment to history taking, the passive–aggressiveness, *is* the diagnosis.

   > The physician may also learn more about the illness from the way the patient tells the story than from the story itself.
   > —James B. Herrick (Herrick, 1949, p 147)

   c. If a mother cannot report the details of her child's development, suspect a passive–aggressive personality disorder, depression, or extreme emotional detachment. If you ask the passive–aggressive mother of a young child "At what age did your child walk?" she will reply, "Oh, I forget to bring in my baby book." She knows full well when her child walked—virtually every mother remembers that—but her psychopathology forces you to work to pry it out of her.

d. Significance of passive–aggressiveness for management
   The passive–aggressive personality forewarns you of a patient likely to misunderstand instructions and to find some reason for not taking any medications prescribed. The patient can't manage to get to appointments for laboratory work or to physical therapy. The physician may have to settle for a supportive relationship through follow-up visits, rather than immediately struggling to recast the patient's entire lifestyle (Lipsitt, 1970).

> There are certain people who behave in a quite peculiar fashion. . . . When one speaks hopefully to them or expresses satisfaction with the progress of treatment, they show signs of discontent and their condition invariably becomes worse. Every partial solution that ought to result, and in other people does result, in an improvement or a temporary suspension of symptoms produces in them for the time being an exacerbation of their illness.
>
> —Sigmund Freud (1856–1939)
> (Freud, 1953–1974, vol 19, p 49)

3. The depressed patient
   Pt 14: This 50-year-old divorced, childless bookkeeper responded with no animation or interest. She spoke slowly, in a soft, low voice, with sighs and downcast eyes. Her face remained blank. She hesitated many seconds before replying to simple, straightforward questions. Her answers, in contrast to those of a paranoid patient, remained relevant and coherent when they came; but she delivered them slowly, indecisively, with no verve or joie de vivre. She reported no energy and no interest in life. She conceded weeping excessively and thinking of self-destruction. These features implicated a major depression (see Table 9–7). On the contrary, some patients mask their depression or anger behind an automatic but wan smile each time they provide an answer.
   Some types of questions may motivate the depressed patient to respond: "When did you last feel well?" or "Describe how things went for you yesterday [or on a typical day in the last week]."

4. The pure paranoid patient

   Pt 15: This 32-year-old laborer also supplied restricted or noninformative answers but to a different end and with a different pattern from passive–aggressive or depressed patients. Profoundly suspicious and distrustful, the paranoid patient discloses as little as possible. When I asked this patient "What brought you in to the hospital?" expecting him to give a medical reason, he responded, "A car brought me," and then he sat in silence, scowling and offering no more. In response to "Tell me why the car was bringing you here," the patient replied, "Because my wife was driving it." In response to "Why did your wife drive you here?" he answered, "Because she wanted me to come." To the next question, "Did she have some reason for bringing you?" the patient replied, "No." without elaborating at all. And so the chase went on, the patient begrudgingly offering bits and scraps of answers.

   The facial expression of these three noninformative responders, the passive–aggressive, the depressed, and the paranoid, usually matches their diagnosis. The passive–aggressive patient may smile as she thwarts the history. The depressed patient has a downcast, emotionless face and a barely audible voice, while the paranoid patient vigilantly, warily watches or glares at you, avoiding every thrust that might penetrate his mental fortress. This patient's pervasive stonewalling unmistakably revealed the paranoia state.

5. The manic patient

   Caught in the manic phase, the manic–depressive patient demands center stage, producing a torrent of words and gesticulating emphatically. The diagnostic clues are the exaggerated mood, pressure of speech, and loud voice declaiming unrealistic fantasies about imagined or projected personal triumphs and grandiose schemes. A few minutes of such hot-wired speech hands you the diagnosis of mania, again on the proverbial platter.

6. The schizophrenic patient

   Pt 16: This 20-year-old man delivered words that had the proper articulation and syntax but with a very flat affect. He attempted to answer questions but could not reach the conversational goal because, in obeisance to his disordered thought processes, he soon detoured into describing radio waves running through his body and visitations by external forces. He heard threatening voices but did not want to describe them. He could not connect events in a logical cause-and-effect relationship. The disease dominated his entire mind, resulting in tangential and bizarre thoughts that obliterated the patient's will. As the history proceeded, the patient laid out the diagnosis of schizophrenia, positive feature by positive feature (delusions, hallucinations, and tangentiality) and negative feature by negative feature (affective blunting and absence of logic).

7. The demented patient

Pt 17: This 81-year-old man, rather than himself requesting an examination, was brought in by his family. His wife stated, "He just doesn't act like himself anymore." The family had noticed a gradual decline in the patient's overall function. Previously well functioning, he was now hesitant, forgetful, and peevish. His face and body seemed to have aged rapidly in the last year. He retained some social poise and automatic phrases, but his inability to answer general questions revealed defects in mentation and memory. When asked to describe what he had done that day, he responded, "Well I got out of bed . . . uh . . . uh . . . I looked for my shoes . . . uh . . . put on my shirt . . ."

Of course, the patient should state simply that he got up, got dressed, and went about his daily activities; but the concrete, terse answers, rather than conveying content, disclosed a vacant mind, a loss of "abstract attitude." Advancing dementia had impaired his ability to instantly abstract and to synthesize the day's activities into one sentence. The patient failed the examination of the sensorium (see Chapter 9, sections IV and V).

8. The nonstop talker (logorrheic) patient

Pt 18: This 48-year-old man with arm pain narrated endless irrelevant details instead of coming to the point. He never censored a single thought in the interest of brevity or relief for the listener but did not show the extreme pressure of speech or grandiosity of the manic patient. The logorrheic patient drowns the listener in a stream of trivialities. When I asked this patient "When did the pain begin?" he replied, "Well, I was sitting on the porch . . . no . . . well, but it was raining outside . . . .and I was thinking of going for a drive . . ."

This patient, like the passive–aggressive patient, will fail in interpersonal relations because he bores and distresses other people. Everyone has met these conversational narcissists who insist on reciting every detail, when you just want to escape gracefully and get on with your day.

9. The obsessive–compulsive patient

Pt 19: The parents brought in their 12-year-old son because he engaged in many elaborate rituals, such as hand washing, counting objects, and arranging them in a particular order. Before going to bed he had to tour the house to insure that the window shades were closed. His schoolmates shunned him. He responded to my inquiries very forcefully, with an overly precise, repetitive, demanding voice and manner. The difficult history clearly suggested obsessive–compulsive disorder, but this patient also displayed multiple facial tics and made excessive throat sounds. The obsessive–compulsive disorder, the high-geared, somewhat abrasive personality, the vocalizations, and the tics, abetted by the seemingly difficult history proclaimed the diagnosis of Tourette syndrome.

10. The hysterical patient (conversion disorder)

Pt 20: This 16-year-old girl arrived in a wheelchair, stating that her legs were too weak to support her. She reported loss of all feeling and movement from her waist down. She accepted her disability stoically and seemed very sincere and cooperative. When trying to move her legs, she made a great show of effort but to no avail. Preservation of bladder and bowel control, normal abdominal reflexes, normal muscle stretch reflexes, and normal plantar responses eliminated an organic cause for the paraplegia. Further questioning disclosed that she had just broken up with a boyfriend of long standing. Within a few days she was walking normally.

The difference between this patient and a malingerer who may present with the same symptoms is that a conversion disorder is presumed to arise at an unconscious level. The patient experiences the paralysis and loss of feeling as a real physical illness, but the malingerer knowingly fakes the illness. In one sense, it does not matter how much of the illness of the chronic pain patient, the malingerer, or the hysteric is conscious or unconscious. All patients require a nonjudgmental physician who will work with them over a period of time to try to resolve the maladaptive illness, whatever its origin.

11. The hypochondriacal patient (*Diagnostic and Statistical Manual of Mental Disorders*, 2000)

    Pt 21: Preoccupation with heart disease dominated this 46-year-old bachelor's thoughts, but it just as well could have been fear of cancer or some other life-threatening malady. The hypochondriacal patient fears that the physician has failed to find some potentially fatal disease. After the workup excludes heart disease, the physician has to extend the history to discover the conscious and unconscious causes for the patient's fears. Encourage the patient to discuss the feared disorder and to disclose, if possible, what brought it to the patient's attention. Did a friend or family member die from it? Did it come from a magazine article or TV program? Or is it a result of unconscious mental mechanisms? If a careful history and subsequent workup confirm the diagnosis of hypochondriasis, the patient often declines psychiatric referral but will come back for follow-up appointments and can be supported by a long-term relationship (Lipsitt, 1970; Monson and Smith, 1983).

    > But if the doctor can assure himself that there is no organic failure sufficient to account for the anxiety of the patient, what is to be done? The physician may feel inclined to say that there is nothing the matter with him. But there must be something the matter with a man who comes to a doctor when there is nothing the matter with him. The anxiety must have a cause. As it is an anxiety about himself, the cause must lie in himself. If it has no observable body correlate, the anxiety itself is a disease, and expresses the patient's sense that something is the matter with his functioning as a human being.
    >
    > —John MacMurray (1952, p 230)

12. Psychophysiological overreactor (somatization disorder)

    Pt 22: The previous patient had a monovalent preoccupation with mainly one disorder, heart disease; but this 26-year-old secretary overreacted to every body sensation or trivial illness and could not accept it philosophically or casually. Everything had cosmic proportions. No pain was ever slight but struck with titanic force. She had no mild diarrhea, always a veritable torrent. Each borborygmus portended rupture of the bowel. Menstrual cramps devastated her. She had migraine headaches, but no one had suffered so much or gotten so little help or relief. She arrived with a long, written description of her headaches and insisted on reading every word. Every category of the review of systems produced positive responses: indigestion, bloating, food intolerances, fatigue, dark circles under the eyes, diarrhea or constipation, sweating, flushing. She experienced hyperventilation and multiple abnormal sensations that had no physical explanation. Again, the patient has presented the diagnosis of somatization disorder (Monson and Smith, 1983) to you on a platter. The recital of symptoms was not so irrelevant and wasteful as it seemed initially. Moreover, the history warns you that the patient may be overly sensitive to medications, which if needed should be started in tiny doses.

The danger always is that a physical disease may lurk behind the barrage of symptoms. The presence of a mental disorder in no way precludes a physical disorder. Moreover, some of the overreaction may result from efforts of the patient to get a hearing from the numerous physicians already consulted. These are indeed difficult histories because the physician does not know which complaints to investigate or to ignore. The following disorders exemplify the difficulty in the differential diagnosis of somatization disorder.

a. Panic attacks

Pt 23: This 28-year-old woman had 30–45 minute attacks of sweating, shortness of breath, heart palpitations, extremity tingling, trembling, dizziness, and feelings of terror, impending doom, and death. She had had five such attacks in the last 6 weeks. Most of the time she felt too cold. Her multiple symptoms again provide a nearly diagnostic history, in this case of panic attacks. About half of these patients have mitral value prolapse.

b. Attacks of hypertension

Pt 24: This 28-year-old female had a stereotyped set of symptoms daily, without specific, discrete attacks.

She had a variety of complaints of headache, palpitations, nausea, abdominal pain, and visual obscurations, which came and went and for which no ready neurological explanation could be found. While the history raised the question of a somatization disorder, this patient had multiple café au lait spots indicative of neurofibromatosis type 1, and she also had hypertension. Urinary screening disclosed high levels of catecholamines, and a computed tomographic scan disclosed a pheochromocytoma of her adrenal region, a lesion known to be associated with neurofibromatosis type 1.

c. Carcinoid syndrome

Another rare disorder causes attacks of confusion, dyspnea, and purple or brilliant scarlet tricolor cutaneous flushing of the head and neck, lasting 1–5 minutes. The patient has abdominal cramping, diarrhea, and episodes of confusion. Ingestion of cheese and alcohol triggers the attacks, a key feature of the history. The lesion is a carcinoid tumor that secretes serotonin and other vasoactive peptides.

> This man was addicted to moanin'
> Confusion, edema, and groanin'
> Intestinal rushes
> Great tricolored flushes
> And died of too much serotonin.

—William Bean, M.D. (Bean, 1958, p 117)

d. Miscellaneous disorders with multiple symptoms

Other disorders that may cause puzzling neuropsychiatric and systemic symptoms include porphyria, collagen-vascular diseases, and multiple sclerosis. Often, the most important management technique for the difficult patient is to make follow-up appointments and extend the history and tests until you have systematically explored the diagnostic possibilities.

13. The hostile patient or hostile informant

A type of patient will arrive with a hostile, angry attitude, bordering on paranoia (Groves, 1978). Although conditioned by the person's own psychodynamics, the anger is often augmented by adverse responses from previous physicians or hassles with health-care organizations or insurance companies. The physician serves as a lightning rod during the early part of the history. Let the patient talk it out, vent his or her spleen as it were, without reacting personally. Defensive remarks will merely fan the flames. Accept the anger as a clinical phenomenon, not as a personal affront. The provocateur seeks to incite you to anger as a way to control and demean you. As in most human interactions, humility and grace serve best. *The message you send is the one returned.* Calmly acknowledge the patient's distress, responding with an open invitation: "I see that you are very upset ["upset" and "distressed" are softer words than "angry"]. We'll go over what's happening and try to find some solutions." Voice no opinion as to the justice or injustice of the patient's anger, but continue to listen until the storm abates. The patient will eventually calm down and become more rational. The withering anger during the medical interview warns that similar anger will erupt in everyday interpersonal relations.

14. The chronic pain patient

Pt 25: Since spraining his back 2 years ago this 28-year-old former factory worker reported that pain plagued him every minute of the day and kept him from sleeping at night. Pain absolutely dominated his life and limited every effort to work or engage in recreational activities. He arrived with a back brace and a cane, outward symbols that proclaim illness. The patient had enlisted his wife and insisted on her presence during the history. Each time after he stated how much pain he suffered and how profoundly it limited his activity, he would turn to her for confirmation. His wife eagerly substantiated and embellished the patient's narrative. He recounted in great detail many failed therapies in spite of valiant efforts to overcome his difficulties. Litigation was in process.

Chronic pain syndromes are compounded of varying mixtures of organic disease, depression, hostility, dependence, conversion disorder, and sometimes overt malingering, particularly if litigation is in process. Some patients simulate chronic pain to get narcotics. Similarly, a patient may simulate narcolepsy, quoting the symptoms verbatim from a textbook, to obtain amphetamines. These manipulative patients gain a perverse reward in duping the physician, but the physician looks beyond such negative considerations to see a human being in distress and tries to work out the best long-term plan of management (Carr et al., 2005; Carson et al., 2004).

15. The Munchausen syndrome/malingering patient
Pt 26: This 28-year-old woman presented time after time at emergency rooms at different hospitals. She usually complained of abdominal pain and has brought in a urine sample to which she has added blood. She has had previous negative exploratory operations for "appendicitis" or "gallbladder disease." She has become well known in the local medical community as having Munchausen syndrome. Munchausen patients repeatedly seek hospitalization for wholly fictitious illnesses, often memorized from a medical text (Feldman and Ford, 1993). They try to baffle or con the learned profession to gain attention, and then they masochistically receive the punishment of painful diagnostic or surgical procedures that assuage the guilt for dissimulating. If confronted or unmasked, the patient reacts hostilely and signs out AMA (against medical advice), threatening to sue everybody.

Pt 27: In the baffling disorder Munchausen syndrome by proxy, the perpetrators present their own child as the ill patient (Galvin et al., 2005). My most extreme personal example involved a professional woman whose boy I saw repeatedly in our hospital emergency room because of hypoglycemic seizures. Repeated workups disclosed no explanation for hypoglycemia. Finally, assay of his blood showed porcine rather than human insulin, that is, insulin given by injection. Some time later, his mother was admitted to another hospital in hypoglycemic coma and found to have porcine insulin in her blood, apparently self-administered.

Pt 28: Another Munchausen by proxy patient in our hospital was a young child with repeated admissions for fever of unknown origin. Blood cultures repeatedly showed coliform septicemia, even while in the hospital and under careful sanitary precautions. The workup disclosed no access from bowel to bloodstream. Secret video surveillance showed his mother injecting his own feces into his IV tubing with a hypodermic needle. Not all parents love their children. The history may initially mislead the physician. The Munchausen or malingering patient usually gives a very convincing story and seems sincere, cooperative, and duly concerned. In coping with malingering, the physician tries simultaneously to serve the patient and the truth. The resolution lies in applying basic principles. First, the physician is not at the service of the patient's wishes but at the service of the patient's health. After taking all due care, including any tests and consultations needed, the physician straightforwardly and calmly informs the patient that the medical workup has not disclosed a disease that would explain the symptoms. Avoid confrontations and allegations of dishonesty. Do offer follow-up appointments in the hope of clarifying the need for fabricating the symptoms. This may fail to placate the patient or resolve the problem, but it may be the best you can do. Notify child protective services for Munchausen by proxy involving children.

16. The deaf patient

    For deaf patients and those who can read but not speak, you can use an interpreter who knows sign language or a booklet that has standard questions printed out.

17. The mute patient (who is not deaf)

    a. Some patients will refuse to talk. They may have elective mutism, as in a 5-year-old who may speak freely at home but not at all in school or in the physician's office. The patient may be a sullen teenager who did not want to visit the physician but who came at the insistence of the parents. Mutism may accompany severe mental illness, including profound depression, dementia, and catatonic schizophrenia.

    b. The physician has to extract as much history from informants as possible. Interview the informants in private because the mute or seemingly deaf patient may understand every word said.

18. The cross-cultural patient

    a. If a practice consists of many patients who speak only a foreign language, the physician has little choice but to learn the language.

  b. Cross-cultural patients require especially careful phrasing of questions and instruction, to avoid misinterpretations (Cuéllar and Paniagua, 2000). Language tests may help to determine whether a patient is competent enough in English to permit a history without an interpreter or to give informed consent or to understand the physician's recommendations for management (Downey and Zun, 2007).

19. The comatose patient

  a. Not uncommonly a patient is brought to the hospital comatose off of the street with no history whatsoever available. After emergency measures have stabilized the patient, learn where and how the patient was found. Survey the patient's clothing, pockets, and body for background clues. Then, search the patient's wallet or pocketbook for a suicide note, street drugs, medications, a card affirming that the patient has some illness that might cause coma—such as diabetes, liver or kidney disease, or epilepsy—and the name, address, and phone number of the next of kin. Telephone or have the police locate the relevant persons and have them come in for an interview.

  b. Focus the interview of the informant on a few pertinent questions to resolve the immediate diagnosis, rather than striving for a complete life history. Because of privacy concerns, the physician uses discretion in revealing specific information about the cause of the coma but at the same time has to insure that the informant will disclose the required history. Ask the informant about the following:

   (1) The overall mental and physical health of the patient

   (2) Whether the patient has any known disorders that affect major organs

   (3) Drug or alcohol abuse and depression

   (4) The patient's behavior and activities during the few hours or days prior to the coma

   (5) Any neurologic disorders that might herald coma, such as headaches or dizziness, nausea and vomiting, weakness, visual complaints, and previous unconscious episodes

B. Obtaining the history and examining an acutely injured but conscious patient suffering severe pain

During a Mediterranean cruise in 1967, my wife, Marian, and I visited the ruins of the Minoan palace at Knossos on the island of Crete. The palace contains the labyrinth where, according to legend, the mythical half-man, half-bull Minotaur lived. It is the site for the story of the thread of Ariadne that she gave to her lover, Theseus, to lead him back out of the labyrinth after he had penetrated it to slay the Minotaur.

Pt 29: While walking on the uneven stone pathway leading to the palace, a stout, fiftyish American woman tripped and fell heavily, suffering a badly sprained left ankle. She was lying on her back on the rough stone, crying loudly from the pain. I was about to step forward and identify myself as a physician, but having practiced only neurology, I felt uncertain about coping with a possible fracture. At that instant, another American stepped forward, identifying himself as a general practitioner. "Thank goodness," I thought. This marvelous GP then proceeded with a masterful demonstration of how to take a history and examine an acutely injured patient who has no apparent head or spinal injury.

The physician gave the woman his name, identified himself as a physician, and asked her name. This reverses the usual procedure of asking first for the patient's name but fit the circumstance. He then addressed her as "Mrs. ____" (not a patronizing "Honey" or "Dolly") and stated that he saw many patients with ankle injuries in his general practice back home in Iowa, thus offering the patient some assurance of his experience and competence. He first retrieved the her purse and very gently placed it under her head, stating that it would make her head comfortable and that she would also know it was safe. This in itself was a wonderful insight because everyone worries about the location of his or her purse or wallet, and in alleviating that concern and making her head comfortable he started to divert her attention from her pain and made contact with the patient as a person, rather than just as an ankle injury. Before placing the purse, he insured that she had no neck pain, and he did not actually flex or displace her neck because the physician avoids that if the patient may have a neck or spinal cord injury. He then asked her to take some deep breaths and to relax and exhale. He reassured her (and himself) that she was breathing well, which of course he already had inferred from her loud crying. He then asked her to flex and extend her arms and to squeeze his fingers, offered to her right and then her left hand, demonstrating to himself and to her that that these parts were intact. He then reassured her that her arms and hands were not injured.

Instead of immediately attending to the injured left ankle, he asked her to lift her right leg, to bend the knee and ankle, to wiggle her toes, and whether she could feel him touch her. He reassured her that this leg was all right. He asked if her back hurt, to which she replied, "Only a little." By this time he had clearly demonstrated that she had not suffered a back or spinal cord injury. Then, he very gently cradled the injured left limb and asked her to bend her thigh and knee and wiggle her toes, and he again said hips, knee, and toes were working fine and that the nerves in the leg seemed intact, increasing the inventory of working parts. Finally, he gently passed his fingers over the injured ankle and said, "This seems to be the only part that is hurt. We'll get you to an X-ray machine to see whether it's broken. In the meantime, I'll splint it just to be safe." He got some ice from a thermos bottle and placed it in a sock over her ankle, stating that it would soothe her pain and swelling. He deftly fashioned a crude splint out of some cardboard, a belt, and a necktie.

By this time the woman knew that she had not suffered any serious injury. Her crying had ceased, without the physician using any medication and without condescending platitudes, such as "There, there, Dearie, you'll be all right. Don't cry now. Be brave." He had treated her as an adult, capable of coping with the situation. He had diverted her attention from the pain by gently leading her to discover for herself that most of her remained intact and that the part that wasn't could be attended to.

With the patient calmed, he asked, "Have you been subject to faints or falls?" to which she replied "No." "Did you trip?" brought a reply of "Yes," thus establishing an etiologic diagnosis and helping to exclude immediate, ominous neurologic or cardiovascular disorders that might recur. He asked, "Do you have any general health problems?" which is the briefest possible review of systems. When she said "No," he still asked about her blood pressure and heart and any previous falls, fractures, or injuries. Then, assuming a more conversational air, he asked whether anyone else was with her, where she lived, and her occupation, reversing the usual order by ending the interview with chitchat and the "face sheet" data, rather than beginning it that way. In just a few minutes he had established rapport and ameliorated her pain and anxiety.

When he had finished, I realized that, as was my habit when observing medical students or residents, I had automatically critiqued his performance and found it perfect. When I returned to our ship, I wrote down the sequence of that perfectly scripted performance because I knew that someday I would write this book and that he had demonstrated, better than anything I could say, the finest art of the physician. I wish I had a videotape of that performance for every medical student to study. I was never prouder of my profession than in observing how this physician, from a little town in Iowa, had brought such comfort to a complete stranger in just a few minutes, employing only his voice, hands, and the best techniques of the medical model. There in the Mediterranean where Western medicine began, the power and glory of the medical model had returned full circle. The legacy had extended over time, some 2000–3000 years, over distance, having spread to Iowa, thousands of miles away, and had returned, reflected back in its pure, original, crystalline form: a gentle voice, thoughtful sequencing of the questions of the history, and the comforting touch of the physician's hands. It occurred to me that Hippocrates and all thoughtful physicians between him and now surely would have done it the same way.

When I congratulated the physician on his skill, he demurred that he had not done much of anything at all. Yet, his humility and grace, his compassionate professionalism had given me a transcendental example of how to practice my own profession: the voice, the demeanor, and the hands—the ultimate secrets of medical practice.

III. Keeping the Difficult Patient on Track During the History
A. Dealing with digressions
   1. The physician has to strike a balance between clinically relevant information and unproductive digression. Too leisurely a pace signals the patient to meander, but if you

ask questions too fast, the patient will balk. To move the dilatory history along, make periodic summaries of the patient's narrative to that point and then introduce an open question to signify the end of that line of inquiry and a transition to the next part of the history. The patient should then understand that you do need to come to closure on each line of inquiry and then move on.

2. If the patient digresses, such as by quoting the opinions of other persons about the symptoms, the disease, or the diagnosis, the physician may respond, "Let's first find out just how the disease is affecting you. Then we'll go on to what others think about it." Some patients use phantom relatives to voice their own fears, "My mother-in-law thinks I might have cancer," rather than stating their fears directly.

3. If a patient hesitates to answer questions for one part of the clinical history, simply set that topic aside for the moment and go on to something else. Do not force the issue. Return to it at a later time, when the patient may feel freer to discuss it.

   a. I asked the mother of a child who had very aggressive outbursts, "How does Eddie get along with his father?" She demurred, "Oh, I find that difficult to describe." This classic temporizing remark really says "You've asked that too fast. I'm not ready to deal with that yet."

   b. You might impatiently want to say "Oh come on now. You're there every day. You've got to have some opinions." The unvoiced issue at that point was the abusive relationship of father to son and to her, which she was not yet able to lay out or admit point blank. Back off, but return to the issue later.

4. Aphorism: What the patient wishes to talk about is often not the real problem. What the patient does not wish to talk about often is.

B. Monitor the quality of your interview technique to insure a good history

Vigilant monitoring of the patient's responses provides the best measure of the quality of your interviewing technique. Monitoring commences as soon as you greet the patient. You have to read each verbal and "body language" response the patient makes to each of your statements and actions. From the beginning, you, the professional, bear the responsibility for controlling the train of events, the transfer of information, and the interchange of feelings and understanding. While monitoring the patient's feelings, you also have to monitor your own. This double monitoring holds the key to success or failure.

IV. **Emotional Interactions Between Patient and Physician that Result in a Difficult History**
  A. What single factor causes the most difficulty in the practice of medicine?
    1. What is the single most important cause for a difficult history?
    2. What is the single most important cause for missing a diagnosis?
    3. What is the single most important reason patients reject appropriate medical management?
    4. What is the single most important cause for failure of the patient–physician relationship?
    5. What is the single most important cause for malpractice suits?
  B. One statement answers all of these questions
    1. Negative attitudes of the physician—anger, irritation, censure, disrespect, or disinterest—cause more trouble in the practice of medicine than any other single factor (Lown, 1996; Vincent et al., 1994).
    2. Typically, these negative feelings arise if you judge the patient as worthless, parasitic, incompetent, or weak-willed and responsible for his or her own ill health and undeserving of medical care (Lipsitt, 1970). You will tend to react negatively to the obese patient who doesn't lose weight; the passive–dependent or hostile patient; addicts, for example, the patient with emphysema or heart disease who continues to smoke; the diabetic who neglects the prescribed diet; and any patient whose lifestyle clashes with the physician's expectations. These patients who respond poorly to management recommendations challenge the physician's self-image as a healer. To focus on the emotional interactions engendered in the physician–patient relationship, psychoanalysts have introduced the concept of "transference" and "countertransference."

C. Definition of transference and countertransference
   1. We all react in some way to everyone we encounter. We cannot avoid some degree of speculation, fantasy, or curiosity. The person always generates some positive and negative feelings of greater or lesser magnitude. A combination of conscious and unconscious factors determines these feelings.
      a. *Transference* refers to the negative and positive emotions, conscious and unconscious, that arise in the patient from contact with the physician. These are the emotions that the patient experiences toward the physician.
      b. *Countertransference* refers to the negative and positive emotions, conscious and unconscious, that arise in the physician by the contact with the patient. These are the emotions that the physician experiences toward the patient.
   2. These broad definitions by Kaplan and Sadock (1991) differ from the original conception of Sigmund Freud (1856–1939), who limited the terms to the feelings generated by unconscious factors (Searles, 1979).
   3. The clinical history and physical examination weave a constantly changing tapestry of transference–countertransference.
D. Conscious determinants of emotional interaction between patient and physician
   1. Obviously, conscious perceptions of face, form, costume, voice, and role may generate positive or negative feelings in the patient or physician. We all automatically make inferences from the overall demeanor and appearance of everyone we meet. These initial perceptions increase or diminish as the two persons continue to interact.
   2. A rigidly judgmental physician may perceive a female patient who drinks, smokes, gambles, and wears low-cut blouses and miniskirts as dissolute or, to the contrary, a rigidly judgmental patient may perceive a cigarette-sucking, beer-guzzling, pot-bellied physician as dissolute.
   3. An outspoken liberal may relate poorly to a strongly conservative person, or someone with strict religious convictions may relate poorly to an atheist. Such differences, if voiced, result in opinionated debates that inevitably detract from the professional relationship. For this reason,

you should deliberately avoid debating or imposing personal political, social, or religious views during the professional relationship because they polarize and divide.

E. Unconscious determinants of emotional responses

1. Why do you, over here, prefer the color blue and you, over there, prefer orange? Why did you choose tennis for a hobby and not golf? Why does one odor repel you but attract someone else? Why does one person's face or body contour attract you?

2. You will find it difficult to explain such preferences. Clearly, factors inaccessible to consciousness determine many of our choices and attitudes. Although conscious stratagems allow us to record and rationally analyze daily events (see Chapter 9, section IV), we have no ready access to the well of unconscious factors that determine basic likes, dislikes, and drives.

3. A patient full of resentment toward authoritarian parents is the classical example of how unconscious transferences influence interpersonal relations. The patient unconsciously or automatically transfers those resentments to any other authority figure encountered, such as a judge, teacher, employer, or physician. The patient unconsciously adopts the new authority figure as a surrogate for the overcontrolling, hated, or feared parent. An authoritarian physician will ignite these old resentments, causing the patient to relate poorly to this physician. When an authoritarian physician and a patient with a rebellious personality clash, neither the patient nor the physician may immediately recognize the origin of their hostility. These unconscious feelings that mistakenly identify a new person or a new experience with previous persons or experiences may damage a relationship even more than conscious factors. By recognizing and anticipating these often powerful emotional intrusions, you will avoid many mistakes in practicing medicine.

4. A basic rule in human interactions is that the message sent is the message returned. If you send humility and grace, you will receive them. If you send hostility, you will get it back. However, even if the physician sends the proper messages, the patient's unconscious determinants or mental illness may distort the message. Precisely here do the skill,

responsibility, and intervention of the physician become critical. Instead of blaming a patient whom you don't like, ask yourself "What life experiences, unconscious determinants, or malfunctions of the brain led the patient to these maladaptive reactions?" and "What characteristics of mine may have augmented the negative response?" In other words, the problem transforms from "I don't like this person" to a game, an exercise in differential diagnosis to discover an explanation.

F. Avoiding excessively strong positive feelings in the physician's countertransference

1. Positive feelings of affection, overidentification, or rescue fantasies will cause errors of judgment and management almost as quickly as hostile feelings. Instead of eliciting hostility, some patients, particularly those with an antisocial (sociopathic) personality, con the unwary physician into strong positive feelings. In the formal setting of the interview or while in prison, the sociopath appears sincere, rational, and highly motivated to improve. The physician anticipates great therapeutic success with this rational, cooperative, likeable person whose misfortunes have only come about through fortuitous external circumstances. If you feel too attracted, stop. The sociopath is a conscienceless exploiter who preys on others by recognizing their vulnerabilities and ego needs. The patient's modus operandi is to con, defraud, and exploit. As an antidote read *The Mask of Sanity* by Hervey Cleckley (1982).

2. Some patients manipulate others by sexual seduction. Regard it as a purely clinical phenomenon and defuse the sexuality. If a sociopathic or sexually seductive patient succeeds in snaring you in his or her psychopathology, you surrender your role as a physician.

G. Avoid excessively strong positive transferences by the patient Physicians should not strive to portray themselves as all-loving, all-knowing saints in an attempt to elicit adoration from their patients: "Oh, you are the best doctor in the world." Such a statement means that the patient has manufactured unrealistic fantasies about you that ultimately you cannot fulfill. If the patient loves you or worships you too much, reexamine your management of the professional relationship. Respect, trust, and gratitude, yes, but adoration, love, and worship, no. The goal is not love or even soul-mate friendship but maximal promotion of the patient's health through rapport and empathy that lead to justifiable trust. The contact between patient and physician should not lead to emotional entanglements by either party.

H. How to cope with strong positive or negative countertransference feelings

1. If you begin to experience strong positive or negative feelings toward the patient, do not attempt to deny, ignore, or suppress the feelings or assume that some magical immunity will protect you. Recognize and acknowledge the emotions as danger signals that warn of impending mistakes. It may help if you work through a checklist to recognize the feelings and to deal with them (Table 12–2). The physician should ask "Why am I reacting this way?" and then proceed with caution to analyze and cope with the feelings (Groves, 1978).

2. To recapitulate: You, the physician, bear the responsibility to anticipate, recognize, and productively manage the transference–countertransference dynamics because this interaction, more than any other, determines the success or failure of the entire patient–physician relationship. I have emphasized all along that the physician must adjust to maximize benefit for the patient (Siegler, 1993). This explicit principle governs clothes, demeanor, office setting, and the

---

Table 12–2. Factors for the Physician to Review to Recognize Strong, Potentially Dangerous Emotional Reactions to a Patient

1. Am I recognizing and coping with my emotions to this patient?
2. Do I look forward to or dread the patient's visit?
3. Do I get extreme pleasure out of seeing the patient?
4. Do I feel sexually attracted to the patient?
5. Is the patient overly seductive?
6. Do I regard the patient as boring or tedious?
7. Does the patient's failure to follow treatment plans (losing weight, continuing to smoke, etc.) strongly irritate me?
8. Do I resent the patient's lifestyle and want to punish the patient for it?
9. Do I strongly oppose the patient's religious or political beliefs?
10. Am I overly impressed with the patient's agreeable personality, rationality, and apparent cooperation? (Beware, a sociopath is conning you.)
11. Does the patient praise me too much or exaggerate my abilities?
12. Is the patient's mental state abnormal enough to warrant psychiatric referral?

techniques for taking the history and doing the physical examination. If strong feelings intrude into the patient–physician relationship, they will alter the questions of the history, the questions you ask and the questions that you don't ask.

I. A checklist of errors in technique by the physician during the history

    1. Table 12–3 summarizes points to check to diagnose the reasons for the difficult history.

    2. Review whether the patient might have had cause to perceive you as indifferent, rushed, preoccupied, judgmental, or hostile. Even subtle factors, such as inadvertent body language and a tenseness of voice, may contribute to alienation.

    3. Review the type of questions asked, tone of voice, and appropriateness of the questions for the stage of the interview. You may have been too directive or mechanical, as if filling out a checklist. You may have used medical jargon, making the questions incomprehensible, or a vocabulary that differed too much from the patient's accustomed speech. Review the ratio of the number of the patient's

Table 12–3. Checklist of Errors by the Office Staff and Physician that Make the History Difficult

    I. Impersonal grilling or interrogation by the receptionist (see Chapter 6)
    II. Improper interview room with respect to size, décor, and privacy; distraction by beepers or telephone calls
    III. Failure to establish contact with the patient as a human by a handshake and preliminary chitchat
    IV. Premature pressure to get the patient to articulate a specific chief concern
    V. Judgmental, condescending, indifferent, rushed, or preoccupied attitude
    VI. Improper questioning
        A. Too many direct and mechanical, rather than open, questions and too much pressure on the patient to produce crisp, prompt answers
        B. Inappropriate introduction of intimate questions, prematurely or out of context
        C. Asking questions with medical jargon or a vocabulary incomprehensible to the patient
    VII. Improper personal characteristics
        A. Inappropriate costume
        B. Improper posture and body language: slouching, standing rigidly
        C. Inappropriate grooming: slovenly or overdone with ostentatious makeup and jewelry, religious or political symbols, or expensive adornments
    VIII. Preoccupation with writing or recording the patient's statements
    IX. Failure to monitor the patient's responses to pick up clues of distress
    X. Failure to monitor the transference–countertransference reactions, resulting in hostile, depreciatory, or negative feelings or an excessive positive attraction

words to yours. It should be high. To best analyze these factors, students should critique videos of their own interviews.

V. **When It's a Question of the Honesty or Accuracy of the History**
   A. Believe the patient until proven otherwise
      At some point during a history the physician may begin to doubt the truth or the reliability of the patient's narrative. The best rule is to accept and record the history as given unless clearly proven false.
   B. Several classical topics raise the question of honesty and accuracy in the clinical history
      1. When the patient describes the amount of food, alcohol, and other drugs ingested. Even with such drugs as laxatives or sleeping pills, patients tend to deny or understate the amount.
      2. When litigation is in progress
      3. When the patient has an ulterior motive, such as giving a false history to get a prescription for amphetamines or narcotics, or the patient wants an excuse from work or attending school
      4. When one divorcing parent tries to align the physician against the other parent in child custody proceedings
      5. When it is a question of child or spousal abuse
      6. When the topic is sexual deviance, such as pedophilia
   C. Complete the doubtful history as if it were true, but requestion the patient later
      Whatever suspicions arise, you should continue through the history in the usual neutral manner, making no accusations and taking no sides. Record what the patient actually reports. Do not make editorial comments, either openly or in writing. After all, the history always constitutes hearsay evidence. Sometimes the patient is honestly mistaken or misremembers some event from the past and contradicts previous statements after reflecting. Encourage the patient to rethink the answers to the questions of the interview and to amend previous statements, if necessary. Even the best patients may contradict themselves on some issues. That does not justify alarm or accusations of dishonesty. Simply requestion the patient about doubtful points during the initial interview or at a later appointment. Above all, avoid arguing with the patient about

the truth of the history. Try to get independent information from a family member.

VI. **When It's a Question of Irreconcilable Differences Between the Patient and the Physician**
   A. Coping with bad chemistry
      1. Call a spade a spade and start over
         a. Rarely, the physician may directly acknowledge an obviously failing history: "I think we both sense that this is not going well. Have I done or said something unwelcome?" Sometimes that question will bring out a simple misunderstanding, a gaffe, or a fear.
         b. That ploy failing, the physician may ask whether the patient might like to come back for another appointment, giving each party a chance to reconsider how to relate better the next time.
      2. Refer the patient to another physician
         Very rarely, the chemistry between patient and physician fails from the start. The personality conflict is too great to resolve. The physician who, after due effort, cannot work with a given patient may choose to withdraw. This problem may arise in questions of sexual attraction, euthanasia, reproductive technology and abortion, sex change, drug use, and diametrically opposed belief systems of patient and physician. Generally, if the physician feels uncomfortable with the relationship, the patient does also and welcomes a referral. The physician, with humility and grace, may say "I find that some other doctors can help you more than I can with the problem you are having [alcoholism, drug abuse, obesity, sexual orientation, etc.]. Let me refer you to someone who is better qualified." This fulfills the Hippocratic admonition of attempting to do only what your training and ability has prepared you for and applies to those patients whom you can't diagnose or help or with whom you cannot agree on management (Veatch, 1995).
   B. The patient who fails to follow the therapeutic program
      1. Sometimes resolution is simple. You failed to explain the diagnosis or management well enough, or the drugs prescribed produce unacceptable side effects. A simple change in medications may resolve the problem.

2. Sometimes in spite of all efforts, resolution fails completely. The patient with obvious psychiatric problems will not consider the possibility of a mental illness and will not accept a psychiatric referral to explore that issue, or the patient will not change detrimental habits. In any event, the physician always has to question whether the history has provided sufficient knowledge of the patient to correctly diagnose and cope with the cause for the patient's self-destructive reactions (Groves, 1978; Lipsitt, 1970; Peschel and Peschel, 1986; Wolberg, 1954).

3. Some patients in spite of all due efforts by the physician remain intransigent or hostile (Groves, 1978). Without gratitude or insight, they absorb the time, stamina, and beneficence of the physician and the health-care system, even when the physician and hospital staff works through the night to pull the patient through one crisis after another. The patient with chronic emphysema who continues to smoke is a common example. Again, the best solution is to consider the failure as a diagnostic problem, not as a deliberate attempt by the patient to vex the physician.

C. Physician get thyself healed

Should more than a very rare patient seem unworkable, refer yourself to a psychiatrist to examine your motivations and fitness to practice medicine. You can't transform yourself alone. The admonition "Physician heal thyself" becomes "Physician get to a healer."

> Don't get mad at your patients if they don't improve with your therapy.
> Don't get mad at patients because of their life style.
> Don't get mad at your patients [at all].
> If you do, get some help.
>
> —Clifton K. Meador (1992, rule 219)

VII. Summary

A. Factors that affect the quality of the history

1. The causes for a poor history fall into three categories

a. Causes intrinsic to the patient (Table 12–1)

b. Causes in the circumstances and techniques of the medical interview

c. Causes in the personal qualities of the physician and patient and the management of the transference and countertransference

2. The quality of the history mostly depends on the physician's ingenuity and technique. If a patient fails to give a straightforward history, avoid anger or exasperation. Explore the reason for the poor history as a clinical puzzle that requires a differential diagnosis and a solution, just like any other clinical puzzle.

3. A mixture of psychiatric and organic symptoms confounds the history.

B. Factors intrinsic to the patient that may interfere with the history

1. Often, a pattern of seemingly noninformative or trivial answers given by the patient points to a specific mental disorder, such as passive–aggressive personality, paranoia, hypochondriasis, or depression, rather than obscuring the diagnosis.

2. Many other special circumstances confound the history, such as cross-cultural differences, deafness, the unconscious patient, or the patient suffering severe acute pain. Specific techniques to garner a history apply to these situations.

C. Dealing with digressions

To rescue the history from unproductive digressions or chatting, the physician should periodically summarize the pertinent material covered and indicate the need to move along by introducing a new open question: "Yes, I understand about that. Now let's see how your vision has been."

D. Emotional currents between patient and physician: transference and countertransference

1. The clinical history has two goals: the search for symptoms and the development of rapport and trust between physician and patient. For the development of rapport and trust the most important factor is to understand the power and importance of the transference and countertransference. *Transference* means the emotion that the patient feels toward the physician, and *countertransference* means the emotions that the physician feels toward the patient.

253

2. Mismanagement of the emotional interactions engendered in the patient–physician relationship causes more grief in the practice of medicine than any other factor.

3. Excessively strong positive emotions are as potentially dangerous as negative ones (Table 12–2). If the history becomes difficult, the physician should check through a list of factors that impair the history (Table 12–3).

E. Accept the history as given unless proven otherwise
Most patients will give mostly accurate histories, but certain circumstances warrant skepticism: when litigation is in process, the use of alcohol and other drugs, child or spousal abuse, and sexual deviance.

F. Managing irreconcilable differences between patient and physician
Very rarely, a patient and physician cannot work together. The physician then refers the patient to someone else known for competence in the area of the patient's needs. Physicians who have irreconcilable outcomes with too many patients should refer themselves for psychiatric help.

References

Bean WB. Vascular Spiders and Related Lesions of the Skin. Springfield, IL: Thomas, 1958, p 117.

Carr DB, Loeser JD, Morris DB. Narrative, Pain and Suffering. Seattle: IASP Press, 2005.

Carson AJ, Stone J, Warlow C, et al. Patients whom neurologists find difficult to help. J Neurol Neurosurg Psychiatry 2004;75:1776–1778.

Cleckley, H. The Mask of Sanity. An Attempt to Clarify Some Issues About the So-Called Psychopathic Personality. New York: New American Library, Mosby, 1982.

Cuéllar I, Paniagua FA, eds. Handbook of Multicultural Mental Health: Assessment and Treatment of Diverse Populations. San Diego: Academic Press, 2000.

Diagnostic and Statistical Manual of Mental Disorders, 4th ed. Washington DC: American Psychiatric Association, 2000.

Downey LVA, Zun L. Testing of a verbal assessment tool of English proficiency for use in the healthcare setting. J Natl Med Assoc 2007;99: 795–798.

Feldman MD, Ford CV. Patient or Pretender: Inside the Strange World of Factitious Disorders. New York: John Wiley, 1993.

Freud, S. Ego and id. In: Strachey J , Freud A. (eds), The Standard Edition of the Complete Psychological Works of Sigmund Freud. London: Hogarth Press and Institute of Psycho-Analysis, 1953–1974, vol. 19, p 49.

Galvin HK, Newton AW, Vandeven AM. Update on Munchausen syndrome by proxy. Curr Opin Pediatr 2005;17:252–257.

Groves JE. Taking care of the hateful patient. N Engl J Med 1978;298: 883–887 (see also Letters to the editor. N Engl J Med 1978;299: 366–367).

Herrick, JB. Memories of Eighty Years, Chicago: University of Chicago Press, 1949, p 147.

Kaplan HI, Sadock BJ. Synopsis of Psychiatry. Baltimore: Williams and Wilkins, 1991.

Lipsitt DR. Medical and psychological characteristics of "crocks." Psychiatr Med 1970;1:15–25.

Lown B. The Lost Art of Healing. Boston: Houghton Mifflin, 1996.

MacMurray, J. A philosophers view of modern psychology. Lancet, 1938: In Roope R, The Quiet Art: A Doctor's Anthology. Edinburgh & London: E. & S. Livingstone Ltd., 1952, p 230.

Meador, CF. A Little Book of Doctors' Rules. Philadelphia: Hanley & Belfus; St. Louis: Mosby-Year Book, 1992, rule 219.

Monson RA, Smith GR. Somatization disorder in primary care. N Engl J Med 1983;308:1464–1465.

Peschel RE, Peschel ER. When a Doctor Hates a Patient and Other Chapters in a Young Physician's Life. Berkley: University of California Press, 1986.

Searles HF. Countertransference and Related Subjects. New York: International Universities Press, 1979.

Siegler M. Falling off of the pedestal: what is happening to the traditional doctor–patient relationship? Mayo Clin Proc 1993;68:461–467.

Veatch RM. Abandoning informed consent. Hastings Center Report 1995;25(2):5–12.

Vincent C, Young M, Phillips A. Why do people sue doctors? A study of patients and relatives taking legal action. Lancet 1994;243:1609–1617.

Wolberg L. The management of untoward attitudes in the therapist counter-transference. In: The Technique of Psychotherapy. New York: Grune and Stratton, 1954, pp 488–493.

Ending the Clinical History, Recording It, and Integrating It with the Physical Examination

13

I. **Three Questions to Close the History, Before the Physical Examination**

A. The first question is "What do you think may have caused your symptoms?" or "Are you worried about any particular disease causing your symptoms?"

1. Such questions may disclose fears of specific disorders such as cancer, heart disease, and AIDS. The patient's symptoms may imitate those of a relative or friend who died of these diseases.

2. From the patient's answers, you plan a workup that will exclude the feared disease, or you will know how best to present the unwelcome news if the patient has the feared disease (Creagan, 1994). I had a compelling experience with the father of the next patient.

Pt 30: The parents brought their 3-year-old son to the Riley Hospital emergency room because he had just had a brief febrile convulsion. As the father narrated the history, his voice quavered and his hands shook visibly. Convulsions in a child always upset parents, but the father's reaction far exceeded the usual. I stopped the progression of questions and said, "I see that something has made you extremely upset. Can you tell me about it?" He said, "When I was 9 years old, I had a puppy that had convulsions, and he died one day, in my arms, having a convulsion."

After finishing the workup of the child, I carefully explained that brief febrile convulsions, in an otherwise neurologically normal child with no family history of convulsions, were generally benign. I also provided him with a photocopy of an article from a professional journal that documented this good prognosis. The article served another purpose: It helped him to understand that, although statistically the prognosis was good, not every individual followed the same benign course. Sometimes the good prognosis fails. Along with hope, you have to convey the truth about the range of outcomes. Wherever possible, demystify medical decisions and medical predictions by citing the evidence upon which you act. This process also educates the patient to understand better the scientific evaluation of evidence in general.

B. The second question is "In what way does your health problem bother you most?" This question shows your concern about the effect of the disease on the patient as a person (Schor et al., 1995) and often brings out a very poignant response.

   Pt 31: A mother brought in her 16-pound, 7-month-old baby for a routine follow-up examination for a resolved, mild brachial plexus birth injury. The 47-year-old grandmother, who had myotonic dystrophy, accompanied them. In simply talking with the grandmother about her disorder, I asked, "What bothers you most about your condition?" She broke into tears as she answered, "My hands are too weak to pick up my grandson and hug him." The infant's mother had not realized the depth of her mother's feeling about this incapacity and responded, "Oh, I didn't know. I'll help you hold him." The mother placed the infant in the grandmother's arms, supporting them as the grandmother hugged her grandson and felt his full presence, body to body, for the first time. The tears of sadness streaming down her face now changed to tears of joy. The revelations from this second question, "What bothers you most?" are often immense.

   A corollary question is "What about your life would you most like to change?"

C. The third question to close the history is "Do you have anything else you want to tell me about?" This question forestalls one of the commonest complaints that the physician did not listen to what the patient wanted to say. This question allows the patient to decide whether to continue (White et al., 1994).

D. Reexploring diagnostic hypotheses when closing the history
   1. During the history, the patient's symptoms will have suggested various diagnoses to the physician. These diagnostic hypotheses will lead to expansion of pertinent areas of the history and remind you of what to focus on during the physical examination. The symptoms that at first seem disconnected may begin to fall into patterns. For example, numbness in the fingers and toes suggests neuropathy; severe abdominal pain may come from

pancreatitis. But how do this patient's periodic blackout spells fit in? The closure period prior to the physical examination provides an excellent time to requestion the patient, in the present instance about alcohol ingestion, which can cause neuropathy, pancreatitis, and amnestic spells. However, you must avoid premature conclusions about the diagnosis—in the preceding example porphyria would be another consideration. Defer any actual discussion of diagnosis, prognosis, and management until the end of the physical examination or after completing any necessary tests.

2. A thorough history suggests what tests to concentrate on during the physical examination.

   a. If the patient complains of fatigability, one diagnostic hypothesis might be myasthenia gravis. To test for the fatigability caused by this disease, the physician would have the patient make 50 repetitive vertical eye movements to check for progressive ptosis of the eyelid or progressive diminution of upward gaze. That test is unnecessary without the complaint of fatigability.

   b. If the patient complains of fainting when arising from a sitting position, test for orthostatic hypotension.

   c. A routine examination of an asymptomatic person would not require either of these two tests.

3. The longer (and better) the history, the shorter (and better) the physical examination because the physician will know what does or does not require extensive testing.

E. A question for the physician to pose to himself or herself
At some point—and this is an appropriate one—the physician may ask, silently, "Have I discovered the real needs of this patient?"

II. Acquiring Additional History

A. The telephone test

1. At the end of an interview with an evasive, mentally ill, or demented patient, you may lack essential information or the information derived may have left more of a puzzle than a solution. If the history requires amplification, ask the patient to bring a spouse or friend to the next session. A face-to-face history with the informant is always the best, but in lieu of that, ask for the patient's permission to

telephone a spouse or friend who can fill in the gaps in the history. Generally, the patient should make the call to introduce the physician to the informant. The physician must phrase the questions even more circumspectly than usual to gain the information required while trespassing as little as possible on the patient's privacy or revealing the diagnoses under consideration.

2. For a child with learning or behavioral difficulties, request signed permission from the parents to contact school officials to release teachers' comments and test results.

3. If the patient reports the diagnosis of a serious disorder by another physician, have the patient sign a release of information form and telephone for faxes of the original records to confirm the accuracy of the patient's report. Faxes from a physician's records or a laboratory frequently can be sent immediately, while the patient is still in the office.

4. If doubts remain, repeat the questions after the physical examination or on a follow-up visit. The patient, after thinking for awhile, may provide better answers when requestioned. Students and interns often are surprised or chagrined when a senior staff physician comes right along after them and gets much more informative answers to the same questions than the first interviewer got. The patient has had some practice and time to think and organize.

B. Summarizing the history prior to the physical examination

1. On closing the history, prior to the physical examination, you may want to summarize the important historical information out loud and again to ask the patient to confirm its accuracy, as described earlier (see Chapter 6, section IX). The second summary is particularly important if the review of systems and additional history substantially alter the interpretation of the chief concern and present illness.

2. For intermittent symptoms, such as headaches, the physician may want to requestion the patient about trigger factors.

C. Avoid extending the history during the physical examination Generally, after having closed the history, you should not ask additional historical questions during the physical examination itself. You have to focus full attention on the technique and findings of the physical examination and on keeping the patient comfortable and informed about what is to come. Let the patient get dressed and regain a modicum of dignity after the poking and prodding and the vaginal and rectal examinations. Then face-to-face again, when not towering over a half-clad, recumbent patient, you will obtain much better answers to any additional questions.

III. **Recording the Clinical History**
  A. Note taking
    1. You may make a few notes such as dates or weights during the interview, but you should not appear to the patient as preoccupied with writing everything down. If the physician hunches over the writing pad, eyes riveted on the paper, the patient will feel ignored or left out or will balk at revealing sensitive information. The paranoid patient will be especially wary.
    2. Contrarily, always construct the pedigree while the patient watches, as explained in Chapter 8.
  B. Format for the permanent medical record
    1. Record the history using the standard outline as given in Tables 1–1 and 1–2.
    2. If at all possible, dictate or type the history immediately at the end of each patient contact. You will find a printed record more readable yourself, and any other physician who has to read the notes will give thanks. Transcription of dictation by a typist leaves one major unresolved problem, confidentiality, until technology allows direct transcription from voice to paper. An alternative is to use a code number when sending the tape to the typist and then for the physician to add the patient's name later.
  C. Word choice in the medical record
    1. Although you do not transcribe an interview verbatim, the record must faithfully reflect the original statements. Use the patient's own words and vocabulary where appropriate.
    2. Medical record librarians will supply you with an accepted list of abbreviations and acronyms.
  D. Statements to avoid in recording the history: never, never land
    1. Never, *never* when recording the clinical history speculate or interpret. It is not the editorial page. Record what the patient said. Write down "The patient describes pain behind the breastbone during exercise," if that is what the patient

said, not "The patient describes anginal pain." The latter is a conclusion or interpretation, almost a diagnosis. Take care to distinguish description or factual statements from interpretations. In spite of ambiguities or the possibility of mistaken or dishonest testimony, the recorded history must faithfully reflect the statements that the patient actually made.

2. Never, *never* replace the patients own words for symptoms with technical terms because they may not mean the same. If the patient complains of dizziness, do not automatically substitute the word "vertigo." "Dizziness" has an endless number of meanings, only one of which is vertigo. If the patient describes pain in the right lower quadrant of the abdomen and has pointed to that region, you may use some technical terms—"The patient reports pain in the RLQ of the abdomen"—but in general the fewer technical terms, abbreviations, or acronyms in the record the better.

3. Never, *never* insert pejorative, derogatory, or snide remarks about a patient.
   a. Even if you know that the patient is untruthful, avoid legalisms like "The patient alleges that. . . ." Use the nonpejorative "The patient states that. . . ."
   b. If the patient cannot report dates accurately for whatever reason, dementia or otherwise, state with dignity that the patient is uncertain, not that the patient is demented, is lying, or has a bad memory. Those are conclusions or interpretations, not accurate descriptions of what transpired.

4. Never, *never* insert pejorative, derogatory, or snide remarks that the patient makes about the quality or the appropriateness of previous medical care. Simply record what the patient reports and the outcome. After all, you weren't there and have heard only one side of the story. The malcontent patient who excessively criticizes previous physicians will add you to the list when he or she abandons you for the next physician.

5. Never, *never* obliterate or black out anything written or recorded in the medical record. If you wish to change something, draw a light line through it or around it, leaving the original still legible. Label it an "error," and add a dated, signed explanatory note. Otherwise, it appears that you may have censored or falsified the record.

IV. Integrating the History and the Physical Examination to Complete the Initial Medical Record

A. Write out a summary of no more than three lines

1. After recording the complete history and physical examination, write out a summary. If you understand the patient's clinical problems, you can summarize even very complicated cases in three or, at most, four or five lines, if you work at it:

> This 53-year-old insulin-dependent, diabetic, hypertensive woman had acute, sudden onset of severe mid-chest pain 2 days ago.

2. When presenting patients to me for staffing, students may try to make an impression by reciting an endless history and an endless list of negative physical findings, but I will ask for a three-line summary first. It takes effort to be brief but comprehensive. Mark Twain once apologized to a friend for writing a long letter by stating that he did not have time to make it a short one. The measure of your potential as a physician is not how many noncritical details you can recite but how well you can summarize the pertinent information.

B. Importance of the summary as the bridge to the diagnosis and management

1. A short but compelling summary well repays the hard work. The summary is the most important cognitive part of the medical encounter because it contains the critical data that rationalize the provisional and differential diagnoses and subsequent management of the patient (review Fig. 4–1). The summary is the bridge, the *pons asinorum*, between the clinical findings and the outcome.

2. Not only does the summary sharpen and focus your attention at the time of creation but reading it later allows you to reacquaint yourself immediately with the clinical problem when you see the patient again after a long interval. Similarly, another physician reading your summary knows immediately the thought process that led to your management decisions.

3. After the full workup finally discloses the correct diagnosis, the summary and diagnostic lists allow you to review your thought processes to discover where your reasoning or

fact-finding succeeded or failed. This self-monitoring and self-correction of your own errors is priceless for your continuing medical education. A review of your summary will generally disclose why you made the right or wrong decisions.

C. Write out a clinical impression (preliminary or provisional diagnosis) and a formal list of differential diagnoses (see, Chapter 4, section V, and Fig. 4–1)
   1. The law of parsimony (Occam's razor)

   > Things ought not to be magnified, except out of necessity.
   > —Sir William of Occam (1285–1349)
   > (Hyman, 1983, p 650)

   This law, attributed to William (but not stated in his extant writings), requires the physician to seek a single diagnosis that most parsimoniously explains the clinical data. The physician then records that diagnosis as the "clinical impression" or "provisional diagnosis" and lists the differential diagnoses.

   > Clinical Impression: Essential hypertension.
   > Differential Diagnosis: Rule out renovascular hypertension and pheochromocytoma.

   2. If you suspect two or more unrelated diseases, list each and its differential diagnosis separately, placing the most important disease first:

   > Clinical Impression:
   > 1. Essential hypertension. Rule out renal disease and pheochromocytoma.
   > 2. Contact dermatitis

D. Discussion of the probable diagnosis and differential diagnosis with the patient
   The history will prepare you to explain the diagnosis in terms of the patient's personal fears and previous medical experiences. A benign diagnosis, for example, "tennis elbow," requires no special skill. "You may have breast cancer" requires maximal compassion (Buckman, 1992; Creagan, 1994).

E. Construct a numbered list of the problems to be addressed and their solution
   If the patient has multiple problems, construct a numbered problem list and state the planned solutions as part of the

overall management. The construction of a list of separate problems should not obscure the thread that unites the symptoms and signs. For example, intermittent fever, bleeding gums, anemia, and weight loss may not be four problems but one: leukemia. Nevertheless, when each problem requires different management, the problem list proves its value. Epstein et al. (2003) give several excellent examples of the use of problem lists.

F. Write out a list of tests and consultations
Select the tests and consultations required to establish the correct diagnosis and to reject the alternative diagnoses. First, order the most critical test or tests that will most directly confirm or reject the clinical impression. Go for the jugular. If the diagnosis remains in question after the initial tests, select additional tests, but test in a stepwise manner, in order of probabilities, rather than immediately ordering every conceivable test.

G. Date the document and sign your name legibly
Nothing excuses an illegible signature. Take the time and trouble to write your name legibly, or at least have the courtesy to print it out underneath your signature or carry a rubber stamp that prints your name and affix it after your illegible signature. This is simple courtesy for the next person and good legal practice. Legibility is especially important when several physicians are writing notes in a hospital chart or when documents, such as prescriptions or forms, require signatures.

V. **Integrating the History and Physical Examination: Analyzing the Commonest Symptom of All, Headaches**

A. A patient with one symptom and no signs has a vast differential diagnosis.

1. Given just one symptom, such as stomachache or headache, the physician faces an endless number of differential diagnoses (see Table 6–11). One symptom by itself rarely makes a diagnosis. That comes from the constellation of positive and negative findings. As the history and physical examination reveal more and more relevant symptoms and signs, the shorter the list of differential diagnoses becomes and the more etiologically specific is the final diagnosis. Even one additional symptom or sign drastically reduces the list of possibilities.

2. The next series of patients, who presented with headaches, will show how each additional finding reduces the differential diagnoses to focus on the correct one.

a. *Pt 32:* This 15-year-old girl reports severe intermittent headaches that began 4 years ago. They now occur two or three times per month, causing her to miss school. They tend to come 1 or 2 days after she stays up very late, but she recognizes no other possible trigger factors.

Her headaches commence with a feeling of slight discomfort behind one eye, usually the left. Then she notices zigzag streaks of orange and white light in her vision, moving from left to right. Within a half an hour, the discomfort increases to an unbearable, throbbing pain. The pain usually remains on the left side but sometimes may affect both sides. She becomes nauseated and frequently vomits. Because light and sound cause unbearable discomfort, she must retire to a quiet, dark room. Any efforts to remain up and active or to exercise worsen the headache. Standard analgesics have little effect, but she can usually go to sleep. She will then awaken feeling exhausted but nearly free of pain.

The patient's mother reports that the patient "looks different" by being pallid before or during the headache. The mother and the mother's sister both have similar intermittent, sick headaches that began during their adolescence. The physical examination, done during a headache-free interval, was completely normal.

b. Analysis of Pt 32

(1) If you interrogate many patients with headaches, a number will have a history that matches this patient's, almost word for word. Sorting through descriptions of headaches, we recognize her attacks as migraine (see Table 6–9). Migraine affects some 5%–10% of the population. One or more close family members usually have similar headaches. The headaches frequently begin in childhood or adolescence. Each additional finding extracted by the history, including the family history, buttresses the diagnosis of migraine, building a pattern rarely matched by any other type of headache. For example, tension headaches usually are generalized, tend to

occur every day instead of intermittently, and often are described as feeling like a constricting band or a bursting type of constant pain (see Table 6–11). They may cause blurred vision but not the typical zigzag or fortification scotomas of classical migraine.

(2) The actual lesion of migraine remains unknown, but an increased thickness of the somatosensory cortex has been associated with long-standing migraine (Alexandre et al., 2007). The history may disclose trigger factors such as alcohol, sleep deprivation, or rarely a food intolerance, as established by keeping a diary. The diagnosis is purely historical. We have no objective tests to confirm or reject the diagnosis of migraine. Nevertheless, given a patient with a classical migraine history, the diagnosis is about as secure as any established by objective tests. About the only differential diagnosis in such a patient is an arteriovenous malformation of the brain. Given a family history and a normal examination, most physicians would not obtain radiographic images of the patient's brain. An atypical clinical pattern and a negative family history would weigh toward imaging, while a neurologic sign of brain dysfunction would mandate imaging. Magnetic resonance imaging (MRI) is the method of choice. The entire burden of diagnosis and management falls on the history.

c. *Pt 33:* This 19-year-old nursing student had noticed increasingly severe generalized headaches for 2 months, generally worse on exertion. She had occasional mild blurring of vision lasting up to an hour. She took no medications or vitamins. No one in her family had similar headaches. The physical examination disclosed bilateral papilledema (swelling of the optic nerve heads) and moderate obesity but no other findings.

d. Analysis of Pt 33

(1) Headache, papilledema, and intermittent obscuration of vision (amaurosis fugax) constitute a syndrome because one pathogenetic mechanism, increased intracranial pressure, lawfully explains all three. While other disorders can cause a syndrome of headache and amaurosis fugax, the papilledema

begins to limit the diagnostic probabilities and focuses the diagnostic search on the probability of an intracranial cause. The papilledema means that the diagnostic search has to focus on secondary headaches, rather than primary ones as in migraine or tension headaches (see Table 6–9).

(2) The physician then makes a descriptive clinical impression and differential diagnoses as follows:

Clinical Impression: Headache secondary to increased intra-cranial pressure presumably idiopathic intracranial hyper-tension (also called pseudotumor cerebri).

Differential Diagnosis: Space-occupying lesion: neoplasm or hematoma

Vascular lesion: venous thrombosis

Intoxication: lead, vitamin A, or tetracycline

Endocrinopathy: steroid, thyroid

Infection/chronic basilar meningitis

(3) To explore these possibilities requires an MRI of the brain with an magnetic resonance venogram (MRV) to rule out or to identify a specific mass lesion that threatens to cause internal brain herniation and death or a vascular lesion. The MRI may clearly establish the etiologic diagnosis such as bilateral subdural hematomas. If normal, the MRI provides critical evidence against life-threatening lesions, such as internal herniation of the brain, hematoma, neoplasm, or obstructive hydrocephalus, which would require surgical treatment. This information excluding diseases proves as essential to diagnosis and management as a positive finding.

(4) The patient's MRI scan showed normal-sized or questionably small lateral ventricles. The MRV showed patent venous sinuses, excluding venous sinus thrombosis. The evidence now suggests that the patient has so-called idiopathic intracranial hypertension (pseudotumor cerebri). The provisional diagnosis narrows the window of diagnostic possibilities but still, in itself, leaves a differential diagnosis (Table 13–1).

Table 13–1. Causes for the Syndrome of Increased Intracranial Pressure Without Localizing Signs

Hydrocephalus
  Intraventricular obstruction
  Aqueductal stenosis
  Extraventricular obstruction
  Colloid cyst of third ventricle
  Choroid plexus papilloma
Metabolic disorders
  Obesity
  Uremia
  Hypophosphatasia
  Vitamin B2 deficiency
  Metabolic megalencephaly
  Alkalosis
  Hypertensive encephalopathy eclampsia
  Vitamin D–deficient rickets
Toxic agents
  Heavy-metal poisoning
    Lead
    Arsenic
  Hypervitaminosis A
  Tetracycline and minocycline therapy
  Nalidixic acid therapy
  Sulfamethoxazole
  Isoretinoin
  Indomethacin
  Nitrofurantoin
  Praxiquantal
  Amiodarone
Cardiovascular–pulmonary insufficiency
  Dural sinus obstruction: thrombotic,
    inflammatory, or neoplastic
  Congestive heart failure
  Pulmonary insufficiency
  Superior vena cava obstruction

Infections or parainfectious diseases
  Otitis media
  Sinusitis/mastoiditis
  Landry Guillain Barre Strohl syndrome (high CSF
    protein)
  Fungal/viral meningoencephalitis
  Parasitic infestations
Endocrinopathies
  Oral contraceptive use
  Pregnancy
  Ovarian dysfunction
  Prolonged steroid therapy
  Steroid withdrawal
  Hyperadrenalism
  Hypoadrenalism (Addison disease)
  Hypothyroidism
  Hyperthyroidism
  Hypoparathyroidism
  Pseudohypoparathyroidism
Blood dyscrasias
  Polycythemia
  Leukemia
  Anemia
  Hemophilia
  Wiskott-Aldrich syndrome
  Thrombocytopenia
Miscellaneous conditions
  Idiopathic intracranial hypertension
    (pseudotumor cerebri)
  Skull dysplasia, such as Paget disease
  Any cause of high CSF protein
  Some demyelinating encephalopathies

CSF, cerebrospinal fluid.

(5) Because of the suspicion of intracranial hypertension, I requestioned the patient about overingestion of vitamin A and about any possible long-term use of tetracycline antibiotics and endocrine drugs such as estrogens or steroids. I ordered thyroid function tests and blood lead levels. Since the MRI had shown no danger of brain herniation, I did a lumbar puncture to exclude chronic meningitis, such as cryptococcal. The workup was designed to identify any treatable proximate causes for increased intracranial pressure

and remove the idiopathic label. A lumbar puncture would not be done in a patient with papilledema unless a computed tomographic (CT) or preferably an MRI scan had excluded a mass lesion that threatened to cause brain herniation. I had a neuro-ophthalmologist measure the patient's visual acuity and chart the visual fields very carefully because chronic papilledema can permanently diminish vision by causing secondary optic atrophy.

(6) In patients with idiopathic increased pressure, in spite of increased intracranial pressure, the MRI shows no consistent changes in ventricular size or diagnostic features. Fairly commonly in medical practice a finding is consistent with a diagnosis but not diagnostic of it. Laboratory findings can be normal, can be consistent with but not diagnostic of the lesion, can positively identify the lesion, or can definitely exclude certain lesions. All of the clinical and laboratory findings in Pt 33 support the provisional diagnosis of idiopathic intracranial hypertension: the disease is commoner in obese, young women. The workup had excluded identifiable intoxications and endocrinopathies, and the MRI had excluded other causes of increased intracranial pressure. Thus, the diagnosis, in this instance based on exclusion of identifiable proximate causes and the conjunction of positive and negative findings, was idiopathic intracranial hypertension.

e. *Pt 34:* This 42-year-old man had noticed increasingly severe headaches for several months. Prior to that, he had suffered only mild headaches two or three times per year. He felt the pain in the front of his head, about equally on both sides. He described the pain as a rather severe but dull ache, somewhat worse in the mornings and increased by straining. He complained of some vague unsteadiness in walking and of some difficulty concentrating on his work. His family reported a tendency for increased irritability. The review of systems produced no significant additional symptoms. The family history disclosed some mild headaches in other family members but no information that clarified the cause of the patient's symptoms.

The general physical examination was normal. The neurologic examination showed questionable weakness on his right side and some slowness in finger tapping on the right, his dominant hand.

f. Analysis of Pt 34

(1) The history of a change in headache pattern, a change in mental state, and a probable neurologic sign led to the provisional diagnosis of an intracranial space-occupying lesion. This hypothesis mandates imaging of the brain as the first critical step in management.

(2) An MRI scan disclosed a butterfly-shaped lesion extending across the corpus callosum. It involved the left cerebral hemisphere a little more than the right. A stereotaxic biopsy disclosed a glioblastoma multiforme.

(3) While headache is a sine qua non for the diagnosis of classical migraine or idiopathic intracranial hypertension, headaches occur in only about half of patients with brain tumors at the time of the diagnosis (Forsyth and Posner, l993). The history discloses no single pattern that separates brain tumor headaches from all others, but patients with increased intracranial pressure tend to have generalized headaches, associated with nausea and vomiting. Headaches tend to reflect the rapidity of growth of the tumor and the degree of midline shift. The pain probably comes from increased pressure or the tension on pain-sensitive structures such as the dura, blood vessels, or cranial nerves. Neurologic symptoms or signs generally accompany a brain tumor headache and draw attention to the fact that the headache is secondary rather than primary (see Chapter 6, section VII, C, 4, and Table 6–9).

B. A headache admonition

New-onset headaches, like any new-onset pain, require an extensive search for definable causes. For example, re-read the protocol for Pt 5 (Chapter 4, section VI), who presented with new-onset headaches.

VI. **Summary**
  A. Summarize the history
    Before moving on to the physical examination, summarize the history out loud to the patient. Ask the patient to modify or correct any inaccuracies.
  B. Close the history with three questions.
    1. First, ask what the patient thinks may have caused the symptoms. This question discloses whether the patient fears a particular disease. The physician can then reassure the patient that the feared disease is not present or can cushion the news if it is present.
    2. Second, ask how the health problem or disease affects the patient's life the most.
    3. Third, ask whether the patient wants to discuss anything more. This question allows the patient to close or to continue the interview as desired.
  C. Acquiring additional historical information
    1. You may need to supplement the patient's narrative by talking to an informant or by getting consent to review school or medical records.
    2. Usually, you should avoid historical questioning during the physical exam because of the necessity to focus all attention on the techniques, the findings, and the patient's comfort. While half-clad or recumbent, the patient will not answer as freely as clothed and face-to-face.
  D. An increase in the number of findings narrows the diagnostic possibilities.
    Diagnosis of one symptom, such as headache or stomachache, with no supporting findings is almost hopeless because of too many possibilities. Each additional bit of historical data and each positive or negative physical or laboratory finding narrows the diagnostic quest. Two findings are easier to diagnose than one, three easier than two, and so on. The diagnosis of disorders such as headaches, which may produce no physical or laboratory signs, depends on the positive and negative findings disclosed by the history, the physical exam, and certain laboratory tests that exclude alternative diagnoses or focus on one.

E. Ending the session

At the end of the history and physical examination, the physician summarizes the findings of the history and physical examination and discusses the diagnosis and appropriate management. Ask whether the patient wants a family member present during this discussion and how much you should disclose.

F. Recording the history

1. Taking some notes during the history is permissible, but focus on the patient, not the writing pad. Extensive recording of everything the patient says will inhibit some patients. Put aside your pencil when taking sensitive parts of the history, such as sexual activity.

2. After dismissing the patient at the end of the visit, write out or dictate the history according to the standard outline (see Table 1–1 and outline of Chapter 1), but use the patient's words and terms, not technical terms. Dictate the history if possible. Otherwise, write legibly.

3. Record the actual information derived. Do not editorialize or speculate. Avoid pejorative or demeaning remarks about the patient or previous medical care.

4. Correct any errors already entered in the medical record by drawing a light line around the error, and write a signed and dated explanatory note. Do not black out any part of the chart.

5. Make a three-line summary. Work hard to make it as brief as possible. It justifies everything to follow (see Fig. 4–1).

6. State a single diagnosis as the clinical impression, in accordance with the law of parsimony. Then add a list of differential diagnoses and a list of tests or consultations. Some tests serve to confirm a suspected diagnosis. Other tests exclude alternative diagnoses, particularly those requiring immediate attention.

7. For a complicated patient, devise a problem list, with the proposed solutions to each problem.

8. List a treatment plan and, where appropriate, a prevention plan and a wellness plan.

9. Date the document and sign it legibly.

e

Stop.

References

Alexandre FM, DaSilva DDS, Hadjikhani N, et al. Thickening in the somatosensory cortex of patients with migraine. Neurology 2007;69:1990–1995.

Buckman R. How to Break Bad News: A Guide for Health Care Professionals. Baltimore: Johns Hopkins University Press, 1992.

Creagan ET. How to break bad news—and not devastate the patient. Mayo Clin Proc 1994;69:1015–1017.

Epstein O, Perkin GD, de Bono DP, et al. Clinical Examination, 3rd ed. Philadelphia: Mosby, 2003.

Forsyth PA, Posner JB. Headaches in patients with brain tumors: a study of 111 patients. Neurology 1993;43:1678–1682.

Hyman A, Walsh JJ. Philosophy in the Middle Ages: The Christian, Islamic, and Jewish Traditions. Indianapolis: Hackett, 1983, p 650.

Schor EL, Lerner DJ, Malspeis S. Physicians' assessment of functional health status and well-being. Arch Intern Med 1995;155:309–314.

White J, Levinson W, Roter D. "Oh by the way . . .": the closing moments of the medical visit. J Gen Intern Med 1994;9:24–32.

The History, Appropriate Management, Informed Consent, and Patient Autonomy

14

I. How the Same Techniques for the Clinical History Evaluate Patient Autonomy and Informed Consent
  A. Summary of the techniques for the clinical history
  Thus far, the text has presented the best techniques for obtaining an optimal clinical history. These techniques consist of
    1. Programming every action or circumstance for the patient's benefit
    2. Appropriate demeanor and dress
    3. Use of open questions
    4. Privacy and confidentiality
    5. Nonjudgmental acceptance of every patient
    6. Respect for the patient's autonomy, goals, and values and avoidance of imposing personal beliefs and proselytizing
    7. Monitoring of the transference–countertransference interactions
  B. Critical factors in informed consent and patient autonomy
    1. Conveniently enough, the best techniques for eliciting the basic clinical history and the mental status also serve best to explore whether the patient has the basis for autonomy and informed consent.
    2. The critical factors in informed consent and true patient autonomy are that the patient has received and understands fully the pros and cons of management options and that the patient has *sapience*, the intellectual power and capacity to decide wisely. In summary, the same techniques blend seamlessly to achieve these goals:
      a. Gathering data for the clinical history per se (see Table 1–1)
      b. Evaluating the mental status (see Table 9–3)
      c. Evaluating whether the patient has the knowledge base and capacity for informed consent by exploring for irrationalities, misinformation, mental illness, or familial or societal pressures that usurp the patient's apparent autonomy

      d. Achieving understanding, compassion, and trust between patient and physician

C. Multiple factors direct patient autonomy and informed consent

  1. When thoughtfully examined, the terms "patient autonomy" and "informed consent" qualify as abstractions that conceal a maelstrom of competing mental forces. Patient autonomy invokes the concept of free will, but is anyone ever truly autonomous or in possession of free will?

  2. One's choices derive from innumerable fortuitous factors such as the date and place of birth; family, peer, and societal pressures; the kaleidoscope of powerful events that impinge on us daily; our IQ and education; our physical and mental health; and the streams of hormones and biochemicals that flood our brain. Relatively little that we experience as conscious selection arises simply from rational thought.

II. Interrelations of Appropriate Management, Informed Consent, and Patient Autonomy

A. What is appropriate management?

  1. At the end of the history and physical, the physician discusses the likely diagnoses with the patient and outlines options for appropriate management, according to evidence-based guidelines. Management includes all aspects of differential diagnosis, therapy, prevention, and patient education (see Fig. 4–1).

  2. Appropriate management meets scientific evidence for validity, safety, and efficacy or, in lieu of evidence-based data, reflects the consensus of experienced physicians. It varies from doing nothing more than a complete history and physical examination to total life support. Physicians should define appropriate management options, not lawyers, judges, and legislators, who lack medical and scientific training and the day-to-day experience of patient care (Annas, 1994).

  3. The physician presents prognosis and risk/benefit ratios in sufficient detail for the patient to give informed consent. Sometimes more than one plan offers about an equal chance of success (e.g., surgical versus medical therapy). If one plan is clearly best, the physician recommends it, such as to biopsy a lump in the breast. Usually, patient and

physician agree on the management and proceed forthwith. Medical ethics and the law require informed consent from either the patient or surrogate for the physician to initiate treatment (see also the discussion in this chapter, section III, C–E).

4. Appropriate management may also include referral to a lay support group or governmental agency.

5. Because many patients today go right from the office visit to the Internet, I forewarn them to consult reliable sites, such as the consensus statements of the various professional organizations and their information booklets for patients and the U.S. Public Health Service. Some patients may benefit from Stephen Barrett's www.quackwatch.org and appraisals of alternative medicine by Bartecchi (2002), Friedland (1998), and the *Nutrition Action Health Letter* (particularly the January 24, 2006 issue, www.cspinet.org).

B. When do informed consent and patient autonomy work best?

1. Patient autonomy works best when a competent physician informs a sapient patient of the valid management choices and their likely outcomes.

2. True patient autonomy for informed consent requires a rational understanding of medical realities. Decisions based on misinformation, irrational fears, mental illness, or societal pressures produce only illusory autonomy, not free choices (Miles, 1991). Freedom is the knowledge of necessity, of medical reality. That is what the physician does, apprises the patient of medical reality.

3. Physicians may fail to recognize incompetence, particularly if the history is substandard. Applebaum (2007) and Etchells et al. (1999) provide detailed criteria for evaluating the patient's competence for informed consent.

C. To base consent on reality, patients should accept appropriate investigation of their illness

1. Patient/physician teamwork imposes obligations on the patient, the necessity to answer questions honestly during the history and to allow the tests required to make the diagnosis. Informed consent can come only from an accurate diagnosis.

2. A patient who has *Pneumocystis jirovecii* (formerly *Pneumocystis carinii*) pneumonia and Kaposi sarcoma needs

testing for AIDS because these conditions virtually never appear together in any other disease. Refusal to allow the investigations that will disclose the real basis for the patient's illness destroys the physician's professional purpose. Obstructive autonomy, "You can't question me about that" or "I won't allow you to test me for diabetes," defeats the very purpose of seeking professional help and destroys any possibility of informed consent.

D. Role of the history in assessing patient preferences, autonomy, and appropriate medical management

1. From the history, the physician learns the patient's beliefs and values in order to reconcile appropriate management with them (Angell, 1984; Inui, 1998; Tauber, 2005). Nevertheless, a physician should act to promote the patient's health, not simply to acquiesce in or pander to what the patient desires (Miles, 1991). Knowing medical realities, most physicians do not passively accept preferences that contradict appropriate management (Brock and Wartman, 1990). The patient may prefer alcohol to treat anxieties or desire a narcotic or amphetamines. Some persons might argue that the patient has merely exercised free choice, but can the addicted, diseased, or misinformed brain exercise free choice?

2. Patient autonomy does not mean sauntering through a medical cafeteria, "I prefer a little of this and some of those, but never any of that." A striking paradox arises in balancing the patient's personal preferences and appropriate management: The physician must offer management that serves the patient's health, not necessarily the patient's desires or the desires of the patient's family or, for that matter, the desires of society at large. This conclusion rests on the fact that numerous factors such as mental illness may dictate the patient's decisions or cultural and governmental demands may prevail, as in the killing of the mentally retarded in Nazi Germany (Burleigh, 1994; von Weizsacker, 1947) or in circumcising pubertal girls. Even the family may not know or be depended on to clarify the patient's preferences (Sulmasy et al., 1998).

3. The physician does not capitulate to an unwise medical decision as if it was simply the patient's political right (Pellegrino, 1993).

> The patient comes to the physician for the best advice about what ought and ought not to be done.... The physician cannot escape his or her responsibility for doing what is medically sound and refusing to do what is not medically sound.
> —Edward Pellegrino
> (see Pellegrino, 1993, p 34)

4. Serving the patient's health, not simply the patient's desires, does not mean ignoring the wishes of the patient and the family. It means just the opposite: An extended history must search for pressures and reasons that result in inappropriate choices (Brock and Wartman, 1990; Lachs et al., 1990).
5. In addition to the pressures on the patient's autonomy from the family and society, health-care plans may further reduce autonomy by restricting choices to an approved list of physicians, hospitals, management choices, procedures, and medications (Burnam, 1984).

E. Use of the standard history to anticipate barriers to accepting appropriate management
1. The history affords several prime opportunities to discover unobtrusively the patient's true attitudes about illness and its management.
   a. During the past clinical history, discern the patient's reactions to previous personal illnesses, hospitalizations, injuries, and operations.
   b. During the family history, discern the patient's reactions to the management of illnesses and deaths of family members.
   c. During the psychosocial history and mental status examination, explore for beliefs that will affect the management.
   d. When closing the history, ask what the patient thinks may have caused the illness (see Chapter 13). The patient may fear that the physician has overlooked some dreaded disease.
2. When discussing management options, learn whether the patient believes in irrational therapies or has irrational attitudes to medications or surgery: "I won't take any pills" or "Nobody is going to cut on me."

F. When is patient preference virtually the only determinant of the management?

1. Sometimes, as in electing to participate in a clinical trial or donation of organs before or after death, the preference of a competent patient must solely prevail (Caplan and Coelho, 1998).

2. Still, the person's choice, especially organ donation by a living donor, is not always free (Ingelfinger, 2005; Steinbrook, 2005; Truog, 2005, 2008). Argani (1999, p 16), a veteran physician involved in transplantation, observed this:

> But I have moved in clinical situations where coercion, or bribery was not so obvious. The unspoken threat of family discord, the possibility of exclusion from loved ones and from a life-style if one did not comply—how many clinicians can detect these hidden motives in a brief interview?
>
> —Sholey Argani

3. Sometimes, as in seeking predictive genetic information, the physician may want to alter the patient's decision. Huntington chorea, an autosomal dominant degenerative brain disease, appears at an average age of 37 years. It causes gradual dementia and incessant twitching. Over many years, the patient declines into a helpless, bed-ridden, demented state. No cure is known. Now, DNA analysis can identify persons at risk. Would you choose at 21 years of age to learn that at 37 you will start to twitch and become demented and helpless, just as you have already seen in a parent or other relatives (Elias and Annas, 1994)? In discussing genetic tests, as for breast cancer, you should explore the patient's likely reaction to the results. If the patient overtly intends to commit suicide if the test foretells the disease, the physician then may try to discourage testing. Two possibilities justify rejecting suicide: the possibility of a change of mind by the patient (Albert et al., 1999; Patterson et al., 1993) and the possibility of the discovery of effective treatment in the interim. Consider referring the patient to an experienced genetics counselor for a thorough explanation of the pitfalls and limitations of genetic testing.

4. In the future, genetic engineering again will involve patient choice. The patient might choose to alter a gene to prevent a heredofamilial disease, but what about altering a gene to change the length of the nose, eye color, or a personality

trait (Mehlman, 2003; Wivel and Walters, 1993)? Here, patient autonomy may have to submit to some societal controls (Fletcher, 1988).

5. In summary, patient autonomy involves a number of gradations from nearly absolute to conditional. Autonomy in regard to newer reproductive technologies and stem cell research elicits polarized debates (Maienschein, 2003) that cannot be resolved here. Kass (2002) presents a cautious view (Bernat, 2003) that many cellular biologists oppose (Holden, 2004).

III. **Extending the History When the Patient Declines Appropriate Management**

A. Practical steps in response to inappropriate preferences

1. If the patient rejects appropriate management, review Table 12–3 for errors in taking the history. Extending the history guides the physician in how to explain the medical necessities and in furthering the patient's education and understanding.

2. If the initial reasoning fails, avoid arguing, but schedule return appointments to extend the history. Sometimes, if the patient agrees to it, a meeting with the spouse or the family resolves the issue. Ultimately, the discovery and resolution of the patient's resistances may require full psychiatric evaluation.

> Whenever the patient cannot see the obvious it is because he needs his blindness.
>
> —Lawrence Kolb, M.D.
> (see Kolb, 1977, p 774)

3. Sometimes the beliefs of physician and patient differ too much for reconciliation. In such circumstances, the physician should avoid authoritarian arguing or proselytizing (Curlin et al., 2007).

4. If all due efforts at resolution of differences fail, the physician may have to withdraw (*recuse*) and refer the patient to another physician, but matters rarely reach such an impasse if a compassionate history has achieved empathy and trust. Surrogate approval for management of mentally ill or retarded patients, who cannot make their own decisions, constitutes a separate issue (Cantor, 2005). The task then becomes one of assessing the

patient's competence (Applebaum, 2007; Etchells et al., 1999).

B. How to avoid paternalism and personal advice
   1. *Paternalism* means pressuring the patient to do it simply because the "doctor knows best."
   2. If the patient asks directly "What would you do if you were me?" one reply is "I would do just what you are doing. I would go to an experienced doctor to learn the medical realities, talk with the people in my life whom I respect, and then decide what is best in my circumstances." This answer gently but firmly divides the physician's role, which is to portray the medical realities, from the patient's role, which is to select appropriate management.

C. Active intervention with noncompliant, infected patients
   1. A thorough compassionate history aimed at reconciliation must precede any interventions to forestall destructive choices.
   2. Some patients with infections like tuberculosis or AIDS refuse treatment and continue to infect others. The physician extends the history to uncover the reason for the irrationality and then tries to get the patient to accept appropriate treatment on ethical and scientific grounds. In the end, in spite of the patient's wishes, the laws governing the reporting and management of infectious disease have to be obeyed.
   3. The management of an AIDS-infected pregnant woman exemplifies the complex intersection of medical ethics, patient autonomy, and legalities. Appropriate drug treatment during the pregnancy greatly reduces the risk of the baby being infected (medical reality). Is treatment then a matter of personal preference by the mother, or should it be legally mandated?
   4. Another profoundly difficult decision arises in whether to force-feed a person dying of anorexia nervosa or a person choosing starvation as a political protest (Glick, 1997).

D. Active intervention when parental preferences constitute child abuse
   1. By law, physicians must report suspected or overt child abuse, whether physical, sexual, emotional, or a matter of neglect.

2. Parents may abuse their child by refusing life-saving treatment, for example, choosing homeopathy or prayer to treat meningitis. No creditable evidence establishes either as effective. While recognizing the parents' right to their beliefs, the law generally prohibits imposing these beliefs when, in reality, the beliefs may lead to the child's disability or death (Asser and Swan, 1998).

3. Sometimes an emergency court order for the appropriate, life-saving management is the last resort.

E. Active intervention when mental illness or a brain disease precludes rational judgment and leads to self-destructive preferences

1. From the history and physical examination, the physician determines whether the patient has an overtly diseased brain or mental illness that nullifies free will and free choice (DeMyer, 2004). Five minutes of history with any symptomatic schizophrenic will quickly disclose that the disease commands the patient's thoughts and nullifies any semblance of free will. You can politicize the patient's refusal of appropriate medical care as an inalienable right, or you can consider Dr. William F. Sheeley's (1975, p 1) plea for social responsibility:

> ... I have these hopes, that is, that others would make decisions for me should disease take my ability to decide for myself.
>
> But . . . I hear of movements to deny me constraint and treatment unless I demand them—that is, if I reject constraint and treatment for whatever reason, I won't get them.
>
> I hear of those who would protect my right to die of brain hemorrhage or diabetes, my right to maim and kill myself from melancholy, my right to fear shadows and to rage at windmills, my right to thirst while lost in old man's confusion under Arizona's desert summer sun, my right bemusedly to starve in flophouse or alley, or my right to spree myself into financial and social rubble.
>
> Does he who does not assume for me the onus of responsible decision-making when I've lost my ability to make it, and who won't allow someone to treat me while I'm too sick to ask for it, thereby deny me my right to his concern and help?

2. This plea reflects the wisdom of a physician schooled by long hours at the bedside, not a cloistered theorist who understands neither mental illness nor how to diagnose and

treat it but charges paternalism against physicians who do so. The danger in intervention always consists of imposing a physician's or family's personal prejudices, societal attitude, or state-defined orthodoxy about what constitutes health and appropriate action. A delicate balance always exists between patient rights and coercive management (Gasner et al., 1999; Kapp, 2000; Kassirier, 1983; Saks, 2002; Schneider, 1998; Tauber, 2005).

> Taking freedom seriously means acknowledging the rights of competent individuals to dispose of their lives in ways that others may judge imprudent.
>
> —H. T. Engelhardt
> (see Engelhardt, 1989, p 79)

F. Active intervention when a patient tries to commit suicide
   1. When a patient is brought to an emergency room, comatose from a barbiturate overdose, with a suicide note in his or her pocket, the physician saves the patient's life, in direct opposition to the patient's expressed wishes. No doubt exists about the patient's intent. The note and the barbiturate ingestion prove intent beyond any doubt. But the physician does not shrug his or her shoulders and say, "Oh, this one preferred to die. Therefore I will respect the patient's right to die." Most physicians do not regard suicide politically, as a right to die, but medically, as an opportunity for prevention by utilizing the history to disclose the causes for the death wish. Survivors often express thanks for medical intervention that has saved their life (Jamison, 1999).
   2. A careful history of suicidal patients may disclose depression, borderline personality disorder, substance abuse (Block and Billings, 1994; Hudgens, 1983; Lesage et al., 1994; Sullivan and Youngner, 1994), and sometimes unexpected underlying systemic or neurologic disease, such as lupus erythematosis or anemia. In the United States, around 30,000 suicidal deaths are reported each year; 90% of the victims have a mental illness (Iglehart, 2004). The history must always explore suicidal thoughts, especially in troubled teenagers.
   3. For the depressed patient with no somatic disease, the history has to distinguish between reactive and endogenous depression. Reactive depression may represent a normal

reaction to circumstances, which the history will disclose. Reactive depression often responds to supportive psychotherapy. Cycles of mania and depression and a family history suggest a bipolar depression. It usually responds to combined psychotherapy, antidepressant drugs, and lithium.

4. Another reason to reject suicide is that follow-up histories disclose that the death wish is not immutable (O'Brien, 1999; Patterson et al., 1993). The patient may have acted impulsively, on the spur of the moment. Survivors usually regret the act, change their mind, and want to live (Chochinov et al., 1995; Jamison, 1999; Patterson et al., 1993; Silverstein et al., 1991).

5. The book *Final Exit* by Humphrey (1992 and earlier versions), a how-to-do-it suicide manual, has promoted the death of individuals who were merely depressed, not terminally ill (Marzuk et al., 1993), who might have changed their mind.

IV. **How Promotion of Elective Cosmetic Surgery of Normal Tissues Biases the History**

A. What motivates requests for purely cosmetic alterations of normal tissues?

1. The skills of today's surgeons border on the miraculous. If the indications are correct, no treatments in medicine exceed surgery for the likelihood of a rapid, successful outcome. This applies particularly to the teams of plastic surgeons; neurosurgeons; ophthalmologists; ear, nose, and throat specialists; and dentists, who recontour malformed or injured faces and now even transplant faces (Dubernad et al., 2007). But when a patient requests surgery to alter a normal contour rather than to correct a true defect, the history should probe why the patient wants it done and what the patient expects it to accomplish.

2. A searching history usually discloses deep insecurities about appearance and acceptability, an underestimation of risks and complications, and an overestimation of the benefits. Although producing temporary or even permanent testimonial satisfaction, cosmetic operations frequently fail to solve the basic lack of esteem that initiated the request (Blum, 2003; Davis, 1995; Haiken, 1997). A year later the

patient, with her altered nose, thickened lips, and bulging breasts, may still suffer from the same self-doubts as before; but now she has endured hours of pain and spent thousands of dollars that could have secured an education or psychotherapy that would genuinely repair self-esteem (McBryde, 1999). A current popular entertainer, starting with a perfectly normal—one might say handsome—face, has had it transformed it into a mélange of unharmonious parts. Had a careful history disclosed why the patient repeatedly requested surgery? Does that patient suffer from body dysmorphic disorder (Phillips et al., 1993)? Did the history explore the patient's real knowledge of risks (Borah et al., 1999; Rothman and Rothman, 2003; Shute, 2004), including increased risk of suicide (McLaughlin et al., 2004)?

B. Integrating the history with surgical principles

   1. One of my professors of surgery, Dr. Jacob Berman, impressed three aphorisms upon my class in 1952. He did it so effectively that, decades later, I still hear his voice:

      a. "Surgery usually means the failure of medical management." Modern surgery has softened but not eliminated this injunction.

      b. "Handle the tissues with loving kindness."

      c. "The body tolerates foreign substances more or less poorly." Again, modern technology has softened, but not eliminated, the injunction.

   2. Physicians who adhere to these three principles would not make perforations for rings in the nose, nipples, or navel or perform mutilating female circumcision, as practiced in some cultures (Allam et al., 1999; Schroeder, 1994; Toubia, 1994). Similarly, most dentists would decline a teenager's request to implant diamonds in the front teeth. The entire training, the raison d'être, of health professionals is to preserve teeth and tissues, not to violate them.

C. How advertising creates demand but curtails and distorts the history, changing its purpose, depth, and the very questions asked

   1. Some ads exploit the insecurities of physically healthy women by touting "free consultations," like the liability attorneys (Margo, 1987). An example of how societal attitudes in synergy with financial incentives for physicians

recruit patients is this ad, paraphrased from an actual one that regularly appeared in an Indianapolis newspaper:

BREAST AUGMENTATION

The _____ Clinic announces a TWO FOR ONE consultation on breast augmentation! When you bring a friend or relative with you to a breast augmentation consultation, the surgeon's fee is at half the normal cost—for both of you.

2. Will that surgeon explore and offer nonsurgical alternatives or take a psychiatric history (Sarwer et al., 2004)? To whom will the patient turn when the breast augmentation fails to alleviate the depression and sexual and personal anxieties that the ads exploit? By shrewd inclusion of some questions and exclusion of others, the history transforms into a vehicle to sell operations or make profit, rather than to discover the best medical management for each person. Numerous studies show that the manner in which an interrogator asks question and offers options and the conditions of the interview strongly influence the choices made (Kahneman and Tversky, 1984; Tauber, 2005.

3. In summary, our ethics determine the purposes, techniques, content, and goals of our histories and our offerings for management. We cannot separate ethics from what we do (Tauber, 2005). Our ethics and goals, good or bad, define us and determine our every policy and action.

D. How inadequate histories that failed to document the extent of informed consent destroyed trust and led to mass action lawsuits

1. Physicians could have avoided the bitter, mass action lawsuits over breast implants by applying Dr. Berman's surgical aphorisms and taking complete histories that accurately gauged the degree of "informed consent" of the women. Did the surgeon's history explore the insecurities of each woman and help her to accept her body as it was without surgery (aphorism 1 of Dr. Berman)? Does slicing open a breast to stuff in a prosthesis constitute handling the tissues with loving kindness (*primum non nocere* and Berman's aphorism 2)? Did the histories disclose whether women fully understood the frequency and type of local complications from the implants (aphorism 3) and that we simply did not know the long-term risks? Now, even though

implants apparently do not cause systemic disease (Kjoller et al., 2001), that was unknown earlier. Around 60% of women considered preoperative information as insufficient (Kulmala et al., 2004). Did the preoperative histories disclose whether the women really knew that they were the experimental subjects, the guinea pigs, from whom any short- or long-term risks would be discovered; and did the women give informed consent to serve as experimental subjects (American Academy of Neurology, 1998b; Truog et al., 1999)? Utilization of the techniques advocated here would have insured truly informed consent, eliminating the sense of violated trust.

2. The illicit trafficking in human organs and tissues, including fetal tissues, illustrates another extreme of commercial exploitation (Andrews and Nelkin, 2001). The physician receiving payment from the buyer is unlikely to have taken a probing history from the donor.

> Under the rule of economism, one may expect to find exploitation wherever there is opportunity.
> —Charles D. Aring, M.D. (1904–1998) (1971, p 180)

3. The physicians who encouraged the market for breast implants and body recontouring do not feel obligated to dig through a long history to find out how to encourage women to feel sufficient about their value and worth as persons, apart from breast size or body contour (Blum, 2003; Davis, 1995).

4. Around 500 years ago Thomas Gale dealt with the ethical concerns about surgery discussed here, including the necessity to insure that the patient had realistic expectations about the outcome:

> The chirugian must also in theis his operations observe five thynges principally. First that he doeth it safelye, and that wythout hurte or damage to the pacient, secondly, that he do not detracte tyme or let slepe good occasions offered in workyng, but with suche spede as arte wyll soffer, let hym finishe his cure. Therdly, that he work jently, courtyously, and wyth so lytle payne the pacient, as conveniently you may, and not roughly, butcherly, rudlye, and wythout a comlenes. Forthly, that he be as free from crafte and deceyte in all his workynges, as the East is from the Weaste. Fiftly, that he taketh

> no cure in the hande for lucre or gaynes sake only, but rather for an honest and competent rewarde, with a godly affection, to doe his diligence. Laste of all, that he maketh no warrantyse of suche sicknes, as are incurable, as to cure a Cancer or ulcerate, or elephantiasis confirmed: but circumspectlye to consider what the effecte is, and promyse no more then arte can performe.
>
> —Thomas Gale, An Institution of a Chirugian, 1563 (1958)

V. The Clinical History, Physician-Assisted Suicide, and Euthanasia

> Do not go gentle into that good night.
> Rage, rage against the dying of the light.
>
> —Dylan Thomas (1914–1953) (2001, p 151)

A. Feelings disclosed by a thorough history in patients who request physician-assisted suicide or euthanasia
  1. The patient facing aggressive, life-threatening disease feels diminished, defiled, debased, and isolated. The ill person undergoes stages of grieving: denial, anger, guilt, depression, and resignation. The patient experiences some resentment and even jealousy at the health of others: "Why, oh why, did this disease attack me?"
  2. The patient feels some guilt, as if personally responsible for the illness, which justly punishes her or him. These feelings interfere with the acceptance of love and comfort and augment a death wish.
  3. Patients who harbor lifelong feelings of inferiority, unworthiness, or guilt cannot tolerate burdening the physician and family or absorbing costly medical resources (Sullivan et al., 2001).
B. Reverence for life and desire for life
  1. Most physicians accept on principle that patients with a healthy mind want to live, even patients with disease-ravaged bodies, even quadriplegic or locked-in patients (Patterson et al., 1993). A wish to die reflects a state of "unease" or "disease" that we can diagnose and treat (Chochinov et al., 1995; Lesage et al., 1994; Sullivan and Youngner, 1994). Physicians in the past have rejected killing as appropriate management. If physicians do not revere

each person's life, who in our society should we rely on to do so?

2. Numerous medical organizations reject physician-assisted suicide, euthanasia, or both: the American Medical Association (2000–2003), the American Academy of Neurology (1998a), the World Federation of Doctors, and many ethicists (Angell, 1997; Foley, 1997; Foley and Hendin, 2002). For discussions of end-of-life policies, see Baird and Rosenbaum (2003), Baergen (2001), Kaufman (2005), Quill and Battin (2004), and Weir (1997). Quill and Battin (2004) and Quill (2007) have long advocated physician-assisted dying, but as yet (2008) only Oregon has legalized physician-assisted suicide. No state has legalized euthanasia, which the Netherlands and Belgium have accepted (van der Heide et al., 2007). For further discussions of assisted suicide see Cohen et al. (1994), Foley and Hendin (2002), Nuland (2000), O'Brien (1999), Snyder and Caplan (2002), and Ulmer (2003). Table 14–1 summarizes the arguments against assisted suicide and euthanasia.

3. The most powerful argument for these procedures is preservation of patient autonomy and the overwhelming desire of patients to retain some control of their lives.

Table 14–1. Reasons Most Physicians Oppose Assisted Suicide and Active Euthanasia

Killing is against the traditional reverence for life.

Secular law in most jurisdictions rejects killing, as do most religions.

The patient's death wish may arise from depression or other treatable conditions.

The wish to die may arise from self blame for the illness or feelings of unworthiness. The right to die may turn into the feeling of an obligation to die.

Patients may change their mind about wanting to die if given time, but death ends patient autonomy.

The diagnosis of a terminal state may be incorrect.

The better the terminal care, the fewer the requests for euthanasia.

Physician and family may have influenced an especially difficult or disliked patient to request death because of unconscious transference–countertransference dynamics.

A cure or at least a palliation may arise for a previously untreatable terminal illness.

The management and control of very ill or terminal patients may fall into the hands of nurses, hospice workers, and physicians who are serial killers.

Sometimes family members will lie to manipulate the physician into killing a disliked or troublesome patient.

Some physicians are incompetent or, worse, purchasable and may become executioners for hire.

After euthanasia, no one can rectify mistakes in diagnosis or judgment as to the permanence of the patient's death wish. The dead patient cannot inform you that you made a mistake— "Damn you. I didn't really want to die."

4. All sides agree that improved terminal care would greatly reduce requests to die (Baird and Rosenbaum, 2003; Field and Cassel, 1997; Foley, 1997). Simply administering sufficient pain medication would reduce many requests to die (Hammack and Loprinzi, 1994; Lamar, 1994). Instead of trying to resolve the debates about assisted suicide and euthanasia here, I will show how to use the techniques of the history to promote the desire to live. The history can be tailored to search for reasons for the patient to die or for reasons to live. If you listen to the chilling death history taken by Dr. Jack Kevorkian (as aired on CBS's *60 Minutes*, November 22, 1998; Hewitt, 2008), you will understand the difference between a life history and a death history.

5. I suggest that the wish to die reflects a failure of optimal management and that often means a failure of the history to establish rapport and trust and full disclosure of the patient's feelings (Buckman, 1988).

> I've noticed this: that no kind of death is so bitter but that it can be endured if one has resolved to die with steadfast mind.
> —Desiderius Erasmus (1466–1536) (1957, p 94)

C. Techniques of the history to encourage the will to live
  1. On each visit the physician may extend the history to encourage the terminally ill patient to reminisce about some happy and rewarding events of the patient's life, instead of just asking whether a bowel movement has occurred.
  2. Assign the patient a task for each visit: "Tomorrow tell me about your wedding day or your hobbies."
  3. Ask the patient to talk about those whom he or she appreciates and respects and, if physically able, to send thank you notes for what that person has contributed to the patient's life.
  4. Arrange for cherished family members to narrate or write to the patient some fond memory. Suggest that the patient and other family members draw up a family pedigree (see Chapter 8) and, where feasible, a family photo album or video. These acts link patients to their predecessors and successors, securing the patient's place and role in the entire human family.
  5. The physician may simply caress the patient's hand or forehead as part of the daily greeting (Connelly, 2004) and

smooth and readjust the pillow and blankets when leaving. In fact, why not apply these policies to every patient? Why withhold kindness until a patient is dying? All in all, patients who have something to look forward to are more likely to choose life and life-supporting measures (Albert at al., 1999).

6. These actions may reduce the death wish by making remaining moments of the patient's life precious. It becomes then not a political question of whether to debate assisted suicide or euthanasia as the patient's right but a medical question of learning how to prevent the conditions that cause patients to choose death (Hendin, 1995).

> . . . the secret of the care of the patient is in caring for the patient.
>
> —Francis Peabody (Straus, p 367)

7. A patient terminal with prostate cancer expressed the need of the dying patient for a compassionate dialogue with his physician this way:

> I wouldn't demand a lot of my doctor's time. I just wish he would brood on my situation for perhaps five minutes, that he would give me his whole mind just once. I would like to think of him as going through my character as he goes through my flesh to get at my illness, for each man is ill in his own way. . . . Just as he orders blood tests and bone scans of my body, I'd like my doctor to scan me to grope for my spirit as well as my prostate.
>
> —Anatole Broyard (2001, p 170)

8. Compassionate care will benefit not only the patient but also the physician, who can achieve fulfillment from aiding people in their time of greatest need (Ogle and Hopper, 2005, p 828):

> . . . the emotional burden of avoiding the patient may be much harder on the doctor than he imagines. . . . A doctor's job would be so much more interesting and satisfying if he would occasionally let himself plunge into the patient, if he could lose his fear of falling.
>
> —(Broyard, 1990)

9. See also in Chapter 16 similar sentiments in the letter from a dying student nurse, "Death in the First Person."

10. Offering helpful interventions and palliative care resulted in a change of mind of patients in Oregon who had requested physician-assisted suicide (Ganzini et al., 2000). Although some hospice patients who chose to hasten death by refusal of food and fluids seemed to have died peacefully (Ganzini et al., 2003), the "death with dignity" slogan carries a peril. It can translate into the "revolutionary suicide" or "peaceful death" that Reverend Jim Jones advocated to cause the suicide-murder of more than 900 People's Temple followers in Guyana, and the "passing over" by suicide of the members of Marshall Applewhite's Heaven's Gate cult (see http://en.wikipedia.org for details of the mass suicides in these cults).

11. Palliative care for dying children is less understood and even more difficult than for adults (Himelstein et al., 2004; Wolfe, 2004).

12. As powerful as the history can be for the still rational patient, it fails with the severely demented, completely mute patient whose personhood has permanently disappeared. What then constitutes appropriate, compassionate management resists any easy solution.

D. Limitations on the history caused by the emotional countercurrents (transferences–countertransferences) surrounding the terminally ill patient

1. The patient who requests assisted suicide or euthanasia may have suffered through a long illness that has discouraged and frustrated everyone, the patient, family, and physician, and has bankrupted the family emotionally and financially (Rosen, 1987). If the patient has an abrasive personality, all of the caregivers may wish him dead. They will, in some degree, communicate death wishes to the patient. The force of unconscious motivations in the transference–countertransference phenomena (see Chapter 12, section VI) among physician, family, and patient may loom even more powerfully during terminal care than in ordinary transactions.

2. The patient is not strictly rational about death. The patient's motivations to die range from feeling unworthy of care because of guilt and shame for the burdens that the illness causes to anger or regret over too much pain and suffering. Patients who are poor bear a greater symptom

burden in the terminal year than patients with a high net worth (Silveira et al., 2005).

3. The family is not strictly rational and altruistic about death. Sometimes family members advocate death to receive their inheritance or to avoid further inconvenience (Schulz et al., 2003). The family may even connive to get the physician to hasten the patient's demise. The family members may differ or be mistaken about the patient's wishes (Sulmasy et al., 1998). Then the issue becomes just how accurately the history can disclose or reconcile the wishes of the family members and the wishes of the patient.

4. The physician is not strictly rational and altruistic about death. Having failed to cure the terminally ill patient and tired of trying to cope with the patient's unsolvable medical, social, and emotional problems, carping attitude, and belligerent family, the physician may overtly or covertly convey negative feelings to the patient.

5. Thus, deathbed decisions do not depend simply on a living will, rationality, or sweetness and light. Powerful subterranean currents compete. The physician and family and hospital setting may subtly promote or even create the patient's death wish (Kaufman, 2005).

6. An insecure or ambivalent patient may broach assisted suicide just to test the waters, probing for assurance that others want the patient to live. The unquestioning acceptance of the patient's death wish by physician and family may tip the balance of a susceptible patient toward death (Smith, 1997). Even the most complete history may fail to unravel the complex factors that lead to the death wish. And finally, some physicians who would have the power to impose or encourage death are simply incompetent or, worse, purchasable, not to mention the rare nurse, aid, or physician who is a serial killer (Iserson, 2002; Miller et al., 1994).

7. The considerations outlined suggest that slogans like "patient autonomy" or "death with dignity," on the one side, and "reverence for life," on the other, severely oversimplify the complex issues involved.

E. Offering suicide or euthanasia becomes a self-fulfilling prophecy, particularly if sanctioned by the way the history is taken

1. Killing ends the hard work, the compassion, dedication, and caring required to encourage the patient to want to live (Lynn, 1994) and reduces the pressure for additional research to find better ways of comforting patients (Doyle et al., 1993; Singer and Siegler, 1990).

2. The taking of a "death history" to justify offering death as appropriate management will ipso facto encourage it: "Here is our euthanasia consultant, Dr. Death. He would like to discuss it with you."

> The fear is that the right to die will become the duty to die and then the coercion to die.
>
> —Cecily Sanders (Brallier, p 131)

F. Serial killers

As a final worry, how will we bar serial killers from assisted suicide and euthanasia programs? Dozens of serial killer health professionals are already known: nurses Charles Cullen, Vickie Dawn Jackson, Orville Lynn Majors, Kristen Gilbert, Rhea R. Henson, and Lucy de Berk and physicians (Iserson, 2002) Dr. Harold Shipman, convicted of 15 murders but suspected of killing as many as 300 people before he committed suicide while in prison, and Dr. Jack Kevorkian, who killed an estimated 130 patients some of whom at autopsy had no organic disease.

VI. **The Clinical History, the Living Will, and Planning for Terminal Care**

A. When is the right time to make terminal care decisions?

1. Undoubtedly, physicians must improve their histories to understand the patients' wishes for management of terminal illness (Bedell and Delbanco, 1984; Emanuel et al., 1991; Morrison and Meier, 2004). Patients' reactions vary from "I don't ever want to go to a hospital" to "Do everything possible to keep me alive." The history has to explore the reasons for such extreme attitudes.

2. Many hospitals require patients upon admission to sign directives about DNR (do not resuscitate) (Youngner, 1995), CPR (cardiopulmonary resuscitation), and terminal care; but such mandates do not solve inherently unsolvable problems and often complicate the management (Menikoff et al., l992). Should physicians

turn off their intelligence to obey directives hastily signed at the front desk? Vague directives help but little, while specific directives may hamstring the physician when trying to balance them against the contingencies of the illness. In fact, the physician generally ends up by fulfilling the usual standard of care (Asch et al., 1995; Danis et al., 1991).

3. Drawing up directives years in advance of need may be too early. Circumstances and practices change, and no one knows what decisions their terminal illness will require. Newly discovered techniques of managing putatively terminal conditions may have been developed, invalidating directives from a living will or previous concepts of futility (Becker et al., 2001; Helft et al., 2000). Without trying it, we sometimes do not know whether an extraordinary measure might tide the patient over and allow survival. Even age is not a barrier (Foerch et al., 2004). Finally, the diagnosis of a terminal illness may be in error (Keswani and Wityk, 2002).

4. Waiting until the patient is hospitalized and emotionally drained by a life-threatening illness or is mentally impaired is too late.

B. Who should draw up living wills and directives about terminal care?

1. Regarding life-and-death decisions as a legal matter or a political right removes medical management from the physician's provenance to the paneled opulence of the lawyer's office or judge's chambers. Legal stipulations and court procedures are unlikely to improve terminal care (Bacon et al., 2007). The law becomes another "third party" intruding into the patient–physician dyad. In the sanitized calm and quiet of the law office, the patient makes decisions divorced from the unknown realities that may require consideration during a terminal illness. What kind of counseling for informed consent can the lawyer provide, without the background of a thorough clinical history? To overstate the issue, the partially informed leads the uninformed to adopt directives governing circumstances as yet unknown. I suggest that to discuss terminal care for truly informed consent requires a physician or nurse or professional with years of experience managing dying patients, experiences that the lawyer, judge, and patient lack.

The apparent freedom of choice is false because the chooser does not know the real conditions to be faced or the real options and probabilities that might apply. How does a lawyer react to a sheath of dos and don'ts from the defendant on how to manage a defendant's murder trial?

2. To apprise the patient of the risks and benefits of procedures, for truly informed consent, the physician must know the real conditions of the illness. What seem extraordinary measures under one circumstance may be ordinary under another, even such seemingly simple procedures as feeding (Steinbrook and Lo, 1988), particularly in respect to the end stages of dementia (Gillick, 2000). Dialysis and transplantation are entirely appropriate procedures in one instance of kidney failure but not in another (e.g., multiple systems failure in a terminal cancer patient). Table 14–2 lists procedures that the physician may approach through the history when circumstances or the patient's illness make such discussions appropriate.

C. Directives should follow a thorough history, not precede it

1. In principle, all medical decisions, certainly life-and-death decisions, should come after a thorough history that discloses the patient's beliefs, knowledge, and mental state. Then, repeated discussions extend the learning process for both physician and patient to reach the level of rapport and trust required (Marquis, 2001; Morrison and Meier, 2004; Steinhauser et al., 2000). The living will and any other directives should emerge as a normal stage in the physician–patient transactions, perhaps during regular office visits and updated as needed (Emanuel and Emanuel, 1994; Sayers et al., 2001), not something signed years in advance or hastily managed in the front office of the hospital.

2. To prepare to discuss directives, the patient should do preliminary study and formulate questions for the physician to answer. Some places to start include Americans for Better Care of the Dying (www.abce.org) and the *Journal of Palliative Care*. Most jurisdictions have laws about terminal decisions and often provide the actual forms. For example, the state of Indiana has the Indiana Health Consent Act (IC 16-36-1), the Living Will Act (IC 16-36-4), and the Powers of Attorney Act (IC 30-5). Colby (2006) reviews the current end-of-life laws.

Table 14–2. Classification of Medical Care According to Ordinary and Extraordinary Procedures

Basic care
Feeding
Temperature control
Physical comfort, cleanliness, and standard nursing care
Intellectual and emotional support appropriate to developmental or mental level
Ordinary medical care
    Electrolyte and metabolic balancing, oral or IV
    Nasogastric feeding
    Antibiotics
    Anticonvulsants
    Suction
    O2 supplementation by endotracheal tube or oropharyngeal airway
    Catheterization of bladder
    Fracture management
    Surgery
        Bowel obstruction
        Appendectomy
        Abscess drainage
        Ventriculoperitoneal shunt
        Invasive diagnostic tests
        Endoscopy
        Biopsy
Extraordinary care
    Tracheostomy
    Artificial respiration
    Gastrostomy tube
    Scoliosis treatment (Harrington rod)
    Central alimentation
    Cardiopulmonary resuscitation
    Cardiac surgery
    Cardioversion
    Dialysis

3. Directives and living wills should contain a final disclaimer that if any provision violates newer developments and the common sense of experienced physicians and surrogates, common sense shall prevail. (For the adjudication of common sense, see Chapter 9, section IV, D.) The most important function of a living will is to provide not a binding list of directives but a careful list of surrogates (Menikoff et al., 1992), who, in lieu of the patient's own competence, will reflect with the physician and make decisions dependent on the real contingencies of the illness.

4. Although one physician has to finally make the decision and write the orders, consultation with other physicians and with a formal ethics committee is frequently helpful

(La Puma and Schiedermayer, 1994) and, in the case of assisted suicide, required by law. However, ethics committees act on secondhand knowledge, which is dependent on the quality of the history and information from the attending physician. No corrective feedback mechanism exists to evaluate the quality of decisions made by a committee (Bernat, 2002; Rubin and Zoloth, 2000).

5. The last and most difficult supportive measures to withdraw are feeding and mechanical ventilation. The key is to find an intersection between the patient's and family's wishes and the physician's professional estimate of medical reality (Mayer and Kossoff, 1999; Wijdicks and Rabinstein, 2007).

D. An ethics, values, and spirituality history

1. An ethics, values, and spiritual history is essential for patient–physician communication in office practice and in terminal illness. Medically pertinent attitudes or beliefs then may be included in the patient's medical record (Das and Mulley, 2005; Sayers et al., 2001). Topics to consider include the following:

a. Attitudes to life support and CPR and DNR directives (see Table 14–2)

b. Disclosure of the nature and prognosis of the patient's illness to the family

c. Surrogates for decision making if the patient becomes incompetent

d. Organ donation

2. Spirituality history

You should inquire about any of the patient's beliefs and general philosophy that may affect management (King et al., 2004; Koenig, 2004). Insure that your own beliefs about spirituality, terminal care, and quality of life do not usurp the patient's autonomy. Listen nonjudgmentally and avoid debating with the patient or proselytizing.

3. Sample questions for this part of the history

a. "Do you hold particular beliefs or convictions that are important to decisions about your health care?"

b. "Do you have a particular group of people, relatives, or friends of special importance to you?"

c. "Do you consider yourself to be religious?"

VII. An Example of How a Knowing History Guided the Care of a Terminally Ill Patient

Does reverence for life and reluctance to accept assisted suicide and active euthanasia mean advocating tubes and machines to the death of the last cell? Every one of us will reach an irreversible state that nullifies therapeutic efforts, but physicians should accept irreversibility only after a direct and repeated personal history and examination of the patient and after exploring all reasonable diagnostic and therapeutic avenues. Legal intrusions and directives then will do little to improve this process, as shown by the next patient.

Pt 35: A newborn infant entered the neonatal intensive care unit at Riley Hospital because of status epilepticus (serial convulsions). The parents belonged to a social group that has for decades brought their seriously ill children to our hospital. The hospital staff knows the people well and recognizes the exemplary care that they give to their ill and elderly members.

The hospital staff for the infant consisted of members of the neonatal faculty, me from pediatric neurology, a physician from the metabolism service, nurses, and medical students. We explored every known cause for the infant's convulsions, including endless chemical tests for errors of metabolism and repeated magnetic resonance imaging (MRI) scans of the brain. We tried every known anticonvulsant from pyridoxine to prolonged barbiturate coma. For days we kept the infant in deep barbiturate coma that completely suppressed all electrical activity of the brain. Each time we reduced the barbiturate dose, the epileptiform activity on the electroencephalogram and the continuous convulsions stubbornly reappeared. Serial MRI scans of the brain disclosed severe, increasing atrophy of the brain.

Throughout 3 weeks of maximum but futile diagnostic and therapeutic efforts, the infant continued to deteriorate and other organs began to fail. One afternoon the mother stated, simply and with finality but no histrionics, "I want to take my baby home now." We knew that she wanted to take her baby home to die there, rather than in the hospital. She knew that we knew that that was her purpose, and we knew from talking to her and her husband every day that they held the same ideals as the other members of her group and that she would provide loving care. She stated that she wanted to hold her baby in her arms in her own home, to provide memories of her baby in her arms there in her home, where she always intended her baby to be. We accepted her decision without remonstrance. We all, medical staff and the parents, understood that our best efforts had failed. Discussions between the physicians, nurses, and parents had occupied many hours in the previous days. All of us had already completed the intensive work that established the basis for trust and appropriate management. The communication by that time reached deeper than words and needed no further embellishment. We did not protest that discharging the baby would surely hasten the death. The parents and we all knew that. We did not remonstrate, file a child abuse form, or ask the parents to sign out against medical advice. We lightened the barbiturate dose and discharged the baby, who then died at home.

In this instance parental preference properly prevailed over futile artificial life support and futile therapy. No formal proceedings, committee debates, or directives would have improved or eased the process. The decisions arose from and evolved gradually from the real circumstances. None of the participants harbored ulterior motives or hidden agendas. Loving parents, trust, and the best judgment of experienced physicians who had taken a thorough history that enabled them to know the parents and their culture and who had personally attended the infant daily resolved the issue as well as their current abilities would allow.

VIII. Summary

A. Appropriate medical management

Only from a history and physical examination, often aided by laboratory tests, can the physician determine appropriate management, based on knowledge of medical reality and the patient's values and attitudes. Appropriate management meets ethical standards of the medical model and scientific standards for safety and efficacy or, in lieu of evidence-based data, reflects the consensus of experienced physicians.

B. Informed consent and patient autonomy

1. Patient autonomy works beneficently when a patient has a normal brain, normal intelligence, normal life

experiences, knowledge of medical reality, and a competent physician. The professional role of the physician is to discern and convey the medical realties. For management options of approximately equal safety and efficacy, the physician summarizes the risks and benefits to insure informed consent and the patient selects the plan. The physician tries to propose appropriate management within the patient's system of values, but if one plan is conspicuously better, such as to biopsy a lump, the physician encourages the patient to accept it.

2. If the patient refuses appropriate management, the physician extends the history to discover and remedy the cause. The physician advocates appropriate management irrespective of the wishes of the patient, the family, or society. This paradoxical conclusion is justified because the patient's misinformation, irrationalities, brain impairment, or mental illness or the wishes of the family or societal pressures may contravene the patient's best interests.

3. Personal preferences that disregard medical reality result in blind choice, not free or informed choice. Free choice does not mean the right to self-destruct because of ignorance or mental illness. In exercising autonomy, the patient should not assume the role of the physician and prescribe his own treatment. In that case, the patient has a "fool for a doctor and a fool for a patient." For children or mentally incompetent patients, the physician may have to get legal authorization for appropriate management.

C. Responsibility of the patient in the patient–physician compact
The patient's role is to answer the questions and to allow the tests required for the physician to determine the diagnosis and the medical realities to be faced.

D. In some instances the physician actively intercedes to change the patient's preferences

1. Physicians do not accept preferences for addictive drugs, suicide, or overt child abuse, such as parental choice for alternative medicine in place of evidence-based treatments (e.g., antibiotics for meningitis).

2. Physicians oppose suicide and euthanasia not from paternalism but because we know that frequently patients who want to die suffer feelings of guilt, unworthiness, or depression that we can often correct. The patient may then

undergo a change of mind and want to live. Some persons argue that choosing death is the ultimate expression of patient autonomy, but others hold that death ends all autonomy by removing any possibility of change of mind. Many physicians regard the death wish medically, as an opportunity to diagnose and correct a diseased state of mind, rather than a political "right to die."

E. Degrees of patient autonomy

Sometimes, patient preference is essentially the only determinant of the management, as in whether to donate organs or whether to test for a genetic disease that may appear in the future. Before ordering genetic tests, the history should explore how the patient may react to adverse genetic information, in particular whether the patient might react by suicide.

F. External pressures by altering the time-honored goals and ethics change the actual techniques and actual questions asked in the clinical history

1. By design, the traditional history discloses the full inventory of health concerns, health problems, and real needs of the patient and builds the rapport and trust for the patient to choose appropriate management.

2. Pressures that threaten the development of rapport and trust include the loss of reverence for each person's life and the commercialization of medicine as a commodity or "product," with beneficence subordinated to profits and advertising to promote elective cosmetic surgery.

G. The living will and terminal care directives

Directives are best drawn up by an experienced health professional who has taken a full history and knows the patient's attitudes to illness and life in general. The physician learns much about the patient's attitudes when the patient describes the death and medical management of relatives during the family history (see Chapter 8). The best solution is few specific directives and careful selection of a competent physician and surrogates who can make decisions based on the medical realities of the terminal illness if the patient becomes incompetent.

IX. Epilogue: A Personal View

Reverence for life is a keystone of traditional medical ethics. Accepting killing will change our medical history from a life history to a death history and, by that shift, nullify the commitment to life that has sustained and defined our profession for millennia. If you suspect your physician of searching for justification to dispatch you, how does that affect trust, the indispensable goal of the history? We as humans have not only a moral sense (Hauser, 2006; Wilson, 1997) but also limbic circuits in our brain. These circuits endow us with an innate repugnance, an abhorrence of death, whether the revolting odor of putrefying flesh, the horrifying sight of a dismembered corpse, or the overwhelming sadness when a loved one dies. Do we need any other reason to revere life or any other guidance than the depth of our own feelings, based on the biology of our brain? Whether you react to death with the visceral repulsion of Baudelaire or the exquisite poignancy of Chivers, death always saddens us:

> Ridiculous corpse, I know your pains full well.
> At sight of your loose-hanging limbs, I felt
> the bitter-flowing bile of ancient grief
> rise up, like a long puke, against my teeth.

> —Charles Baudelaire (1821–1867)
> (Morgan, 1987, p 193)

> And after he had felt her pulseless wrist,
> And prest the cold indifference of the palm
> Of her unsocial hand with his, he laid,
> With cautious ease, the stiffening fingers back . . .

> —Thomas Holley Chivers, M.D. (1809–1858)
> (see also Sandler, 1973)

The traditional medical ethics devoted the history and all subsequent medical transactions to insuring no harm, to discovering ways to improve the patient's health, and to preserving life (Rogers, 1994). If the ethics change, the very technique of taking the history—its function, form, and the very questions we ask—will change because the goals change from serving the patient's health to serving extraneous financial or societal goals (Hafferty and McKinley, 1993). Violation of any one of the ethics in Table 4–1 creates problems and slips us further and further into the abyss. If we abandon the time-proven ethics, we transform and destroy the defining characteristics of physicians as beneficent healers (Rothman, 1987). All of the instruction about taking a history given here will become useless. Perhaps that is the future of medicine, but if physicians lose their reverence for and advocacy of each person's life and health, no one will have security or value.

References

Albert SM, Murphy PL, Del Bene ML, et al. A prospective study of preference and actual treatment choices in ALS. Neurology 1999;53: 278–283.

Allam MFA, De Irala-Estevez J, Navajas RF-C, et al. Students' knowledge of and attitudes about female circumcision in Egypt. N Engl J Med 1999;341:1552–1553.

American Academy of Neurology. Position statement. Assisted suicide, euthanasia, and the neurologist. Neurology 1998a;50:596–598.

American Academy of Neurology. Position statement. Ethical issues in clinical research in neurology 1998b;50:592–595.

American Medical Association, Council on Ethical and Judicial Affairs. Code of Medical Ethics, Current Opinions with Annotations. Chicago: American Medical Association, 2002–2003.

Andrews L, Nelkin D. Body Bazaar: The Market for Human Tissue in the Biotechnology Age. New York: Crown Publishers, 2001.

Angell M. Respecting the autonomy of competent patients. N Engl J Med 1984;310:1115–1116.

Angell M. The Supreme Court and physician-assisted suicide—the ultimate right. N Engl J Med 1997;336:50–53.

Annas GJ. Asking the courts to set the standard of emergency care—the case of baby K. N Engl J Med 1994;330:1542–1545.

Applebaum PS. Assessment of patients' competence to consent to treatment. N Engl J Med 2007;357:1834–1840.

Argani S. From transplant clinic. Pharos 1999;62(winter):16.

Aring CD. The Understanding Physician. Detroit: Wayne State University Press, 1971, p 180.

Asch D, Hansen-Flaschen J, Lanken PN. Decisions to limit or continue life-sustaining treatment by critical care physicians in the United States: conflicts between physicians' practices and patients' wishes. Am J Respir Crit Care Med 1995;151:288–292.

Asser SM, Swan R. Child fatalities from religion-motivated medical neglect. Pediatrics 1998;101:626–629.

Bacon C, Williams MA, Gordon J. Position statement on laws and regulations concerning life-sustaining treatment, including artificial nutrition and hydration, for patients lacking decision-making capacity. Neurology 2007;68:1097–1100.

Baergen R. Ethics at the End of Life. Belmont, CA: Wadsworth Group, Thomson Learning, 2001.

Baird RM, Rosenbaum SE, eds. Caring for the Dying: Critical Issues at the End of Life. Buffalo, NY: Prometheus Books, 2003.

Bartecchi CE. The Alternative Medicine Hoax. West Palm Beach, FL: Merit, 2002.

Becker KJ, Baxter AB, Cohen WA, et al. Withdrawal of support in intracerebral hemorrhage may lead to self-fulfilling prophecies. Neurology 2001;56:766–772.

Bedell SE, Delbanco TL. Choices about cardiopulmonary resuscitation in the hospital. When do physicians talk to patients? N Engl J Med 1984;310:1089–1093.

Bernat JL. Ethical Issues in Neurology, 2nd ed. Boston: Butterworth-Heinemann, 2002.

Bernat JL. Book review. Fresh look at new genetic, reproductive, and life-sustaining technologies: a required read for physicians and scientists. Neurol Today 2003;(February):22–23.

Block SD, Billings JA. Patient requests to hasten death: evaluation and management in terminal care. Arch Intern Med 1994;154:2039–2047.

Blum VL. Flesh Wounds. The Culture of Cosmetic Surgery. Berkeley: University of California Press, 2003.

Borah G, Rankin M, Wey P. Psychological complications in 281 plastic surgery practices. Plast Reconstr Surg 1999;104:1241–1246.

Brallier JM. Medical Wit and Wisdom: The Best Medical Quotations from Hippocrates to Groucho Marx. Philadelphia: Running Press, 1993, p 131.

Brock DW, Wartman SA. When competent patients make irrational choices. N Engl J Med 1990;322:1595–1599.

Broyard A. Doctor, talk to me. In: Reynolds R, Stone J (eds), On Doctoring, 3rd ed. New York: Simon and Schuster, 2001, p 170.

Buckman R. I Don't Know What to Say: How to Help and Support Someone Who Is Dying. Toronto: Key Porter Books, 1988.

Burleigh M. Death and Deliverance: Euthanasia in Germany. New York: Cambridge University Press, 1994.

Burnam JF. The unfortunate case of Dr. Z: how to succeed in medical practice in 1984. N Engl J Med 1984;310:729–730.

Cantor NL. Making Medical Decisions for the Profoundly Mentally Disabled. Cambridge, MA: MIT Press, 2005.

Caplan AL, Coelho DH, eds. The Ethics of Organ Transplants: The Current Debate. Amherst, NY: Prometheus Books, 1998.

Chochinov HM, Wilson KG, Enns M, et al. Desire for death in the terminally ill. Am J Psychiatry 1995;152:1185–1191.

Cohen JS, Fihn SD, Boyko EJ, et al. Attitudes toward assisted suicide and euthanasia among physicians in Washington State. N Engl J Med 1994; 331:89–94.

Colby W. Unplugged: Reclaiming Our Right to Die in America. New York: AMACOM, 2006.

Connelly JE. The power of touch in clinical medicine. Pharos 2004; 67(spring):11–13.

Curlin FA, Lawrence RE, Chin MH, et al. Religion, conscience and controversial clinical practices. N Engl J Med 2007;356:593–600.

Danis M, Southerland LI, Garrett JM, et al. A prospective study of advance directives for life-sustaining care. N Engl J Med 1991;324:882–888.

Das AK, Mulley GP. The value of an ethics history? J R Soc Med 2005;98: 262–266 (see also Letters to the editor. J R Soc Med 2005;98:442).

Davis, K. Reshaping the Female Body. The Dilemma of Cosmetic Surgery. New York: Routledge, 1995.

DeMyer WE. Technique of the Neurologic Examination, 5th ed. New York: McGraw-Hill, 2004.

Doyle D, Hanks GWC, MacDonald N. Oxford Textbook of Palliative Medicine. New York: Oxford University Press, 1993.

Dubernard J-M, Lengelé B, Morelon E, et al. Outcomes 18 months after the first human partial face transplantation. N Engl J Med 2007;357: 2451–2460.

Elias S, Annas GJ. Generic consent for genetic screening. N Engl J Med 1994;330:1611–1613.

Emanuel EJ, Barry MJ, Stoeckle JD, et al. Advance directives for medical care—a case for greater use. N Engl J Med 1991;324:889–896.

Emanuel EJ, Emanuel LL. The economics of dying. The illusion of cost savings at the end of life. N Engl J Med 1994;330:540–544 (see also Letters to the editor. N Engl J Med 1994;331:477–488).

Engelhardt HT. Freedom vs. best interest: a conflict at the roots of health care. In: Kliever LD (ed), Dax's Case: Essays in Medical Ethics and Human Meaning. Dallas: Southern Methodist University Press, 1989, p 79.

Erasmus D. Ten Colloquies. Translated by CR Thompson. New York: Liberal Arts Press, 1957, p 94.

Etchells E, Darzins P, Silberfeld M, et al. Assessment of patient capacity to consent to treatment. J Gen Intern Med 1999;14:27–24.

Field MJ, Cassel CK, eds. Approaching Death: Improving Care at the End of life. Washington DC: National Academy Press, 1997.

Fletcher JF. The Ethics of Genetic Control. Amherst, NY: Prometheus Books, 1988.

Foerch C, Kessler KR, Stechel DA, et al. Survival and quality of life outcome after mechanical ventilation in elderly stroke patients. J Neurol Neurosurg Psychiatry 2004;75:988–993.

Foley KM. Competent care for the dying instead of physician assisted suicide. N Engl J Med 1997;336:54–57.

Foley KM, Hendin H. The Case Against Assisted Suicide: For the Right to End-of-Life Care. Baltimore: Johns Hopkins University Press, 2002.

Friedland DJ, ed. Evidence-Based Medicine: A Framework for Clinical Practice. Stamford, CT: Appleton & Lange, 1998 (see also http://www.cochranelibrary.com/cochrane/).

Gale, T. An institution of a chirugian. 1563. Reprinted by permission from Coope R. The Quiet Art: A Doctor's Anthology. Baltimore: Williams & Wilkins, 1958.

Ganzini L, Goy ER, Miller LL, et al. Nurses' experiences with hospice patients who refuse food and fluids to hasten death. N Engl J Med 2003;349:359–365.

Ganzini L, Nelson HD, Schmidt TA, et al. Physicians' experiences with the Oregon Death with Dignity Act. N Engl J Med 2000;342:557–563.

Gasner MR, Maw KL, Feldman GE, et al. The use of legal action in New York City to ensure treatment of tuberculosis. N Engl J Med 1999; 340:359–366 (see also Letters to the editor. N Engl J Med 1999;341: 130–131).

Gillick MR. Rethinking the role of tube feeding in patients with advanced dementia. N Engl J Med 2000;342:206–209.

Glick SM. Unlimited human autonomy—a cultural bias? N Engl J Med 1997;336:954–956.

Hafferty FW, McKinley JB. The Changing Medical Profession: An International Perspective. New York: Oxford University Press, 1993.

Haiken E. Venus Envy: A History of Cosmetic Surgery. Baltimore: Johns Hopkins Press, 1997.

Hammack JE, Loprinzi CL. Use of orally administered opioids for cancer-related pain. Mayo Clin Proc 1994;69:384–390.

Hauser MD. Moral Minds: How Nature Designed Our Universal Sense of Right and Wrong. New York: Ecco, 2006.

Helft PR, Siegler M, Lantos J. The rise and fall of the futility movement. N Engl J Med 2000;343:293–296.

Hendin H. Selling death and dignity. Hastings Center Report 1995; (May–June):19–23.

Hewitt, D. (Executive Producer). (1998, November 22). 60 Minutes (CBS News Transcript). New York. Retrieved November 4, 2008 from http://web.lexis-nexis.com/universe.

Himelstein BP, Hilden JM, Boldt AM, et al. Pediatric palliative care. N Engl J Med 2004;350:1752–1762.

Holden C. Researchers blast U.S. bioethics panel shuffle. Science 2004; 303:1447.

Hudgens RW. Preventing suicide. N Engl J Med 1983;308:897–898.

Humphrey D. Final Exit. The Practicality of Self-Deliverance and Assisted Suicide for the Dying. New York: Dell, 1992.

Iglehart JK. The mental health maze and the call for transformation. N Engl J Med 2004;350:507–514.

Ingelfinger JR. Risks and benefits to the living donor. N Engl J Med 2005;353:447–449.

Inui TS. Establishing the doctor–patient relationship: science, art or competence? Schweiz Med Wochenschr 1998;128:225–230.

Iserson KV. Demon Doctors: Physicians as Serial Killers. Tucson: Galen Press, 2002.

Jamison KR. Night Falls Fast: Understanding Suicide. New York: Knopf, 1999.

Kahneman D, Tversky A. Choices, values, and frames. Am Psychol 1984;39:341–350.

Kapp MB. The right to die mad. Pharos 2000;63(winter):10–11.

Kass LR. Life, Liberty and the Defense of Dignity. The Challenge for Bioethics. San Francisco: Encounter Books, 2002.

Kassirer JP. Adding insult to injury. Usurping patient's prerogatives. N Engl J Med 1983;308:898–901.

Kaufman SR. . . . And a Time to Die: How American Hospitals Shape the End of Life. New York: Scribner, 2005.

Keswani SC, Wityk R. Don't throw in the towel! A case of reversible coma. J Neurosurg Neurol Psychiatry 2002;73:83–84.

King DE, Blue A, Mallin R, et al. Implementation and assessment of a spiritual history taking curriculum in the first year of medical school. Teach Learn Med 2004;16:64–68.

Kjoller K, Friis S, Mellemkjaer L, et al. Connective tissue disease and other rheumatic conditions following cosmetic breast implantation in Denmark. Arch Intern Med 2001;161:973–979.

Koenig HG. Taking a spirituality history. JAMA 2004;291:2881.

Kolb LC. Modern Clinical Psychiatry, 9th ed. Philadelphia: WB Saunders, 1977, p 774.

Kulmala I, McLaughlin JK, Pakkanen M, et al. Local complications after cosmetic breast implant surgery in Finland. Ann Plast Surg 2004;53: 413–419.

Lachs MS, Sindelar JL, Horwitz RI. When competent patients make irrational choices. N Engl J Med 1990;322:1595–1599.

Lamar TJ. Treatment of cancer-related pain: when orally administered medications fail. Mayo Clin Proc 1994;69:473–480.

La Puma J, Schiedermayer D. Ethics Consultation: A Practical Guide. Boston: Jones and Bartlett, 1994.

Lesage AD, Boyer R, Grunberg F, et al. Suicide and mental disorders: a case-control study of young men. Am J Psychiatry 1994;151:1063–1068.

Lynn J. Letter to the editor. N Engl J Med 1994;331:1657.

Maienschein J. Whose View of Life? Embryos, Cloning, and Stem Cells. Cambridge, MA: Harvard University Press, 2003.

Margo CE. Selling surgery. N Engl J Med 1987;314:1575–1576.

Marquis DK, ed. Advance Care Planning: A Practical Guide for Physicians. Washington DC: American Medical Association Press, 2001.

Marzuk PM, Hirsch CS, Leon AC, et al. Increase in suicide by asphyxiation after the publication of Final Exit. N Engl J Med 1993;329: 1508.

Mayer SA, Kossoff SB. Withdrawal of life support in the neurological intensive care unit. Neurology 1999;52:1602–1609.

McBryde L. The Mass Market Woman: Defining Yourself as a Person in a World that Defines You by Your Appearance. Eagle River, AK: Crowded Hour Press, 1999.

McLaughlin JK, Wise TN, Lipworth L. Increased risk of suicide among patients with breast implants: do the epidemiologic data support psychiatric consultation? Psychosomatics 2004;45:277–280.

Mehlman MJ. Wondergenes: Genetic Enhancement and the Future of Society. Bloomington: Indiana University Press, 2003.

Menikoff JA, Sachs GA, Siegler M. Beyond advance directives—health care surrogate laws. N Engl J Med 1992;327:1165–1169.

Miles SH. Informed demand for "non-beneficial" medical treatment. N Engl J Med 1991;325:512–515.

Miller FG, Quill TE, Brody H, et al. Regulating physician-assisted death. N Engl J Med 1994;331:119–122.

Morgan F (ed). Poems: New and Selected. Champaigne, IL: University of Illinois Press, 1987, p 193.

Morrison RS, Meier DE. Palliative care. N Engl J Med 2004;350:2582–2590.

Nuland SB. Physician-assisted suicide and euthanasia in practice. N Engl J Med 2000;342:583–584.

O'Brien M. In the name of compassion. A lawyer fights assisted suicide. An interview with Wesley J. Smith. The Sun 1999;278:9–17.

Ogle KS, Hopper K. End-of-life care for older adults. Prim Care 2005;32:811–828.

Patterson DL, Miller-Perrin C, McCormick TR, et al. When life support is questioned early in the care of patients with cervical-level quadriplegia. N Engl J Med 1993;328:506–509.

Pellegrino ED. Can the doctor's burden be shifted to the patient? Pharos 1993;56(spring):34, p 34.

Phillips KA, McElroy SL, Keck, Jr. KE, et al. Body dysmorphic disorder: 30 cases of imagined ugliness. Am J Psychiatry 1993;150:302–308.

Quill TE. Legal regulation of physician-assisted death—the latest report cards. N Engl J Med 2007;356:1911–1913.

Quill TE, Battin MP, eds. Physician-Assisted Dying: The Case for Palliative Care and Patient Choice. Baltimore: Johns Hopkins Press, 2004.

Rogers DE. On trust: a basic building block for healing doctor/patient interactions. Pharos 1994;57(spring):2–6.

Rosen DH. Casualties of the health care system: patients depressed by medicine's "moral dilemmas." Pharos 1987;50(summer):19–20.

Rothman DJ. Ethics and human experimentation. Henry Beecher revisited. N Engl J Med 1987;317:1195–1199.

Rothman SM, Rothman DJ. The Pursuit of Perfection: The Promise and Perils of Medical Enhancement. New York: Pantheon, 2003.

Rubin SB, Zoloth L. Margin of Error: The Ethics of Mistakes in the Practice of Medicine. Hagerston, MD: University Publishing, 2000.

Saks ER. Refusing Care: Forced Treatment and the Rights of the Mentally Ill. Chicago: Chicago University Press, 2002.

Sandler SG. Thomas Holley Chivers, M. D. (1809–1858) and the origin of Edgar Allan Poe's "The Raven." N Engl J Med 1973;289:351–354.

Sarwer DB, Zanville HA, LaFossa D, et al. Mental health histories and psychiatric medication among persons who sought cosmetic surgery. Plast Reconstr Surg 2004;114:1927–1933.

Sayers GM, Barratt D, Gothard C, et al. The value of taking an ethics history. BMJ 2001;27:114–117.

Schneider CE. The Practice of Autonomy: Patients, Doctors, and Medical Decisions. New York: Oxford University Press, 1998.

Schroeder P. Female genital mutilation—a form of child abuse. N Engl J Med 1994;331:739–740.

Schulz R, Mendelsohn AB, Haley WE, et al. End-of-life care and the effects of bereavement on family caregivers of persons with dementia. N Engl J Med 2003;349:1936–1942.

Sheeley WF. Advisor's Viewpoint: I hope someone will help me. Clinical Psychiatry News, Nov 1975, p 1.

Shute N. Makeover nation. U.S. News & World Report, May 31, 2004, 136.

Silveira MJ, Kabeto MU, Langa KM. Net worth predicts symptom burden at the end of life. J Palliat Med 2005;8:827–837.

Silverstein MD, Stocking CB, Antel JP, et al. Amyotrophic lateral sclerosis and life-sustaining therapy: patients' desires for information, participation in decision making, and life-sustaining therapy. Mayo Clin Proc 1991;66:906–913.

Singer PA, Siegler M. Euthanasia—a critique. N Engl J Med 1990;322:1881–1883.

Smith WJ. Forced Exit: The Slippery Slope from Assisted Suicide to Legalized Murder. New York: Times Books/Random House, 1997.

Snyder L, Caplan AL. Assisted Suicide: Finding Common Ground. Bloomington: Indiana University Press, 2002.

Steinbrook R. Public solicitation of organ donors. N Engl J Med 2005;353:441–444.

Steinbrook R, Lo B. Artificial feeding—solid ground, not a slippery slope. N Engl J Med 1988;310:286–290.

Steinhauser KE, Christakis NA, Clipp EC, et al. Factors considered important at the end of life by patients, family, physicians, and other care providers. JAMA 2000;284:2476–2482.

Straus MB (ed). Familiar Medical Quotations. Boston: Little Brown, 1968, p 367.

Sullivan AD, Hedberg K, Hopkins D. Legalized physician-assisted suicide in Oregon, 1998–2000. N Engl J Med 2001;344:605–607.

Sullivan AD, Youngner SJ. Depression, competence, and the right to refuse lifesaving treatment. Am J Psychiatry 1994;151:971–978.

Sulmasy DP, Terry PB, Weisman CS, et al. The accuracy of substituted judgment in patients with terminal diagnoses. Ann Intern Med 1998;128:621–629.

Tauber AI. Patient Autonomy and the Ethics of Responsibility. Boston: MIT Press, 2005.

Thomas D. Rage, rage against the dying of the light. In: Reynolds R, Stone J (eds), On Doctoring, 3rd ed. New York: Simon and Schuster, 2001, p 151.

Toubia N. Female circumcision as a public health issue. N Engl J Med 1994;331:712–716.

Truog RD. The ethics of organ donation by living donors. N Engl J Med 2005;353:444–446.

Truog RD. Consent for organ donation—balancing conflicting ethical obligations. N Engl J Med 2008;358:1209–1211.

Truog RD, Robinson W, Randolph A, et al. Is informed consent always necessary for randomized, controlled trials? N Engl J Med 1999;340: 804–807.

Ulmer DD. Two books on physician assisted suicide. Pharos 2003; 66(summer):47–50.

van der Heide A, Onwuteaka-Philipsen BD, Rurup ML, et al. End-of-life practices in the Netherlands under the euthanasia act. N Engl J Med 2007;356:1957–1964.

von Weizsacker V. Euthanasie und Menschenversuche. Heidelberg: L. Schneider, 1947.

Weir RF, ed. Physician Assisted Suicide. Bloomington: Indiana University Press, 1997.

Wijdicks E, Rabinstein AA. The family conference. End of life guidelines at work for comatose patients. Neurology 2007;68:1092–1094.

Wilson JQ. The Moral Sense. New York: Free Press, 1997.

Wivel NA, Walters L. Germ-line modification and disease prevention: some medical and ethical perspectives. Science 1993;262:533–538.

Wolfe L. Should parents speak with a dying child about impending death? N Engl J Med 2004;351:1251–1253.

Youngner SJ. Beyond DNR: fine-tuning end-of-life decision-making. Neurology 1995;45:615–616.

The Clinical History of the Medical Model Compared to Alternative Models

15

I. The Science-Based Clinical History

A. Why practitioners of alternative medicine cannot use the history and thought processes of the medical model

1. By design, the clinical history discloses symptoms that relate to a scientific understanding of brain and body functions and disease. The clinical history searches for scientifically verifiable causes of disease, such as exposure to microbes or toxins, heredity, autoimmune reactions, and stress. Beyond the science, the art of the clinical history explores the essence of the patient. Because alternative practitioners reject scientific explanations of causality and pathogenesis, they couch their histories in terms that sell their belief system and their products. Each alternative system, such as homeopathy, faith healing, and the plethora of miracle diets, flatly contradicts the others, claims the crown of righteousness for itself, and deprecates the medical model (see www.quackwatch.org; Whorton, 2002).

2. If you can diagnose and cure something by incantation, popping a vertebra back into place, or sticking a needle into an ear lobe, why bother with a lengthy, science-based history, physical examination, and laboratory tests? One simplistic explanation and one simplistic therapy do it all.

> A pseudoscience consists of a nomenclature, with a self-adjusting arrangement, by which all positive evidence, or such as favours its doctrines, is admitted, and all negative evidence, or such as tells against it is excluded. It is invariably connected with some lucrative practical application.
> —Oliver Wendell Holmes, M.D. (1809–1894)
> (Morgan, 1987, p 193.)

3. To the contrary, osteopathic medicine has joined in advocating scientific evaluation and evidence-based practice (Gevitz, 2004), as have some practitioners of chiropractics. Most of the health food ("nutraceutical") industry and

    other branches of alternative medicine still strongly resist scientific evaluation.

B. Integration of the history, physical examination, and laboratory examinations in the science-based medical model

  1. To diagnose and treat a patient who has a cough, physicians do not supplicate deities or search for unbalanced energy flows. Our history searches for symptom patterns indicative of various known respiratory diseases, such as infections, asthma, and emphysema, and for exposure to scientifically demonstrable respiratory pathogens, such as allergens and microorganisms. Then, after a science-based physical examination, we may get a chest radiograph, measure pulmonary function, culture the sputum for microorganisms, and do bronchoscopy to get a tissue sample for culture or histologic analysis. After an etiologic diagnosis, we select therapy that has been previously established as effective by objective trials. We adhere to this sequence not because we perversely ignore or actively suppress alternative systems of thought but because no approach other than the science-based consistently discloses the cause for a cough and leads to its successful therapy (Buckman, 1995; Relman, 1998). If the disease requires active intervention, anything beyond the placebo effect or simply time, no other procedures regularly prove effective.

  2. To fully appreciate the difference in the outcome of a patient managed by the medical model, review Patient 5 in Chapter 4, section VI. Suppose that this patient with headache and polycystic kidney disease had visited an alternative practitioner who, instead of a thorough, rational history, examination, and pedigree based on science, only manipulated necks, stuck needles in ear lobes, or prescribed herbs. Alternative practitioners could not have taken the history or offered the management that led to the correct diagnosis and the many beneficial results for the patient and relatives.

C. Limitations of the testimonial history as proof of cure

  1. Having lauded the history as the prime and best means of patient–physician communication, I must emphasize one serious limitation in historical data. When questioned, people will testify to cures from every imaginable treatment, from manipulations and developmental patterning to

colonic rinses, therapeutic touch, and miracle diets. Similarly, some persons will testify to mental telepathy, psychokinesis, fortune telling, astrology, palmistry, Big Foot, the Loch Ness monster, the Bermuda triangle, UFOs, abduction by aliens, ghosts, and communication with the dead (Shermer, 1997). Testimony obtained through the history is not proof of reality.

2. Safeguards in the clinical history and objective tests have to distinguish whether the testimony is based on real events or fantasies, hallucinations, illusions, delusions, the placebo effect, or simple dishonesty. Any testimony that a therapy has worked always requires replication and objective verification that the putative illness actually existed and that a cure actually happened (see www.quackwatch.org; Bartecchi, 2002). How can alternative practitioners claim to have cured multiple sclerosis or cancer when they cannot even take the history or do a physical examination or interpret the laboratory tests that will objectively establish the diagnosis? How can they claim to cure blindness if they cannot distinguish hysteria from diseases of the retina or optic nerve?

> The sound of a flute will cure epilepsy and a sciatic gout.
> —Theophrastus (ca. 371–287 BCE)
> (Connolly, 1999, p 239)

3. Which paranormal phenomena, alternative treatments, or therapeutics of Theophrastus are true? The roadway through alternative medicine is littered with inadequately tested or failed nostrums (Angell and Kassirer, 1998; Helfand, 2002; Bartecchi, 2002; American Society of Health-System Pharmacists, 2008; Ryu and Chien, 1995; Wolfe, 2003; Wolfe et al., 2005; Zeisel, 1999; see also the *Nutrition Action Health Letter* at www.cspinet.org). When paranormal phenomena and most of alternative medicine are studied under conditions that eliminate fraud, observer bias, and self-delusion (i.e., are more objective, scientific, fraud-proof and fool-proof), the less successful they prove (Oken, 2004; Randi, 1989). Scientific evaluation of many of the most highly touted alternative treatments demonstrates only a placebo effect or at best mild success and that they cause significant side effects. The list of failures includes saw

palmetto for prostatic hyperplasia (DiPaola and Morton, 2006), St. John's wort for depression (www.quackwatch. org), chondroitin sulfate and glucosamine for arthritis (Clegg et al., 2006), and antioxidant vitamins to prevent colorectal cancer (Greenberg et al., 1994). In the treatment of backache, manipulative therapy and acupuncture are little different from simply making the patient remain active (Carragee, 2005).

D. The power of time, the placebo effect, and the inability of individual, anecdotal histories to establish causality

1. The commonest symptoms for which patients seek medical care include headache, backache, joint or belly pain, anxiety, dizziness, fatigue, depression, and insomnia. These predominantly subjective disorders require a searching history from an often disgruntled patient whom the physician cannot honestly promise to cure. These are precisely the patients who may provoke negative reactions in the unwary or stressed physician (see Chapter 12).

2. A patient with a backache who goes to an alternative practitioner often feels better after the manipulation or needle insertion. Therefore, the claim is made that the treatment caused the improvement, establishing the validity of the theory and the therapy. The patient might also have responded to biofeedback, homeopathy, prayer, application of animal dung, massage, bed rest and aspirin, exercise and aspirin, or doing nothing but waiting until the next morning (Carragee, 2005). The variables are simply the passage of time and, most of all, the belief that the therapy will work (Ott, 1999).

> Most things get better by themselves. Most things, in fact, are better by morning.
> —Lewis Thomas (Lewis, 1978; Lewis, 1974, p 85)

> It is part of the cure to wish to be cured.
> —Seneca (4 BCE–65 CE)

II. Definition of Alternative Medicine

A. Why a therapy remains classed as alternative

Alternative medicine is any medical theory or treatment that has failed to pass or has not yet passed objective, scientific standards for validity, safety, and efficacy. This definition also clearly applies to any new treatment initiated by conventional physicians. Each new treatment must pass rigorous tests for safety and superiority over the old treatments or of no treatment (www.quackwatch.org; Butler, 1992; Friedland, 1998; Guyatt and Rennie, 2002; Hamilton, 2005; Oken, 2004). After scientific validation establishes the safety and efficacy of an old or new therapy or the reality of a new etiologic agent, it becomes mainstream medicine and the history correspondingly is altered to search for the new etiologic agent.

> There are not two kinds of medicine, one conventional and the other unconventional that can be practiced jointly in a new kind of "integrative medicine." Nor . . . are there two kinds of thinking, or two ways to find out which treatments work and which do not . . . all proposed treatments must be tested objectively. In the end, there will only be treatments that pass that test and those that do not. . . . Can there be any reasonable "alternative?"
> —Arnold S. Relman (1998, p 37)

> There is only medicine that has been adequately tested and medicine that has not. . . .
> —Angell and Kassirer (1998)

> How prone to doubt, how cautious are the wise.
> —Homer (ca. 800 BCE)

B. A summary of alternative practices that violate the medical model (Table 15–1)
C. Role of the history in the continuous reevaluation of all medical concepts, conventional and alternative
  1. In fact, all practices and assumptions of mainstream and alternative medicine require continuous reappraisal (Friedland, 1998; Hur, 1995; Silverman, 1998; Silver, 1995; Wolfe, 2003). However, the nutritional supplement industry and herbalists have successfully lobbied to exempt their products and claims from Food and Drug Administration regulation and objective testing (www.quackwatch.org; Nutrition Action Health Letter, www.cspinet.org; Zeisel, 1999).

Table 15–1. Deficits Common to Alternative Systems of Medicine

Failure to take histories that disclose known patterns of disease based on scientific pathophysiology and scientific understanding of cause and effect
Failure to utilize family histories and genetics
Failure to do adequate physical examinations
Failure to define norms
Failure to subject theories and outcomes to objective verification, instead invoking vague notions of skeletal misalignments and unbalancing energy flows that cannot be objectively documented or measured
Failure to validate diagnoses by corrective feedback from scientifically valid laboratory tests and autopsies
Failure to separate organic disease from mental illness in judging "cures," for example, differentiating hysterical paraplegia from spinal cord disease
Failure to validate therapeutic claims objectively and failure to separate the placebo effect: reporting testimony as proof of cures, not reporting failures, and not matching objectively diagnosed patients against a control group
Failure to objectively document and publish 1-, 5-, and 10-year cure rates

2. Unfortunately, geographical variations in the frequency of various mainstream treatments in regard to race, sex, and socioeconomic status show that science does not completely govern mainstream practice either (Blumenthal, 1994; Williams, 2007), but that is the goal.
3. The standard clinical history is the beginning point for all clinical research. All research efforts must mesh with public safety and the public interest (Callahan, 2003; Wood and Darbyshire, 2006), rather than promoting merchandising and private gain. Special safeguards are necessary for children, who cannot themselves give informed consent (Bax, 1992; Glodin and Glantz, 1994). A careful history that leads to accurate diagnosis and asks the proper questions to insure informed consent about risks (see Chapter 14) must precede enrolling any patient in experimental trials.

III. **Accomplishments of Physicians Who Adhere to the Medical Model**
A. What advances have physicians made who adhere to the medical model?
1. Since so many groups attack the medical model, the student must understand that basic to all of the advances of modern medicine is the evolution over millennia of the current clinical history, which integrates compassion with science-based physical examinations and science-based

tests that disclose the real causes of disease and the cures that actually work. It is scientific medicine, not alternative, that can accomplish the actual, demonstrable, and reproducible miracles, such as transplanting organs (Tilney, 2003), the face (Dubernard et al., 2007), and hands (Lanzetta and Dubernard, 2007); reattaching severed limbs; clearing clogged arteries; and curing some cancers. It is we who can make the lame walk by removing the lesion that compresses the spinal cord or the blind to see by removing cataracts. It is we who—by CPR, not mumbo-jumbo—can bring back the near-dead.

2. Medical scientists discovered germs as the cause of infectious diseases, leading to their prevention or eradication and cure by immunization or antibiotics and their control by identification and isolation of disease carriers, water purification, proper sewage disposal, pasteurization, and food preservation.

3. Medical science has wiped out smallpox and greatly curtailed poliomyelitis and measles. Now, whooping cough and flu B meningitis are waning. In fact, the discovery of vaccination by Dr. Edward Jenner (1798), which he announced freely without commercial exploitation, has saved more lives than we have sacrificed in all of our wars. Smallpox once killed 25% of the population of towns hit by an epidemic and once scarred the face of virtually every person, as observed by Samuel Pepys (1633–1703) as he walked along London streets. By 1975 science-based public policy had completely eradicated the scourge of smallpox, our first such triumph (Koplow, 2003), and poliomyelitis is on the wane.

4. Medical science discovered the human sperm and ovum, leading to control of reproduction; decoded the genome and recognized genetic and inherited diseases; and developed intravenous therapy, treatment of hypertension and occlusive vascular disease, antipsychotic and anticonvulsant medications, immune system stimulation or suppression, and hormone replacement or suppression.

5. These feats demonstrate some of the power and the glory of the medical model's insistence on science-based histories and procedures (see Table 4–1).

B. Best examples of the medical model
Many physicians and organizations who exemplify the best of
the medical model stand in direct contrast to the
commercialization of medicine (Leaning et al., 1999). These
physicians do not use the history to sell products and
procedures.

Outstanding examples are organizations and programs for
global health care (Panosian and Coates, 2006) and many
efforts by individuals: Dr. Carl E. Bartecchi (2007) in Vietnam;
Dr. Norman Bethune in Spain, Canada, and China (Allen,
1959); Dr. Paul Farmer in Haiti (Brust, 2004; Kidder 2003);
Dr. Eugene Helveston (see ehelveson@ny.orbis.org and www.
cybersight.org and many others on Orbis and Cyber-Sight);
http://telemedicine.orbis.org; Doctors Without Borders
(Médecins sans Frontières); Interplast.com, which provides
free plastic surgery to children and adults; the Red Cross; the
Alvie Heskowitz and Victoria Hale Institute for OneWorld
Health to provide pharmaceuticals to poor countries; and the
Kenya Outreach program of the Indiana University School of
Medicine, for the treatment of HIV, run by Dr. and Mrs.
Joseph Mamlin, Dr. Bob Eintertz, and numerous associates
(http://medicine.iupui.edu/kenya).

C. What has alternative medicine accomplished?
In comparison to the cornucopia of accomplishments of
scientific medicine, alternative systems of medicine have
changed but little and added but little. Why didn't
chiropractors, faith healers, homeopaths, acupuncturists,
or herbalists discover the cause and cure of infectious diseases
or the effective treatment of endocrine and metabolic diseases?
To identify and fight AIDS, severe acute respiratory syndrome
(SARS), or bovine encephalitis, we did not depend on gurus in
natural healing but upon histories and procedures based on
science (Soares, 2004).

D. The necessity for improvement
1. Our profession requires many improvements, foremost of
all to provide more time for compassionate histories that
restore trust in our ethics and motives. Economic pressures
mistakenly seek to reduce costs by reducing the time we can
devote to our patients, when in fact more time allotted to

the history would lead to better and quicker diagnosis and reduce the need for costly laboratory procedures, many of which are now ordered simply to rule out disorders that a better history would have eliminated. In fact, probably one of the most effective ways to reduce medical costs would by for third-party payers to allocate more time for the clinical history and to compensate physicians adequately for the time. Thus, we do not finance medical care in a way for physicians to practice the best medicine and for all persons to receive the best care (Anders, 1996; Bartlett and Steele, 2004; Fuchs, 2002; Ginzberg et al., 1997; Shaffer, 2000).

2. We react too slowly to abuses (Rothman, 2000). We allow the drug companies too much leeway in biomedical research, academia, advertising, and marketing (Angell, 2000a, 2000b, 2004; Blumenthal, 2003; Bodenheimer, 2000; Consumer Reports, 2004; Drazen, 2003; Greider, 2003; Hawthorne, 2003; Horton, 2004; Krimsky, 2003; Rosenthal et al., 2002; Schulman et al., 2002; Wolfe et al., 2005) and in co-opting continuing medical education (Relman, 2003).

3. Too many preventable errors occur in hospitals and private practice (Berwick, 2003; Sharpe and Faden, 1998; Wolfe et al., 2005).

4. Recent commercial practices threaten the free dissemination of medical knowledge. Today, academicians seek to patent DNA, mice, and life itself (Magnus et al., 2002), ignoring the fact that their discoveries rest on generations of predecessors who gave their knowledge freely and that public funds support much of their research. Recall that Dr. Edward Jenner gave his discovery of smallpox vaccination freely.

5. The other side of the coin is the concept of intellectual property rights and fair ways of rewarding entrepreneurship. Somewhere is a balance between intellectual rights, intellectual obligation, private gain, public good, and the question of what is the basic mission of science and academia (Azoulay et al., 2007; Moses et al., 2002) (see Chapter 4, section III).

IV. Epilogue

I defend the medical model and its history techniques based on science and compassion (see Chapter 4) so vigorously because its practitioners have accomplished so much and its detractors so little. It shows what we can accomplish when we function with the history based on traditional ethics and the objectivity and power of modern science. The medical model advocates the equal value of every person and a probing but nonjudgmental history designed to disclose both the real causes of disease and the essence of the patient. Operating at its best, it is the most beneficent system humans have created. It constitutes one of our most precious heritages. By advocating reverence for life and optimal care for everyone, it enshrines and reflects the best of our human nature—and it all begins with that indispensable, pivotal transaction, the clinical history, which brings the physician's and the patient's minds into compassionate communion and beneficence.

Competency

After all, it comes down to this:
The doctor and patient,
door closed, curtain drawn.
Here the ancient art begins;
history unfolds in
spoken word,
ritual touch,
poultice and purge,
a foretaste of
the blade itself.
And what have we taught them?
What shall we teach them?
This and nothing less:
the gentle gaze,
the discerning heart,
the healing spirit,
the love that begins
with science and ends
in this room, for all our sakes.

—David L. Scheidermayer, M.D. (reproduced by permission from *The Pharos* 1991;54[fall]:37)

References

Allen T. The Scalpel, the Sword: The Story of Dr. Norman Bethune. New York: Cameron, 1959.

American Society of Health-System Pharmacists, Consumer Reports. Consumer Drug Reference. Yonkers, NY: Consumer Reports Books, 2008.

Anders G. Health Against Wealth: HMOs and the Breakdown of Medical Trust. Boston: Houghton Mifflin, 1996.

Angell M. Is academic medicine for sale? N Engl J Med 2000a;342: 1516–1518.

Angell M. The pharmaceutical industry—to whom is it accountable? N Engl J Med 2000b;342:1902–1904.

Angell M. The Truth About the Drug Companies. New York: Random House, 2004.

Angell M, Kassirer JP. Alternative medicine—the risks of untested and unregulated remedies. N Engl J Med 1998;339:839–841.

Azouley P, Michigan R, Sampat BN. The anatomy of medical school patenting. N Engl J Med 2007;357:2049–2056.

Bartecchi CE. The Alternative Medicine Hoax. West Palm Beach, FL: Merit, 2002.

Bartecchi CE. A Doctor's Vietnam Journal. Bennington, VT: Merriam Press, 2007.

Bartlett DL, Steele JB. Critical Condition: How Health Care in America Became Big Business. New York: Doubleday, 2004.

Bax M. Alternative methods. Dev Med Child Neurol 1992;34:471–472.

Berwick DM. Errors today and errors tomorrow. N Engl J Med 2003;248:2570–2572.

Blumenthal D. Academic–industrial relationships in the life sciences. N Engl J Med 2003;349:2452–2459.

Blumenthal D. The variation phenomenon in 1994. N Engl J Med 1994;331: 1017–1018.

Bodenheimer T. Uneasy alliance: clinical investigators and the pharmaceutical industry. N Engl J Med 2000;342:1539–1543.

Brust JCM. Paul Farmer: one doctor's quest to cure the world. Neurol Today 2004;(February):66.

Buckman R. Magic or Medicine? An Investigation of Healing and Healers. Amherst, NY: Prometheus, 1995.

Butler K. A Consumer's Guide to "Alternative Medicines": A Close Look at Homeopathy, Acupuncture, Faith-Healing, and Other Unconventional Treatments. Buffalo, NY: Prometheus, 1992.

Callahan D. What Price Better Health? Hazards of the Research Imperative. Berkeley: University of California Press, 2003.

Carragee EJ. Persistent low back pain. N Engl J Med 2005;352:1891–1898.

Clegg DO, Reda DJ, Harris CL, et al. Glucosamine, chondroitin sulfate, and the two in combination for painful knee osteoarthritis. N Engl J Med 2006;354:795–2006.

Connolly K, Martlew M. Psychologically Speaking: A Book of Quotations. London: Blackwell Publishing. 1999, p 239.

Consumer Reports. Dangerous supplements still at large. 2004;(May): 12–17.

DiPaola RS, Morton RA. Proven and unproven therapy for benign prostatic hyperplasia. N Engl J Med 2006;354:632–634.

Drazen JM. Inappropriate advertising of dietary supplements. N Engl J Med 2003;348:777–778.

Dubernard J-M, Lengelé B, Morelon E, et al. Outcomes 18 months after the first human partial face transplantation. N Engl J Med 2007;357: 2451–2460.

Friedland DJ. Evidence-Based Medicine: A Framework for Clinical Practice. Stamford, CT: Appleton & Lange, 1998 (see also http://www. cochranelibrary.com/cochrane/).

Fuchs VR. What's ahead for health insurance in the United States. N Engl J Med 2002;346:1822–1824.

Gevitz N. The DO's: Osteopathic Medicine in America. Baltimore: Johns Hopkins Press, 2004.

Ginzberg E, Berliner H, Ostow M. Improving Health Care of the Poor: The New York City Experience. New Brunswick, NJ: Transaction, 1997.

Glodin, MA, Glantz LH. Children as Research Subjects: Science, Ethics, and Law. New York: Oxford University Press, 1994.

Greenberg ER, Baron JA, Tostesen TD, et al. A clinical trial of antioxidant vitamins to prevent colorectal adenoma. N Engl J Med 1994;331: 141–147.

Greider K. The Big Fix: How the Pharmaceutical Industry Rips Off American Consumers. New York: Public Affairs, 2003.

Guyatt GH, Rennie D. Users' Guide to the Medical Literature. A Manual for Evidence-Based Clinical Practice. Chicago: AMA Press, 2002.

Hamilton J. Clinicians' Guide to Evidence-Based Practice. J Am Acad Child Adolesc Psychiatry 2005;44:494–498.

Hawthorne F. The Merck Druggernaut: The Inside Story of a Pharmaceutical Giant. New York: John Wiley and Sons, 2003.

Helfand WH. Quack, Quack, Quack: The Sellers of Nostrums in Prints, Posters, Ephemera and Books. New York: Grolier Club, 2002.

Horton R. The dawn of McScience. New York Review of Books 2004; 51(March 11):7–9.

Hur JJ. Review of research on therapeutic interventions for children with cerebral palsy. Acta Neurol Belg 1995;91:423–432.

Kidder T. Mountains Beyond Mountains. New York: Random House, 2003.

Koplow DA. Smallpox. The Fight to Eradicate a Global Scourge. Berkeley: University of California Press, 2003.

Krimsky S. Science in the Private Interest: Has the Lure of Profits Corrupted Biomedical Research? Lanham MD: Rowman and Littlefield, 2003.

Lanzetta M, Dubernard J-M. Hand Transplantation. Milan: Springer, 2007.

Leaning J, Briggs SM, Chen LC. Humanitarian Crises: The Medical and Public Health Response. Cambridge, MA: Harvard University Press, 1999.

Lewis T. The Lives of a Cell: Notes of a Biology Watcher. New York: Viking Press, 1978, 1974, p 85.

Magnus D, Caplan A, McGee G. Who Owns Life? Amherst NY: Prometheus, 2002.

Morgan F (ed). Poems: New and Selected. Champaigne, IL: University of Illinois Press, 1987, p 193.

Moses H, Braunwald E, Martin JB, et al. Collaboration with industry—choices for the academic medical center. N Engl J Med 2002;347: 1371–1375.

Oken BS, ed. Complementary Therapies in Neurology: An Evidence-Based Approach. New York: Parthenon, 2004.

Ott SM. Physical therapy, chiropractic manipulation, or an educational booklet for back pain. [Comment. Letter] New Engl J Med. 1999:340: 389–90.

Panosian C, Coates TJ. The new medical "missionaries"—grooming the next generation of global health workers. N Engl J Med 2006;354: 1771–1773.

Randi JR. The Faith Healers. Buffalo, NY: Prometheus, 1989 (see also www.randi.org).

Relman AS. A trip to Stonesville. New Republic; 1998:219(24):28-37. (see also www.quackwatch.org).

Relman AS. Defending professional independence: ACCME's proposed new guidelines for commercial support of CME. JAMA 2003;289: 2418–2420.

Rosenthal MB, Berndt ER, Donohue JM, et al. Promotion of prescription drugs to consumers. N Engl J Med 2002;346:498–505.

Rothman DJ. Medical professionalism—focusing on the real issues. N Engl J Med 2000;342:1284–1286.

Ryu SJ, Chien YY. Ginseng-associated cerebral arteritis. Neurology 1995; 45:829–830.

Scheidermayer DL. Competency. Pharos 1991;54(fall):37.

Schulman KA, Seils MD, Timbie JW, et al. A national survey of provisions in clinical-trial agreements between medical schools and industry sponsors. N Engl J Med 2002;348:1335–1341.

Shaffer ER. Breast cancer and the evolving health care system: why health care reform is a breast cancer issue. In: Kasper AS, Ferguson SJ (eds), Breast Cancer: Society Shapes an Epidemic. New York: St. Martin's Press, 2000, pp 89–151.

Sharpe VA, Faden AI. Medical Harm: Historical, Conceptual, and Ethical Dimensions of Iatrogenic Illness. New York: Cambridge University Press, 1998.

Shermer M. Why People Believe Weird Things: Pseudoscience, Superstition, and Other Confusions of Our Time. New York: WH Freeman, 1997.

Silver LB. Controversial therapies. J Child Neurol 1995:10(Suppl 1): 96–100.

Silverman WA. Where's the Evidence? Debates in Modern Medicine. New York: Oxford University Press, 1998.

Soares C. A strategy of containment. Sci Am 2004;290:48–49.

Tilney NL. Transplant: From Myth to Reality. New Haven, CT: Yale University Press, 2003.

Whorton JC. Nature Cures: The History of Alternative Medicine in America. New York: Oxford University Press, 2002.

Williams RA. Eliminating Healthcare Disparities in America: Beyond the IOM Report. Totowa, NJ: Humana Press, 2007.

Wolfe SM. Ephedra—scientific evidence versus money/politics. Science 2003;300:437.

Wolfe SM, Sasich LD, Lurie P, et al. Worst Pills, Best Pills: A Consumer's Guide to Avoiding Drug-Induced Death or Illness. New York: Pocket Books, 2005.

Wood AJJ, Darbyshire J. Injury to research volunteers—the clinical research nightmare. N Engl J Med 2006;354:1869–1871.

Zeisel SH. Regulation of "Nutraceuticals." Science 1999;285:1853–1855.

Fostering Empathy and Compassion

16

for all of us, observers all
who live and strive to see beyond the masks
—Harvey Stanbrough
(see Stanbrough, 2005, p 151)

Discovering the Patient's Personhood

Yes, beyond the mask and the daily costume we wear resides a sentient being, a vortex, always hoping, striving, yearning, and finally surrendering a last breath. To discover what's behind the patient's mask, the best physicians listen skillfully and display warmth, modesty, humility, and grace. They compassionately, nonjudgmentally accept every patient (Stevenson, 1971). They shift from a doctor-centered catalogue of symptoms to a patient-centered interview that explores the patient's reactions, feelings, and values to pursue concerns rather than simply complaints (see Chapter 6). Beyond analysis of the symptoms, the history aims at empathy, compassion, and trust. *Empathy* means to understand the patient's feelings and perspectives and to communicate that understanding to the patient. Without empathy and compassion, we just turn out robots who can do procedures or tie surgical knots but cannot act as physicians (Adson, 1995; Benbassat and Baumal, 2004; Coulehan et al., 2001; Crawshaw, 2002; Tauber, 2006).

You can assimilate some of the requisite attributes from a formal ethics course or fortuitously on rounds with a mentor. For your full development two further steps will help. First is the integration of ethics in the history-taking course because they will direct and determine the context within which questions are asked and will strongly influence the decisions the patient will make (Benbassat and Baumal, 2004; Tauber, 2006). Second, by practicing the specific exercises outlined next, you will gain greater and greater access to that bond between us all, where, as the poet Wilfred Owen said, "we share the eternal reciprocity of tears". (Owen, 1973, pp 54–59.

Experiences in Compassion

I suggest that you establish a late evening routine, a ritual which will enhance your feelings about the value of your own life and the life of every person. The ritual involves systematically recapitulating your own day and reading how others have recapitulated their similar experiences. Particularly, choose evenings after you have attended a seriously ill, dying, difficult, perplexing, or rewarding patient. Wait until you are alone and free from distraction, best perhaps fairly late at night and after subduing your sensory avenues of touch, sight, smell, and sound, to clear out your mind; best perhaps if you soften the lights and sit in your most comfortable chair; best perhaps after listening to your favorite music, whether classical or a touching modern or country ballad, whatever music mellows you and opens your heart. As preparation for a session, you might try other relaxation techniques, such as concentrating on your breathing or conscious relaxation of successive muscle groups from the neck down. Although I suggest trying the sessions alone at first, you may want to include a spouse or significant other.

As to actual procedure, after you have cleared your mind and created the ambience, remind yourself of the stark fact that each evening, as you recapitulate your day, you—your patients and each of us—now have one less day to live. Another day's worth of breaths, heartbeats, thoughts, and hopes, another precious, irreplaceable 24 hours have passed from your life, gone forever, except as memory. To experience this feeling of the transience and preciousness of each day, you might start each session by communing with Rupert Brooke, who died when just 28 years old.

Day That I Have Loved
Tenderly, day that I have loved, I close your eyes,
And smooth your quiet brow, and fold your thin
    dead hands.
The gray veils of the half-light deepen; colour dies,
I bear you, a light burden, to the shrouded sands,

Where lies your waiting boat, by wreaths of the sea's making
Mist-garlanded, with all grey weeds of the water
    crowned.
There you'll be laid, past fear of sleep or hope of
    waking;
And over the unmoving sea without a sound

Faint hands will row you outward, out beyond our
    sight,

Us with stretched arms and empty eyes on the
    far-gleaming
And marble sand....
Beyond the shifting cold twilight,
Further than laughter goes, or tears, further than
    dreaming,

(We found you pale and quiet, and strangely
    crowned with flowers,
Lovely and secret as a child. You came with us,
Came happily, hand in hand with the young dancing
    hours,
High on the downs at dawn!) Void now and
    tenebrous.

Close in the nest is folded every weary wing
Hushed all the joyful voices; and we, who held
    you dear,
Eastward we turn and homeward, alone, remembering…
Day that I loved, day that I loved, the Night is
    here!

—Rupert Brooke (1887–1915)
(see Brooke, 1915, pp 23–24)

Next, review your patients for that day. Let your mind range free and think over what you did say and could have said that might have brought more comfort to the troublesome or dying patient or the family. Did your history elicit just a litany of illnesses, grievances, and failures; or did you review any of the patient's interests, positive experiences, and successes in life? Did you shake hands when leaving the bedside or pass your hand across the patient's brow or readjust the pillows to a more comfortable position (Connelly, 2004)? If a patient has died, think about what you might have said to comfort the family or might say in a letter of condolence to the family, a practice once common but now lost (Bedell et al., 2001); and then why not actually write one? Keep a diary to jot down your actual feelings and reactions. Write out some things you might have said or done to bring the patient comfort. Review the circumstances during that day where your contact with patients proved particularly moving, rewarding, or troubling.

After you have created a contemplative mood, read and reread the next two extracts, "Death in the First Person" and "Unbefriended," the first by a student nurse who was dying and the second the meditations of a physician at the side of a brain-dead man. These serve as models to start your own compassion diary.

Death in the First Person

I am a student nurse. I am dying. I write this to you who are, and will become, nurses in the hope that by my sharing my feelings with you, you may someday be better able to help those who share my experience.

I'm out of the hospital now—perhaps for a month, for six months, perhaps for a year—but no one likes to talk about such things. In fact, no one likes to talk about much at all. Nursing must be advancing, but I wish it would hurry. We're taught not to be overly cheery now, to omit the "Everything's fine" routine, and we have done pretty well. But now one is left in a lonely silent void. With the protective "fine, fine" gone, the staff is left with only their own vulnerability and fear. The dying patient is not yet seen as a person and thus cannot be communicated with as such. He is a symbol of what every human fears and what we each know, at least academically, that we too must someday face. What did they say in psychiatric nursing about meeting pathology with pathology to the detriment of both patient and nurse? And there was a lot about knowing one's own feelings before you could help another with his. How true.

But for me, fear is today and dying is now. You slip in and out of my room, give me medications and check my blood pressure. Is it because I am a student nurse, myself, or just a human being, that I sense your fright? And your fears enhance mine. Why are you afraid? I am the one who is dying!

I know you feel insecure, don't know what to say, don't know what to do. But please believe me, if you care, you can't go wrong. Just admit that you care. That is really for what we search. We may ask for why's and wherefore's, but we don't really expect answers. Don't run away—wait—all I want to know is that there will be someone to hold my hand when I need it. I am afraid. Death may get to be a routine to you, but it is new to me. You may not see me as unique, but I've never died before. To me, once is pretty unique!

You whisper about my youth, but when one is dying, is he really so young anymore? I have lots I wish we could talk about. It really would not take much more of your time because you are in here quite a bit anyway.

If only we could be honest, both admit of our fears, touch one another. If you really care would you lose so much of your valuable professionalism if you even cried with me? Just person

to person? Then it might not be so hard to die—in a hospital—
with friends close by.

—Anonymous student nurse (Anonymous, 1970, p 356)
(reproduced by permission from Am J Nurs 1970;70:356)

Remember that Anatole Broyard's deathbed plea echoed an identical
sentiment (see Chapter 14, section V).

This next quotation describes the reflections of Dr. Michael Williams
(2006) upon attending a patient's death. Dr. Tom Inui (2002) reported a
similar experience.

Unbefriended

He was brain dead (almost) when I came on the ICU service
Monday morning. A man whose name we knew, and whose
history and medical records we had, and yet, he had no one
with him. "Homeless" is how most people would describe him.
"Unbefriended" is how my closest ethicist colleague termed it.

He was transferred from another hospital to the NeuroICU
on Sunday to have his severe intracerebral hemorrhage treated.
By the time he arrived, it was too late. He was herniating. The
ICU team and the neurosurgeons made every effort to save
him, including emergency surgery. It was too late.

The ICU team from Sunday was frustrated, even angry, that
because there was no family or friends to get permission from,
they had to go through the whole process of brain death determination instead of withdrawing life-sustaining therapies.
"What a waste," I was told at changeover, hearing the contempt
in their voices.

"What a waste." As if his unbefriended-ness was an imposi-
tion on us. That is how he was presented to me when I took
over as the ICU service attending. After rounds, I examined
him. Nothing. I knew we would pronounce his death later in
the day after a second, confirmatory brain death examination.
I directed the team to seek out family or friends. No luck.

The transplantation coordinator came and went. He was
not a candidate.

Hours passed and I performed the second brain death
examination, and then pronounced his death. The ventilator
breathed. His heart beat.

We waited longer, hoping someone who missed him would
appear. The ICU got busier and busier. Finally, we could
wait no more; we needed his ICU bed for another patient. We
withdrew the ventilator, and the pressors, and all the other
therapies.

As his last breath escaped, his nurse and I quickly turned off the IV pumps, disconnected lines and tubes, put things away, and started to make him presentable, as we always do, for the family.

We stopped suddenly and looked at one another, shaken out of our rituals by the unspoken simultaneous realization, "Family?"

"I'll stay," I said.

She nodded her head. We finished attending to him, cleaning his face and straightening the sheets and blankets, and then waited quietly together at the bedside.

We didn't have to stay. He was already dead. I had pronounced it. I teach others about brain death, and know what it means, and why. He was already dead.

It wasn't denial, or cognitive dissonance. My memory was flooded with images of the many times I had stood in sadness at the bedside with families as we removed the ventilator from patients who were brain dead, and waited and watched for the heart to stop, and the family's grieving to start a second time.

I stood in sadness again, and it was different. Worse. Sadness not only for his death, but also for the absence of family or friends. No one who knew him . . . knew. No one who knew him . . . grieved. How long had he been unbefriended? As easy as it would have been to walk away, something wouldn't let me. Respecting in death a person who may not have been respected in life.

I stood at the foot of the bed silent. No breaths. No movement. EKG still bouncing and blood pressure waning. I placed my hands on the tops of his feet. He was warm, and getting cooler.

The ICU whirled about me. His nurse was called away. Someone came in the room and took the warming blanket for another patient. Someone else came in and took the IV pump. Each of them paused and gave me a curious look, then shrugged and turned away wondering, I was sure, "Doesn't he have something more important to do?" I glanced back, remembering the morning and thought to myself, "What a waste? No. What a shame. No one's death should be unwitnessed in the presence of so many."

Finally, his heart stopped. And although unbefriended, he had not died alone. Removing my hands, I let him go, and hoped he would find reunion.

—Michael A. Williams, M.D. (2006, p 2088) (reproduced by permission from Neurology 2006;67:2088)

Why not also in extending compassion include yourself and all of us trapped as humans on this earth? We may be the only creatures who know for sure that each of us must die. We are all limited by being vertebrate bipeds, co-organisms built of serial somites, with skeletomuscular levers, glands, and tubes: a neural tube, gastrointestinal tube, pulmonary tubes, genitourinary tubes; and we even insert a tube within a tube to reproduce. We constantly seek satisfactions but often fail. To top it off, we are confined to a biosphere that is only a few miles thick as we whirl around on our earth, an obscure planet, the "third rock out from the sun."

Suggestions for Additional Sessions

Study of two poems, one by Wilfred Owen and the other by Algernon Swinburne, will enlarge your understanding of the pathos of being human, increase your bond with all who live, and enhance your appreciation of your own life. Wilfred Owen, a British infantry lieutenant and poet, fought in the trenches in France in World War I. At just 25 years of age, when helping his men to cross the Sambre Canal in northeastern France, a German bullet killed him, at water's edge, on November 4, 1918. Just 7 days later, on November 11, 1918, the armistice silenced the guns. Fate had refused to spare him for just 7 more days. His poems arose out of his direct observation of death on the battlefield. They constitute perhaps the most powerful antiwar and antideath poems ever written.

Futility

Move him into the sun—
Gently its touch awoke him once,
At home, whispering of fields unsown
Always it woke him, even in France,
Until this morning and this snow.
If anything might rouse him now
The kind old sun will know.

Think how it wakes the seeds,—
Woke, once the clays of a cold star.
Are limbs, so dear-achieved are sides,
Full-nerved—still warm—too hard to stir?
—Oh what made fatuous sunbeams toil
To break earth's sleep at all?

—Wilfred Owen (1893–1918)
(see Lewis, 1965, p 58)

Man

Before the beginning of years,
There came to the making of man
Time, with a gift of tears;
Grief, with a glass that ran;
Pleasure, with pain for leaven;
Summer, with flowers that fell;
Remembrance fallen from heaven,
And madness risen from hell;
Strength without hands to smite;
Love that endures for a breath;
Night, the shadow of light
And life, the shadow of death.

From the winds of the north and the south
They gathered as unto strife;
They breathed upon his mouth,
They filled his body with life;
Eyesight and speech they wrought
For the veils of the soul therein,
A time for labor and thought,
A time to serve and to sin;
They gave him light in his ways,
And love, and a space for delight,
And beauty and length of days,
With his lips he travaileth;
And night, and sleep in the night.
His speech is a burning fire;
In his heart is a blind desire,
In his eyes foreknowledge of death;
He weaves, and is clothed with derision;
Sows, and he shall not reap;
His life is a watch or a vision
Between a sleep and a sleep.

—Excerpted from *Atlanta in Calydon*
by Algernon Swinburne (1837–1909)
(Gosse and Wise, 1925–1927, pp 15–16)

For one night's exercise, get the Museum of Modern Art's photo album *The Family of Man*, created by Edward Steichen and with a prologue by Carl Sandburg (Steichen, 1955). Linger over each picture and contemplate the captions and themes. It will connect you with all of our human family. You'll find it in public libraries or online bookstores. If you do nothing else suggested in this section, get this book. It is transformative in its compassion.

Another evening look up and peruse Hamlet's soliloquy, "To be or not to be. . . ." It directly addresses the question of death versus life. Then place it in context with Enright's (1983) compilation of comments about death.

Get a copy of Meador's *A Little Book of Doctor's Rules* I & II (1992, 1999) and make a practice of reading several pages a session. It contains more condensed wisdom about the practice of medicine than any other source that I have found.

Look over the references at the end of this chapter and pick out some that interest you. Some are books, but you can finish many of the journal or magazine references in one evening. These references will change you. At present, you may regard cystic fibrosis as a genetic disorder that causes pulmonary failure; but read how it affects the person, and you will never again think of it as a just a genetic lung disease (Curtis, 1995; Rothenberg, 2003). Surgery may be simply a matter of cutting and stitching until you read the account by Lainsbury (2003), who endured a lifetime of necessary operations to correct congenital bladder extrophy. These two articles are in a magazine called *The Sun*, and again they are transformative, provide insights not to be found elsewhere, and are well worth the effort to locate.

If you are at all into poetry, devote some sessions to William Carlos Williams (see Rosenthal, 1966), Watts (1999), Stone (1990, 1998), and Campo (2003).

When you try the exercises I have suggested, enlist other students and ask what moved them. Takakuwa et al. (2006) compiled a book of such reflections. Start a "compassion club" and talk over your own compassion program and other students' because enlarging your capacity for compassion will make you a far better historian and physician than anything I can teach you. . If we all recorded those experiences of our lives, those contacts with each other, with art, literature, and music, those transcendental moments when our compassion soars out to bond us with all of life, we would compile the most valuable textbook of medicine ever written; but it would contain hardly a word about the specifics of anatomy, biochemistry, pathology, pharmacology, or disease entities.

My own acquaintance with these techniques for expanding compassion began in 1963, about 11:00 one night. My wife, Marian, and our three children were already sleeping and "not a creature was stirring not even a mouse." Marian had just given me a recording of Benjamin Britten's new composition *War Requiem*, in which he set to music the antiwar poetry of Wilfred Owen, whose poems I already knew. That night I reclined on a couch and began casually to listen to the recording, unprepared for the effect. The singers were Galina Vishnevskaya, a soprano from the Soviet Union; Peter Pears, a tenor from Britain; and Dietrich Fischer-Dieskau, a German baritone, thus joining three persons from nations that had just been trying to annihilate each other in World War II. In fact, Germany had conscripted Fischer-Dieskau in 1943 to serve in the Nazi army, just as I myself, also 18 years old in 1943, was conscripted into the U.S. Air Force. He served on the Russian and Italian fronts and ended as a prisoner of war.

From Britten's music and the alternation of singers, Owen's phrases began to overwhelm me. Here were human beings at their practiced best, consummate artists from three nations that had striven to annihilate each other in a war of supreme brutality, three former enemies, joined to display the beauty humans can achieve when they reject killing and come together to celebrate their reverence for life. Each singer had survived in a culture that had reached the depths of degradation by engaging in mass killing, but now they collaborated to produce the heights of compassion. I felt a union with each human who had ever lived or would live, with the struggle of all living things to survive, an elemental connection with all who had ever walked or would walk on our planet.

It was an unforgettable experience. Oddly enough, I have not played the records again, although I keep them and finger them once in a while. I don't want to dispel the magic or dilute the power of that experience. I have only to think of that night to relive it. Perhaps attention to some of the exercises here will give you the same epiphany.

Feeling an Affinity for the Past of Our Profession

To further your maturation as a physician, you should experience the continuity of your educational struggles with that of your predecessors. To that end, read the treatise by Rufus of Ephesus (ca. 98–117 CE) entitled "On the Interrogation of the Patient." Devote one or two whole evenings to it. You will immediately identify with his struggles to understand his role as a physician and the lasting insights he often achieves, as well as his mistakes. Make the effort to take this journey 2000 years backward in time. Rufus's treatise is in Brock (1929).

References and Further Sources

Space limits this list to a fraction of the many excellent references available.

Narratives by Patients and Caregivers

Adamson K. Kate's Journey: Triumph Over Adversity. Redondo Beach, CA: Nosmada Press, 2004 (by a patient paralyzed with locked-in syndrome; see also Bauby, 1997, and Jennings, 2003).

Adamson K. Paralyzed but Not Powerless: Kate's Journey Revisited. Redondo Beach, CA: Nosmada Press, 2007.

Anderson R. The Aftermath of Stroke: The Experience of Patients and Their Families. New York: Cambridge University Press, 2006.

Anonymous. Death in the first person. Am J Nurs 1970;70:356 (letter written by a student nurse who was dying).

Bauby J-D. The Diving Bell and the Butterfly: A Memoir of Life in Death. New York: Vintage Press, 1997 (A magnificent paean to the human spirit from a patient with locked-in syndrome, an infarct in the basis pontis that caused complete paralysis, except for eyelid elevation. He died just 2 days after publication of his book. See following section for a movie based on his illness and entitled the same as the book. For three other books on the triumph of the human spirit over near total paralysis, see Jennings, 2003, and Adamson, 2004 and 2006.)

Broyard A. Doctor talk to me. New York Times Magazine, August 26, 1990.

Cole M. When the left brain is not right the right brain may be left: report of personal experience of occipital hemianopia. J Neurol Neurosurg Psychiatry 1999;67:169–173 (a narrative by a neurologist who suffered an occipital lobe infarction).

Curtis M. Saying its name. The Sun 1995;239:12–16 (a patient's account of the difficulty of accepting the diagnosis of cystic fibrosis).

Flaherty AW. The Midnight Disease: The Drive to Write, Writer's Block, and the Creative Brain. Boston: Houghton Mifflin, 2004 (account of a neurologist trying to deal with hypergraphia).

Harrison J. Returning to Earth. New York: Grove Press, 2007 (an account in the form of a novel of the family interactions of a patient dying with amyotrophic lateral sclerosis).

Hilden JM, Tobin DR, Lindsey K. Shelter from the Storm: Caring for a Child with a Life-Threatening Condition. Cambridge: Perseus, 2003.

Hull JM. Touching the Rock. New York: Pantheon, 1991 (account by a patient who went blind in his 40s, like John Milton, the author of *Paradise Lost*, who went blind at the same age).

Jamison KR. Night Falls Fast: Understanding Suicide. New York: Knopf, 1999 (written by a suicide survivor).

Jennings S. Locked In Locked Out. Saint John, N.B., Canada: Dreamcatcher Publishing, 2003 (written by an M.D. who suffered locked-in syndrome; see also Bauby, 1997, and Adamson, 2004 and 2007).

Lainsbury J. Control. The Sun 2003;238:36–40 (the problems of a patient enduring multiple operations for correcting congenital bladder extrophy).

Levine C. The loneliness of the long-term caregiver. N Engl J Med 1999; 340:1587–1590 (caregiver's account of the problems of caring for a brain-impaired spouse; see also Parker, 2000).

Middlebrook C. Seeing the Crab: A Memoir of Dying. New York: Basic Books, 1996.

Parker S. And Jill came tumbling after. The Sun 2000;289:38–46 (the experience of a wife burdened with the long-term care of a quadriplegic husband).

Rothenberg L. Breathing for a Living. New York: Hyperion, 2003 (the life of a woman who died from cystic fibrosis).

Rucker A. The Best Seat in the House: How I Woke Up One Tuesday and Was Paralyzed for Life. New York: HarperCollins, 2007 (a narrative by a writer who became paraplegic at the age of 51 and faced it with dignity, humor, and insight).

Williams MA. Unbefriended. (thoughts of a neurologist while completing a brain-death protocol on a homeless patient). Neurology 2006;67: 2088.

Movies

For reviews of movies with medical themes, see Malmsheimer R. Doctors Only: The Evolving Image of the American Physician. New York: Greenwood Press, 1988, and Dans PE. Doctors in the Movies: Boil the Water and Just Say Aah! Bloomington, IL: Medi-Ed Press, 2000. Dr. Dans has long reviewed movies for The Pharos.

Beyond Silence (1998), starring Sylvie Testud, Howie Seago, and Emmanuelle Laborit, a subtitled German film that sensitively explores the effect of deafness in a family.

Dark Victory (1939), starring Bette Davis, George Brent, Humphrey Bogart, Geraldine Fitzgerald, and Ronald Reagan, deals with a patient who has a malignant brain tumor and her reactions to it and to physicians and medical care.

Marvin's Room (1996), starring Diane Keaton, Meryl Streep, and Leonardo DiCaprio, deals with a family taking care of an elderly member.

Matter of Life and Death (1946), starring David Niven and Kim Hunter, a love story in which one of the protagonists struggles with complex partial seizures. The patient had olfactory hallucinations as a component of the seizures. (The film is discussed by Friedman DB. A matter of fried onions. Seizure 1992;1:307–310.)

Ponette (1996), a subtitled French film, starring 4-year-old Victoire Thivisol and Marie Trintignant, exploring the reactions of a child to the accidental death of her mother in a motor car in which both were riding.

Something the Lord Made (HBO, 2004), starring Mos Def, Alan Rickman, Kyra Sedgwick, Gabrielle Union, and Mary Stuart Masterson, the inspiring story of developing the operative procedure to correct the tetralogy of Fallot, pioneered by Alfred Blalock and his African American associate, Vivien Thomas. The Andrea Kalin PBS documentary narrated by Morgan Freeman, Partners of the Heart, is historically more accurate. See the autobiography by Thomas, 1985, in the following section.

The Diving Bell and the Butterfly (2007), a subtitled French film starring Mathieu Amalric and Emmanuelle Seigner, a true story based on a patient who was nearly completely paralyzed by a pontine infarct but fully conscious. For the patient's autobiographical book describing the ordeal, see Bauby, 1997, in previous section.

The Third Man (1949), starring Joseph Cotton, Alida Valli, and Orson Welles, has an intriguing subplot about a black market in penicillin shortly after its introduction.

What's Eating Gilbert Grape? (1993), starring Johnny Depp, Juliette Lewis, and Leonardo DiCaprio, one of the few films to explore obesity, mental retardation, and family dynamics.

Wit (2001), starring Emma Thompson, Christopher Lloyd, Eileen Atkins, Audra McDonald, and Jonathan M. Woodward. Emma Thompson plays a medieval scholar, a professor of English literature, who had specialized in John Donne but is dying of ovarian cancer.

General Annotated Bibliography for Compassion and Empathy

Ackerman D. A Natural History of the Senses. New York: Vintage Press, 1991 (a paean in appreciation of the various senses, lyrically written).

Adson MA. An endangered ethic—the capacity for caring. Mayo Clin Proc 1995;70:495–500.

Arnold P. Gold Foundation, http://humanism-in-medicine.org (this foundation offers programs and grants for promotion of humanism in medical education).

Bedell SE, Cadenhead K, Graboys TB. The doctor's letter of condolence. N Engl J Med 2001;344:1162–1163 (the authors suggest revival of a lost custom).

Benbassat J, Baumal R. What is empathy and how can it be promoted during clinical clerkships? Acad Med 2004;79:832–839.

Brock AJ, ed. and tr. Greek Medicine, Being Extracts Illustrative of Medical Writers from Hippocrates to Galen. London: JM Dent & Sons, 1929 (see Majno, 1975).

Broks P. The sea horse and the almond. A neuropsychologist describes the travails and emotions of a patient during pre-surgical evaluation for temporal lobectomy for intractable seizures. Granta 2001;75 (autumn):237–255.

Brooke R. The Collected Poems of Rupert Brooke. New York: Dodd, Mead and Company, 1915, pp 23–24.

Campo R. The Healing Art: A Doctor's Black Bag of Poetry. New York: Norton, 2003.

Campo R. Just the facts. N Engl J Med 2004;351:1167–1169.

Chen PW. Final Exam: A Surgeon's Reflections on Mortality. New York: Vintage, 2008 (a message for physicians to become more engaged with their patients).

Coles R, Testa R, eds. A Life in Medicine. A Literary Anthology. New York: New Press, 2002.

Connelly JE. The power of touch in clinical medicine. Pharos 2004; 67(spring):11–13 (review Patient 29, Chapter 12, section II when reading Connelly's article).

Coope R. The Quiet Art: A Doctor's Anthology. Baltimore: Williams and Wilkins, 1958.

Crawshaw R. Compassion's Way: A Doctor's Quest into the Soul of Medicine. Bloomington, IL: Medi-Ed Press, 2002.

Coulehan JL, Platta FW, Egener B, et al. "Let me see if I have this right…" Words that build empathy. Ann Intern Med 2001;135:221–227.

Davis C, Schaefer J, eds. Between the Heartbeats: Poetry and Prose by Nurses. Iowa City: University of Iowa Press, 1995.

Duffy K. Model Patient: My Life as an Incurable Wise Ass. New York: HarperCollins, 2001 (the author, a model for Revlon cosmetics, living in the fast lane, is stricken with a rare form of sarcoidosis that affects the central nervous system).

Enright DJ, ed. The Oxford Book of Death. Oxford: Oxford University Press, 1983 (quotations from observers throughout the centuries).

Frank AW. The Renewal of Generosity: Illness, Medicine, and How to Live. Chicago: University of Chicago Press, 2004.

Gosse E, Wise TJ, eds. Swinburne, Algernon Charles. Complete Works, 20 vols. London: Heinemann, 1925–1927, pp 15–16.

Hojat M. Empathy in Patient Care: Antecedents, Development, Measurement, and Outcomes. New York: Springer, 2007 (more technical and didactic than most of the other sources here, for evidence-based buffs).

Inui TS. The length of our journey: care near the end of life (teaching and learning moments). J Med Educ 2002;77:1107 (compare Dr. Inui's experience with that of Williams, 2006, in previous section).

Klass P. Treatment Kind and Fair: Letters to a Young Doctor. New York: Basic Books, 2007.

Klitzman R. When Doctors Become Patients. New York: Oxford University Press, 2008 (when doctors become ill, they view illness from the patient's perspective).

Lewis CD, ed. The Collected Poems of Wilfred Owen. New York: New Directions Books, 1965, p 58 (see also Stallworthy J. Wilfred Owen. London: Oxford University Press, 1974, and see the poem "To my sons and daughters for Wilfred Owen," in Stanbrough, 2005).

Lown B. The Lost Art of Healing. Boston: Houghton Mifflin, 1996.

McDonough ML. Poet Physicians. An Anthology of Medical Poetry Written by Physicians. Springfield, IL: Charles C. Thomas, 1945.

Majno G. The Healing Hand: Man and Wound in the Ancient World. Cambridge, MA: Harvard University Press, 1975 (a description of how knowledge emerged from folklore and superstition in promoting wound healing. This is a companion for Rufus (see Brock, 1929) for the student's entrée into the history of medicine.)

Meador CK. A Little Book of Doctors' Rules. I: A Compilation. Philadelphia: Hanley & Belfus, 1992.

Meador CK. A Little Book of Doctors' Rules. II: A Compilation, 2nd ed. Philadelphia: Hanley & Belfus, 1999

Montagu A. Touching: The Human Significance of the Skin. New York: Columbia University Press, 1971.

Ofri D. Incidental Findings: Lessons from My Patients in the Art of Medicine. Boston: Beacon Press, 2005.

Owen W. Insensibility. In: Larkin P (ed), Oxford, Oxford Book of Twentieth-Century English Verse, 1973 pp 54–59.

Reynolds R, Stone J, eds. On Doctoring: Stories, Poems, Essays, 3rd ed. New York: Simon & Schuster, 2001.

Rosenthal ML, ed. The William Carlos Williams Reader. London: New Directions, 1966.

Sachs O. Musicophilia: Tales of Music and the Brain. New York: Knopf, 2007 (presents music as human communication that has a neurologic basis).

Stanbrough H. Beyond the Masks. Albuquerque, NM: Central Avenue Press, 2005, p 151 (a book of poetry about the human condition).

Steichen E, ed. The Family of Man. New York: Museum of Modern Art, 1955 (a collection of the greatest photographs ever taken of humans, selected by Edward Steichen, prologue by Carl Sandburg, with captions. Be sure to view this book—it will touch your heart, page after page.).

Stevenson I. The Diagnostic Interview. New York: Harper & Row, 1971.

Stone J. In the Country of Hearts: Journeys in the Art of Medicine. New York: Bantam Doubleday Dell, 1990 (by a cardiologist).

Stone J. Where Water Begins: New Poems and Prose. Baton Rouge: Louisiana State University Press, 1998.

Takakuwa KM, Rubaschkin N, Herzig KE, eds. What I Learned in Medical School. Personal Stories of Young Doctors. Berkeley: University of California Press, 2006.

Tauber AI. Patient Autonomy and the Ethics of Responsibility. Boston: MIT Press, 2006.

Thomas VT. Pioneering Research in Surgical Shock and Cardiovascular Surgery: Vivien Thomas and His Work with Alfred Blalock: An Autobiography by Vivien T. Thomas. Philadelphia: University of Pennsylvania Press, 1985 (see also *Something the Lord Made* in the movie list).

Watts D. Taking the History. Troy, ME: Nightshade Press, 1999 (a book of poems).

Whitman W. The Complete Poetry and Prose of Walt Whitman. Garden City, NY: Garden City Books, 1954 (reprint of the original deathbed edition, prepared by Whitman himself).

Young A. What Patients Taught Me. Seattle: Sasquatch Books, 2004.

Addendum

An extensive list of medically relevant literature and movies can be accessed by Google: Health and Human Experience through Literature (http://www.gannon.edu/faculty_staff/faculty/moore/litandmed.htm). If you like medically themed novels, consider the recommendations by Coles and Testa (2002) of *Middlemarch* by George Eliot, *Tender Is the Night* by F. Scott Fitzgerald, *Arrowsmith* by Sinclair Lewis, and *Love in the Ruins* by Walker Percy.

Index

Note: Page numbers followed by *f* and *t* indicate figures and tables, respectively.